Ophthalmic Fundamentals: Glaucoma

OPHTHALMIC FUNDAMENTALS:
GLAUCOMA

Edited by
Joseph W. Sassani, MD
Departments of Ophthalmology and Pathology
Penn State Geisinger Health System
Penn State University
Hershey, Pennsylvania

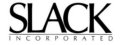

SLACK
INCORPORATED

6900 Grove Road, Thorofare, NJ 08086-9447

Publisher: John H. Bond
Editorial Director: Amy E. Drummond
Assistant Editor: Elisabeth DeBoer
Illustrator: Ira Grunther, CMI
Copyright © 1999 by SLACK Incorporated

Ophthalmic Fundamentals: glaucoma/edited by Joseph W. Sassani.
    p. cm.
    Includes bibliographical references and index.
    ISBN 1-55642-384-5 (alk. paper)
    1. Glaucoma. I. Sassani, Joseph W. II. Title: Glaucoma.
    [DNLM: 1. Glaucoma.   WW 290 0615 1999]
RE871.O644   1999
617.7'41--dc21
DNLM/DLC
for Library of Congress   99-2000   99-16294
                                 CIP

Printed in the United States of America.
Published by: SLACK Incorporated
                  6900 Grove Road
                  Thorofare, NJ 08086-9447 USA
                  Telephone: 856-848-1000
                  Fax: 856-853-5991
                  Website: http://www.slackinc.com

Contact SLACK Incorporated for more information about other books in this field or about the availability of our books from distributors outside the United States.

Authorization to photocopy items for internal or personal use, or the internal or personal use of specific clients, is granted by SLACK Incorporated, provided that the appropriate fee is paid directly to Copyright Clearance Center, 222 Rosewood Drive, Danvers, MA 01923 USA, 978-750-8400. Prior to photocopying items for educational classroom use, please contact the CCC at the address above. Please reference Account Number 9106324 for SLACK Incorporated's Professional Book Division. For further information on CCC, check CCC Online at the following address: http://www.copyright.com.

Last digit is print number: 10 9 8 7 6 5 4 3 2 1

DEDICATION

To my wife, Gloria, who makes everything possible, with love.

CONTENTS

ACKNOWLEDGMENTS

Ophthalmic Fundamentals: Glaucoma is the result of the expertise and commitment of 24 authorities in the various aspects of glaucoma. I am most grateful to each of these very busy individuals for their shared vision, and for their diligence and patience in making this text a reality. I am very proud to be associated with them.

I suspect that information regarding glaucoma accrues to most clinicians in waves. As residents we amass a great many details and the structural underpinnings onto which clinical experience will add relevance. Those of us who take further training in the field, I think, become impressed by the gaps in our knowledge more than by a feeling of omniscience. All of us, no matter what our level of training, accrue a great debt to the professionals and patients who have contributed to our knowledge base in glaucoma. As editor, I am privileged to thank some of the individuals who have taught me.

As a resident, Drs. William C. Frayer, David M. Kozart, Harold G. Scheie, and Richard A. Stone provided a foundation and sparked my interest in glaucoma. During a sabbatical year I had the honor of working as a fellow with Dr. David Epstein and his staff at the Massachusetts Eye and Ear Infirmary, and with Drs. Robert Ritch and Jeffrey Liebmann, and their staff at the New York Eye and Ear Infirmary. Others with whom I had a close professional relationship during this period were Drs. Rand Allingham, A. Robert Bellows, B. W. Morton Grant, B. Thomas Hutchinson, Annelies de Kater, Bernard Schwartz, and Bradford J. Shingleton. I owe them my gratitude as inspirational role models of the caring clinician and committed scientist.

Since starting my practice at the Hershey Medical Center, I have come to work closely with Dr. Ali Aminlari, who is a kind friend and a gifted glaucoma clinician. I would also like to thank my other colleagues and staff at Penn State University and the Milton S. Hershey Medical Center of the Penn State Geisinger Health System for their support, as well as the many clinicians with whom I have worked over the years. Drs. Patricia J. Mc Laughlin and Ian S. Zagon have provided instruction, inspiration, and support as research colleagues.

I also would like to thank John Bond, Jennifer Cahill, Debra Christy, Betsy DeBoer, Amy Drummond, and Viktoria Kristiansson, at SLACK Incorporated for their enthusiastic support of our concept and for their diligence in bringing it to fruition.

Finally, but most importantly, my family, Gloria, Lauren, and Bill, have been understanding and supportive of my publishing interests and adventures. They remain the center of my universe.

ABOUT THE EDITOR

Joseph W. Sassani, MD has been a practicing clinician for 19 years. He received his Bachelor of Science in Biology cum laude from Villanova University in 1969, and his medical degree from Jefferson Medical College in Philadelphia in 1973. He completed an internship and 1 year Surgery residency at the Hospital of the University of Pennsylvania, followed by an Ophthalmic Pathology fellowship and Ophthalmology residency at the Scheie Eye Institute in the Department of Ophthalmology of the University of Pennsylvania. Dr. Sassani joined the staff of the Departments of Ophthalmology and Pathology at Penn State's Milton S. Hershey Medical Center (now the Penn State Geisinger Health System) in 1980. He is currently Professor of Ophthalmology and Pathology within Penn State University.

Early in his clinical career, Dr. Sassani developed an interest in glaucoma, which he was able to pursue in greater depth during sabbatical fellowship experiences at the New York Eye and Ear Infirmary and Massachusetts Eye and Ear Infirmary during the academic year 1989 to 1990. During that time he had the opportunity to work with many inspiring glaucoma clinicians who continue to influence him to this day and to whom he is most grateful.

On returning to Hershey, Pennsylvania in 1990, Dr. Sassani began a long and rewarding research association with Drs. Ian S. Zagon and Patricia J. McLaughlin of the Department of Neuroscience and Anatomy at Penn State. Their association has resulted in research funding from the National Eye Institute, and the production of a number of papers related to a novel opioid growth regulatory system and the eye.

Dr. Sassani has been active in numerous professional organizations including the Pennsylvania Academy of Ophthalmology, for which he served in various capacities including President, the Eastern Ophthalmic Pathology Society, the Verhoeff-Zimmerman Ophthalmic Pathology Society, and the American Association of Ophthalmic Pathologists for which he served as Secretary-Treasurer. He has joined in the writing of over 60 scientific publications, edited two books, and written several book chapters.

For many years, Dr. Sassani has been active in the Boy Scouts of America in which he has held local and regional offices and been the recipient of several awards. Currently he is complementing his clinical experiences by pursuing a Masters of Health Administration as an evening student at Penn State University. Dr. Sassani will soon celebrate his 30th wedding anniversary with his wife, Gloria. Their two children, Lauren and Bill, attend college.

CONTRIBUTING AUTHORS

Ali Aminlari, MD, FACS
Penn State Geisinger Health System
Penn State University
Hershey, Pennsylvania

Iftikhar M. Chaudhry, MD
New England Eye Center
New England Medical Center
Tufts University School of Medicine
Boston, Massachusetts

Evan Benjamin Dreyer, MD, PhD
Scheie Eye Institute
University of Pennsylvania
Philadelphia, Pennsylvania

Thomas F. Freddo, OD, PhD
Boston University School of Medicine
Boston Medical Center
Boston, Massachusetts

Madhu S. R. Gorla, MD
Scheie Eye Institute
University of Pennsylvania
Philadelphia, Pennsylvania

Richard A. Hill, MD
University of California, Irvine
Irvine, California

Hiroshi Ishikawa, MD
The New York Eye and Ear Infirmary
New York, New York

L. Jay Katz, MD, FACS
William and Anna Goldberg Glaucoma Service
Wills Eye Hospital
Jefferson Medical College
Philadelphia, Pennsylvania

Paul Lee, MD, JD
Department of Ophthalmology
Duke University Medical Center
Durham, North Carolina

Jeffrey M. Liebmann, MD
New York Medical College
Valhalla, New York
Glaucoma Service
The New York Eye and Ear Infirmary
New York, New York

Jonathan S. Myers, MD
William and Anna Goldberg Glaucoma Service
Wills Eye Hospital
Jefferson Medical College
Philadelphia, Pennsylvania

Jody R. Piltz, MD
Glaucoma Service
Scheie Eye Institute
University of Pennsylvania
Philadelphia, Pennsylvania

John S. Ray, OD, MS
Assistant Professor
Pennsylvania College of Optometry
Elkins Park, Pennsylvania
Private Practice
Lansdale, Pennsylvania

Robert Ritch, MD
New York Medical College
Valhalla, New York
Glaucoma Service
The New York Eye and Ear Infirmary
New York, New York

Robert F. Rothman, MD
New York Medical College
Valhalla, New York
Glaucoma Service
The New York Eye and Ear Infirmary
New York, New York

Mansoor Sarfarazi, PhD
Molecular Ophthalmic Genetics Laboratory
Surgical Research Center
Department of Surgery
University of Connecticut Health Center
Farmington, Connecticut

Joseph W. Sassani, MD
Departments of Ophthalmology and Pathology
Penn State Geisinger Health System
Penn State University
Hershey, Pennsylvania

Joel S. Schuman, MD
New England Eye Center
New England Medical Center
Tufts University School of Medicine
Boston, Massachusetts

Annapurna Singh, MD
Scheie Eye Institute
University of Pennsylvania
Philadelphia, Pennsylvania

George L. Spaeth, MD, FACS
William and Anna Goldberg Glaucoma Service
Wills Eye Hospital
Jefferson Medical College
Philadelphia, Pennsylvania

Ivaylo Stoilov, MD
Molecular Ophthalmic Genetics Laboratory
Surgical Research Center
Department of Surgery
University of Connecticut Health Center
Farmington, Connecticut

Nasreen A. Syed, MD
Scheie Eye Institute
University of Pennsylvania
Philadelphia, Pennsylvania

Elliot B. Werner, MD
Hahnemann University
Philadelphia, Pennsylvania

PREFACE

Glaucoma represents a spectrum of disorders that may be the source of considerable vexation for both the patient and the clinician. It can be difficult to explain to a patient that they have one of a group of diseases for which there is considerable controversy relative to both the diagnosis and treatment. Normal pressure glaucoma, for most patients, is an oxymoron that may strain both patient credulity and the doctor-patient alliance. All of these elements are particularly confounding for the individual who is first approaching the study of the glaucomas. Even experienced clinicians may be overwhelmed as they attempt to glean the "pearls" from the mass of publications regarding these disorders.

Ophthalmic Fundamentals: Glaucoma is intended for the individual first approaching the study of glaucoma and for the busy clinician seeking a readable review of the topic. We believe that the book can be read during a clinical rotation or over a reasonable number of evenings stolen from clinical practice. Nevertheless, our contributing authors have covered the spectrum of information on glaucoma, including epidemiology; socioeconomic impact; genetics; anatomy and pathophysiology; gonioscopy; diagnostic ultrasound biomicroscopy; optic neuropathy; optic nerve imaging and morphometric analysis; visual fields; clinical features; congenital and pediatric glaucomas; pharmacology and therapeutics; nonincisional and incisional surgeries; and visual rehabilitation and low vision therapy. The authors for each chapter have been chosen for their expertise in their areas. They have condensed the information in their fields to what they believe is relevant to our purposes.

We hope you find *Ophthalmic Fundamentals: Glaucoma* both informative and enjoyable reading. Please feel free to contact me with suggestions as to how we may better serve your needs.

Joseph W. Sassani, MD
June 3, 1999

Chapter One

EPIDEMIOLOGY AND SOCIOECONOMIC IMPACT OF GLAUCOMA

Paul Lee, MD, JD

Glaucoma is the leading cause of blindness among adult African-Americans and the second leading cause of blindness among adult Americans ages 18 to 65.[1] An estimated 80,000 Americans are legally blind from glaucoma (best visual acuity of worse than 20/200 or best visual field of less than 20 degrees).[1] It has been estimated that the costs of caring for glaucoma, including the indirect costs of transfer payments for those disabled due to glaucoma in federal and state government programs, exceeded $2.4 billion in 1992 and is likely to increase significantly in the future.[2,3] Nevertheless, it has also been estimated that half of all patients with glaucoma do not know that they have it and are thus not receiving treatment that may prevent vision loss in many of them.[1]

In order to make sense of this situation and to determine if glaucoma is a significant health concern we need to clearly understand several issues:

• How many people have glaucoma, which depends in large part on how one defines glaucoma.

• What is the natural history of glaucoma, treated and untreated?
• Does everyone with glaucoma *need* treatment?
• What factors influence how we can best deliver treatment for glaucoma if it is warranted?

HOW MANY PEOPLE HAVE GLAUCOMA?
Defining Glaucoma

Glaucoma has become a descriptive term, like congestive heart failure, that identifies a group of clinical conditions as opposed to a specific disease entity with a specific etiology. The term *glaucoma* today encompasses a large number of disparate conditions united by a final common pathway of damage to the optic nerve.[4] Yet, traditionally, glaucoma has been typically organized not by mechanisms of damage to the optic nerve but by the mechanisms that cause an elevation of intraocular pressure (IOP). Thus, there are two major categories based upon where obstruction to aqueous outflow occurs (open-angle or closed-angle, also called angle-closure), further subdivided by whether the cause was primary or secondary. Understanding the differences between the traditional and the newer terminology of glaucoma is essential to placing the epidemiological and socioeconomic data about glaucoma in their proper context.

Under the traditional system, *angle-closure glaucoma* consists of those conditions in which the iris occludes the trabecular meshwork, thus impeding outflow. Although pupillary block is the major mechanism underlying primary angle-closure glaucoma (PACG), there are other conditions in which the iris secondarily occludes the meshwork. Damage to the optic nerve in angle-closure glaucoma often results from extreme elevations in IOP causing direct or indirect injury to the optic nerve. *Open-angle glaucoma* refers to those conditions in which the iris does not occlude the meshwork and the presumed primary difficulty is impediment to outflow in the trabecular meshwork.

In a break with the traditional categorization of the glaucomas, the new American Academy of Ophthalmology (AAO) definition of primary open-angle glaucoma (POAG) states that the disease is multifactorial in origin but that it primarily affects the optic nerve. IOP is an important element of the group of putative causes of damage to the optic nerve, but it is not the only one. As such, the new definition of POAG has no IOP criterion. It requires only optic nerve damage that is consistent with the clinical syndrome to be present in order for a diagnosis of glaucoma to be made.[4] Characteristic findings include thinning of the neuroretinal rim, notching, asymmetry, progressive thinning of the neuroretinal rim, or nerve fiber layer defects. Furthermore, by definition, early glaucoma has *no* associated visual field loss. Instead, the presence of any characteristic glaucomatous field loss automatically makes the glaucoma of at least moderate severity. This definition has since been adopted by other organizations in the field, including Prevent Blindness America, whose screening program based on perimetric screening is targeted toward detecting moderately advanced or worse glaucoma.[1] Several authors have proposed organizing concepts to encompass the range of potential factors that may affect the development and progression of abnormal loss of optic nerve structure and function.

The rationale for the new definition of glaucoma centers on three important clinical observations. First, optic nerve changes precede visual field damage in the vast majority of patients with glaucoma.[5,6] Second, all prior studies using IOP criteria are subject to significant measurement error for not including adjustments for corneal thickness, which can introduce significant artifact relative to the accurate measurement of IOP.[7] Indeed, the entire concept of a normal IOP is based on a statistical distribution of IOP among studied populations.[8] Third, studies have repeatedly shown that the IOP at any one reading is within the normal range in between 30% and 50% of patients with demonstrated glaucoma by optic nerve and visual field criteria.[8]

Thus, the major focus today is not on the drainage pathways of the eye but on injury to the optic nerve and how best to prevent or even reverse such injury. The reader should expect that the definitions and terminology used in glaucoma will change over the next few years.

Determining People Currently Under Care for Glaucoma

One method of determining how many people have glaucoma is to ascertain the number of people being treated for glaucoma in the United States. Data from the RAND Eye Care Workforce study, based on analyses from representative samples of the physicians and institutions providing care maintained by the National Center for Health Statistics, indicates that nearly 2 million people in 1994 were carrying the diagnosis of glaucoma of all types (including suspects) and receiving care.[9]

Use of this approach can further identify the proportion of the different forms of glaucoma in five broad categories similar to the overall clinical categories noted above:
1. POAG
2. Secondary open-angle glaucoma (SOAG)
3. Angle-closure (both primary and secondary)
4. Congenital
5. Suspect

As seen in Table 1-1, the proportions clearly indicate that POAG is the predominant form of glaucoma in the United States, as far as the work demanded of eye care providers.[9]

This approach is unsatisfying for several reasons. First, we cannot tell how each case is being identified

Table 1-1

Proportions of Provider Work Required to Care for Different Forms of Glaucoma Under Care in 1994

POAG	80%
SOAG	3%
Angle closure (all forms)	5%
Congenital	<1%
Glaucoma suspects	11%

by the treating practitioner. Prior work by Lichter and Varma has identified a high degree of variability in the interpretation of optic nerve head appearance, a critical feature in every diagnostic definition of glaucoma.[10,11] As a result, many patients being seen by eye care providers could either be mistakenly diagnosed as having glaucoma or as being free from glaucoma when they actually have glaucoma. Second, using the estimates of individuals currently receiving treatment ("demand") is particularly concerning in understanding the "glaucomas" because of the high degree of unidentified cases not receiving treatment or monitoring by eye care providers at all.[1] Thus, it would be much better to use estimates based on population-based epidemiological studies of the rates and numbers of people with glaucoma rather than those currently being cared for with glaucoma. The reader should evaluate studies carefully as to whether reported rates reflect those under treatment or those ascertained on the basis of population-based methods.

Population-Based Estimates of the Prevalence of Glaucoma

POAG

Fortunately, data from several population-based studies provide varying estimates of the numbers of people with POAG in diverse populations. Unfortunately, each of these studies—Beaver Dam in Wisconsin[12]; the Baltimore Eye Survey[13]; and studies in other countries, such as Blue Mountains in Australia,[14] Rotterdam in the Netherlands,[15] and St. Lucia in the Caribbean[16]—use different definitions to identify a case of glaucoma. In addition, these studies generally have insufficient sample

sizes to draw reliable conclusions about the numbers of people with secondary forms of glaucoma. Thus, any such population-based estimates generally are based on extrapolations from the POAG data. Finally, these estimates are further muddied by the recent change in definition of open-angle glaucoma in the AAO Preferred Practice Pattern (PPP) for POAG noted earlier.

The essential implication of the new definition of glaucoma is that the rates of glaucoma reported in the published population studies need to be reassessed, because all case definitions of POAG used in those studies required the presence of optic nerve, visual field, and, in some, IOP abnormalities. When the published data are re-analyzed to allow for either optic nerve or visual field criteria to be sufficient, the rates of POAG in the population increase significantly. Indeed, it has been estimated that over 15 million Americans in 1993 would be classified as having glaucoma if optic nerve head criteria alone were used, as they are in the new PPP.[17]

Table 1-2 summarizes the prevalence rates from several published population-based studies on the different forms of glaucoma and the definitions used in each study. As noted earlier, every study except aspects of the Baltimore Eye Study uses a definition of POAG that requires optic nerve damage, however defined, *and* another element, either IOP or visual field. In these studies, the prevalence rate of glaucoma would be significantly higher utilizing the new definition of glaucoma. For example, the prevalence rate of the Beaver Dam population would increase 31%, while the already tremendously high rate among blacks noted in the Barbados Eye Study would be increased by 55%.[18] Thus, if one were to use the new definition of glaucoma, the published studies on population-based rates of POAG underestimate prevalence rates of glaucoma by at least one third, and perhaps even more, depending upon the exact optic nerve or visual field defects one would include as being characteristic of glaucoma.

PACG

Far fewer population-based studies have examined the rates of angle-closure glaucoma, as indicated in Table 1-2. In these studies, case identification depended upon the gonioscopic identification of occludable drainage angles together with either elevated IOP or characteristic optic nerve/visual field

Table 1-2

Glaucoma Studies Around the World

Study Site	Reference	Definition of POAG	Population Minimum Age	Overall Rate	Youngest Group	Oldest Group	PACG Rate	Secondary Glaucoma Rate	Other Notes
Beaver Dam	12,19	2 of 3 VF/IOP/ON	≥43	2.1	0.9 (43-54)	4.7 (75+)	0.04		
Baltimore	13	VF or ON	≥40	4.2 black 1.3 white	1.23 black 0.92 white (40-49)	11.26 black 2.16 white (80+)			
Framingham	37,70	VF and IOP/ON or history	≥52	1.4	0.5 (55-59)	4.4 (80-84)			
Blue Mts, Australia	14	VF and ON	≥49	3	0.4 (49-59)	11.4 (80+)			
Rotterdam	15	VF and IOP or ON	≥55	1.1	0.2 (55-59)	3.3 (85-89)			Narrow angles—2.2%
Barbados	18	VF and ON	≥40	7.0 black 3.3 mixed 0.8 white	1.4 (40-49)	23.2 (80-86)			
St. Lucia	16	VF and ON	≥30	8.8					
Melbourne	71	VF and ON	≥40	1.7	0.1 (40-49)	9.7 (80-89)	0.1	0.2	
Egna-Newmark, Italy	72	2 of 3 VF/IOP/ON	≥40	2			0.6		
Ponza, Italy	73	VF and IOP or ON	≥40	2.51			0.97	0.29	
Mongolia	74		≥40	0.5			6.4		
NW Alaska	22		≥40				2.65		Occludable angles in 17% of ≥50

IOP=intraocular pressure
ON=optic nerve
VF=visual field

findings of glaucoma. This definitional specificity is vital because the prevalence rates of potentially occludable angles alone would be expected to be significantly greater than if elevated IOP or glaucomatous damage are also required for the diagnosis of angle-closure glaucoma.[19] Furthermore, one must keep in mind that even glaucoma specialists may disagree as to what is an occludable angle in a given patient.

Indeed, there might be far different rates of PACG if the definition were one based on biometric measurements of anterior chamber depth or angle configuration on ultrasound assessment.[20] Finally, care must also be taken to distinguish studies based on true population-based ascertainment methods as opposed to those that rely upon physician diagnoses in office settings.

The relationship of PACG to refractive error and axial length has been well defined; eyes that are hyperopic or shorter are more likely to have PACG, while eyes that are myopic are far less likely to have an angle configuration susceptible to PACG. As such, population-based studies must be carefully interpreted relative to the distribution of refractive error in that population. This fact is of critical significance in studies outside of Europe and North America, where rapid economic development has transformed the population distribution of refractive error from one of hyperopic predominance to myopic dominance within a generation in a country such as Taiwan.[21] Thus, studies reporting higher rates of PACG among those above age 50 in such populations may not be valid in the future as today's younger, far more myopic adults reach those age thresholds.

Risk Factors for POAG and PACG

No matter how strictly one defines POAG, there are several important risk factors for the development of POAG that have been documented in virtually every study. First, older age is a tremendous risk for developing glaucoma in every study that has examined it. Comparing those in their 40s to those in their 80s, the Baltimore Eye Study found that rates increased in whites nearly 2.5-fold, from 0.92% to 2.16%, while that of blacks increased more than 10-fold, from 1.23% to 11.26%.[13] The Rotterdam Study found over a 16-fold increase, from 0.2% among those 55 to 59 years of age to 3.3% among those in their late 80s.[15] Finally, the Blue Mountains Study in

Australia found almost a 30-fold increase in POAG, from 0.4% among those in their 50s to 11.4% among those in their 80s.[14]

Age plays a similar risk factor for the development of PACG, with older individuals much more likely to have PACG than younger cohorts. Among native populations in North America and Africa, the risk is as much as eight times greater in those over the age of 70 compared to those in their 40s.[22]

Second, race is also an important glaucoma risk factor. Blacks and those with darker pigmentation are more likely to develop POAG and to do so at an earlier age. Data from a direct comparison in the same geographic area as the Baltimore Eye Study demonstrates a 4- to 5-fold increase among blacks.[13] Similarly, the rates in the Barbados Eye Study showed a nearly 9-fold difference between whites and blacks, with an intermediate rate for the mixed race subpopulation.[18]

Ethnic or racial differences similarly appear to exist for PACG. Native populations of Asian descent are reputed to have greater rates of PACG than whites; however, such differences may have more to do with socioeconomic contexts than an underlying racial predisposition. As economic development has increased educational opportunities in Asia, the population distribution of refractive error has shifted from hyperopia to myopia,[21] so that future rates of PACG may be no greater than that of whites. Indeed, over 80% of young adults in Taiwan and other newly developed countries are myopic, perhaps supporting the finding that biometric measurements of anterior chamber depth and axial length among residents of Taiwan do not differ significantly from white means.[20]

Third, those with diabetes have higher rates of POAG than those without the disease, *and* those with glaucoma have higher rates of diabetes than those who do not have glaucoma. Although the initial report from the Baltimore Eye Study found no relationship between POAG and self-reported history of diabetes,[23] three other population-based studies, which were based on laboratory tests of diabetes, found a 2-fold increase in both directions.[24-26] No similar finding has been found among those with PACG.

Fourth, there is a suggestion that men may be more likely than women to have glaucoma. Although most population-based studies have found no difference by gender, both the Rotterdam Study and the Barbados Study found a greater likelihood of glaucoma in men.[15,18]

Finally, IOP remains a strong risk factor for the development of POAG. Mathematical models suggest that at IOPs of 28 to 30 mmHg or greater, the probability of having or developing glaucoma exceeds 50%.[8,27-30] Further, population-based studies have repeatedly identified IOP as a significant risk factor in the subsequent development of glaucomas according to the case criteria used in those studies.

Although most of these glaucoma risk factors are probably so significant that they would persist even with the recent changes in the case definition, the reader should be attuned to potential changes due to re-analysis of study results. Indeed, one should be particularly alert to potential *new* risk factors arising from new case definitions altering the case identification within even these completed studies.

THE NATURAL HISTORY OF GLAUCOMA— TREATED OR UNTREATED?

POAG

Little data currently exist on the natural history of POAG followed in a scientifically rigorous fashion without treatment.[4] The only controlled trial to date is the Collaborative Normal-Tension Glaucoma Study Group (CNTGSG) results which indicate that therapy initiated with the intent to lower IOP by 30% from baseline was associated with a reduction of 50% in the rate of progression of visual field loss over 5 years.[31,32] However, such a survival benefit was found only after removing the effect of cataracts from the analyses. The performance of surgery to lower the IOP sufficiently was associated with a higher rate of cataract progression, which adversely affected visual acuity endpoints. As such, significant questions remain to be answered. Additional knowledge is currently being gained as part of a no-treatment arm in a randomized controlled trial of the benefits and side effects of the medical treatment of early POAG in Scandinavia.

Instead, knowledge of the history of glaucoma is derived from anecdotal experiences of providers (eg, in published consecutive series cases) or from trials (eg, a few randomized, controlled) of the efficacy of different kinds of interventions. In addition, re-analyses of existing data sets such as the Baltimore Eye Study and the Olmstead County Registry in Minnesota are providing important new insights.[33]

POAG, even under treatment, historically has been associated with measurable rates of progression of visual field loss. Published studies indicate that between 3% and 8% of patients under care by an ophthalmologist may suffer progressive field damage on an annual basis.[34-36] Indeed, in a study of patients followed longitudinally in Olmstead County in Minnesota, who were cared for at least 20 years, 27% became legally blind in at least one eye and 9% became legally blind in both eyes.[37] Such rates of progression of disease, even under treatment, have led some to wonder whether treatment is even effective for POAG and whether these rates represent the natural history of glaucoma.

Evidence collected by the AAO in preparing its PPP, however, indicates that progression rates over 5 years rise with higher IOP levels, such that more than 60% of those who have IOPs of 20 mmHg or greater after surgery progress, compared to less than 16% of those with IOPs of 14 mmHg or less.[1] Thus, it appears that the clinical course of even the treated history of POAG may be marked by progressive loss of vision in a significant portion of patients.

In contrast, analysis of progression rates from many studies show that the rates of progression to POAG from glaucoma suspects are significantly lower, and that less than 1% of ocular hypertensives have any visual field progression each year.[38,39] In contrast, the above data should be compared to the rate of blindness in the Olmstead County data, which would average to more than 1% per year of blindness incidence.[37] What is the true rate?

The answer is that both rates are probably correct. When one considers that the low rates are based on a population study of ocular hypertensives and suspects, and the higher rates are based on care provided generally at academic referral centers, the difference can most likely be explained on the basis of population biases in the populations being reported upon. The lower rate indicates that most suspects do well over time. In comparison, the published literature clearly identifies a subset of treated patients who do very poorly over the long term and have significantly higher rates of progression. In addition, many of the published rates of progression represent older paradigms of treatment. One would expect that, given the newer modalities of treatment and the more aggressive stance of glaucoma surgical intervention encoded in the new AAO PPP, current progression rates should be lower than the historical rates. Such a supposition, of course, is based on the predicate that treatment for POAG is effective.

PACG

In contrast to POAG, the natural history of untreated PACG is well-known from historical antecedents. Untreated, this bilateral condition is likely to cause blindness in both eyes, often through painful acute attacks, but also commonly through quiet, relatively asymptomatic, intermittent episodes. Studies have demonstrated that up to 75% of individuals with acute PACG in one eye will suffer a similar PACG attack in the fellow eye over 5 to 10 years, even under treatment with miotic drops.[40]

The current standard of treatment is to perform definitive surgery to relieve the anatomic predisposition for such attacks through the creation of an iridotomy or iridectomy, through either laser or incisional surgery. Such therapy definitively relieves the mechanism of PACG, though residual damage to the trabecular meshwork from previous angle-closure attacks may result in a secondary form of glaucoma that requires continuing care.

DOES EVERYONE WITH GLAUCOMA NEED TREATMENT?

The clear implication of the studies on disease progression are that not every patient with glaucoma, however defined, may require treatment. As indicated in Figure 1-1, modified from figures by Spaeth, Quigley, and others, many patients will die before they have significant visual field loss. In a recent analysis, Quigley demonstrated that although visual field progression can be as high as 8% per year on a population basis, most patients will not go blind even at this rate of progression.[35] We also now have preliminary data on what amounts of visual field loss are required to create significant effects on patient quality of life and vision-related functioning. In other words, there are at least two distinct parts to answering this question. First, how likely is any particular person to develop loss of vision functioning, defined as visual field, visual acuity, contrast sensitivity, or some other physiological variable? Second, how much loss of

physiological functioning is required before an individual begins to have an associated loss of visual abilities or overall quality of life?

Understanding the Likelihood of Loss of Vision Functioning

In Figure 1-1, we can see that the loss of optic nerve fibers must occur for a period of time before measurable visual field deficits are detected.[6] Newer visual field techniques such as blue-on-yellow perimetry (short wavelength automated perimetry, or SWAP) may identify visual field loss at an earlier stage of disease.[41] Once loss has occurred, though, additional nerve fiber degeneration is likely to be associated with an accelerating course of visual field loss for the same absolute amount of nerve fiber loss. This fact can easily be understood by the mathematical notion that each equivalent additional quantitative amount of nerve fiber layer loss is a greater proportionate or percentage amount of the remaining tissue (see Figure 1-1). Thus, a 5000 nerve fiber layer loss at 50,000 remaining fibers (10%) is likely to have less devastating consequences than the same 5000 nerve fiber loss at 15,000 remaining fibers (33%). This simple mathematical relationship may well account for the clinical observations that underlie the axiom that the greater amount of nerve damage, the more susceptible the nerve is to additional damage. Indeed, if the mechanisms of damage are unaltered, one might expect the same amount of nerve fiber loss per unit of time, but the relative effects of such loss would be progressively more pronounced as the remaining amount of nerve tissue declines.

At this time we cannot identify that subgroup of patients who are likely to have steeper slopes of nerve loss, and thus are likely to progress to significant vision loss or blindness prior to death. As such, our goal is to treat every person so that that the smallest possible minority of patients lose vision prior to death. Such a philosophy is consonant with medical therapeutics in other fields of medicine, especially systemic hypertension.[42] Without natural history data on an untreated population basis, it is currently not practical to model the relative risks and benefits of treatment. Thus, it should be among our highest priorities to identify factors that would allow us to better differentiate high risk individuals who should be treated from lower risk individuals who may be able to be followed without treatment until progression suggestive of misclassification occurs.

Fortunately, we do have tantalizing glimpses at some potential methods of identifying those at greater risk. First, the extent of fluctuation of IOP in an eye may indicate those eyes at higher risk.[43] Indeed, larger fluctuations in IOP can be found in those with glaucoma rather than those without glaucoma.[44] Such findings can be understood in the context that connective and other tissues in the human body are possibly more susceptible to injury by dynamic stress rather than static loads.

Similarly, those with vasculopathic diseases, such as diabetes and hypertension, have also been found in some studies to be at higher risk of developing glaucoma. The apparent conflict among studies regarding hypertension may well have to do with the inadequate definitions of hypertension and with its characterization (eg, the need to use mean arterial pressure), and to confounding effects of medications on systemic blood pressure, as well as to the potential effects of hypotension.[45,46]

Third, we already know that there are certain IOP levels that are so high that intervention is warranted. In neovascular glaucoma or acute angle-closure glaucoma (primary or secondary), blindness can result in weeks or months if the pressure and underlying causes are not adequately treated. In congenital glaucomas, untreated elevations in pressure lead to blindness in all cases over time. Experience and mathematical models indicate that those with IOPs of over 28 to 30 mmHg have a 50% probability of having glaucoma, defined using older clinical paradigms (which, as noted above, have a higher threshold for diagnosis).[28-30] From these situations, it is clear that significantly elevated IOP levels are associated with vision loss and that intervention, therefore, is warranted.

If we are better able to broaden this ability to characterize those who suffer faster rates of progression from those who suffer much slower rates of progression of nerve fiber loss (and hence visual field and other performance measures), then we can begin to tailor both the need for and the intensity of treatment. Even a relative risk of 3 or 4 could help identify those at greatest need for intensive treatment and follow-up. Thus, much more research is warranted to better characterize these subpopulations of patients with glaucoma.

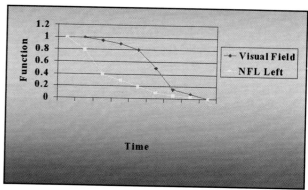

Figure 1-1. Relationship of nerve loss and functioning.

Quality of Life Impact of Visual Loss in Glaucoma

Impaired vision is associated with increased rates of falls, hip fractures, and decreased physical mobility.[47,48] Visual symptoms, such as trouble seeing or blurred vision, are associated with measurable decrements in general quality of life measures such as the SF-36 and instrumental activities of daily living.[49,50] Self-rated quality of vision has a clear relationship to general health functioning. Indeed, vision is a vital aspect of our lives, and decrements in vision can be directly related to decrements in general well-being and quality of life. Nevertheless, merely having a disease such as cataract or glaucoma is not independently associated with general quality of life measures, once the appropriate adjustments for demographic factors and medical and ocular comorbidities are included.[51,52]

Decrements in vision also are directly related to difficulties in performing vision-related or vision-specific tasks.[48,53,54] Not surprisingly, such relationships are stronger and more easily seen relative to vision-specific quality of life than general quality of life measures. As in the analyses of general quality of life, adjustments for demographic differences, visual acuity, and comorbid medical and ocular conditions need to be made. In the case of visual fields, such adjustments reduce but do not eliminate the statistical or clinical significance of visual field decrements in vision-related functioning, as measured by validated instruments.[52,55]

The critical query then becomes one of how much visual field loss needs to occur before a clinically significant decrement in vision-related functioning can be measured. Such a seemingly simple inquiry is complicated, however, by important questions of how we can best quantitate and classify visual field loss, if field loss should be measured binocularly or can be imputed through the visual field loss in the better eye (with the worse eye having more and deeper field loss), and what the method of field measurement should be (central fields or full fields). Such questions will need to be addressed and techniques further modified in future investigations.

Using the information we do have available, however, we can begin to assess the impact of field loss on vision functioning using two common field grading systems—the Advanced Glaucoma Intervention Study (AGIS) grading scale and the Esterman binocular visual field grading system.[52,55] In a pilot study using Esterman fields, Parrish found that there appeared to be a linear relationship between field loss and decrements in the National Eye Institute—Visual Functioning Questionnaire (VFQ).[52] Nevertheless, analysis of many of the scatter plots of results suggests that perhaps not all of the VFQ subscales are directly linear in nature, but additional investigation is needed. In a multi-site study, Gutierrez et al found that better eye AGIS scores were similarly linearly related to VFQ scores.[55] Although the data presented in this study more strongly support a linear relationship, evaluation of the results suggests that many if not most of the VFQ subscales have steeper rates or slopes of loss with more severely affected fields, suggesting a potentially non-linear but inverse parabolic relationship. Put together, these results suggest that it is the loss of field in the better eye that generally drives vision functioning, and that even early loss in the better eye may not be associated with truly significant clinical decrements in quality of life. In other words, individuals probably do not notice a meaningful impact on their lives until relatively noticeable visual field loss has occurred in both eyes, excluding special situations (eg, the professional athlete's or professional truck driver's peripheral vision).

Implications for Treating Glaucoma

Current standards of care call for treatment of all patients who have glaucoma. Clearly, all patients with PACG or who are susceptible to PACG should be treated, given the natural history of those without treatment. The AAO PPP for POAG clearly enables eye care providers and other physicians to diagnose and treat individuals with glaucoma who have no field loss and no elevations in IOP, but do have characteristic optic nerve or nerve fiber layer loss. Such characteristic loss includes: defects in the nerve fiber layer, asymmetry between the two eyes, asymmetry above and below in the same optic nerve, notches in the optic nerve rim, optic nerve hemorrhages, or enlarged cups. In addition, individuals with elevated IOP beyond a "safe" range, generally 28 mmHg or higher, also usually are treated. As estimated from the Baltimore Eye Study results, such a treatment protocol could potentially place upward of 15 million Americans on treatment for POAG.[17]

The evidence cited here suggests that this strategy could be modified significantly if additional data could be generated in the areas of risk factors analyses for *progression* (as opposed to risk factors for *having* glaucoma) and *pace* of progression. Additional data also need to be generated to better identify the degree of physiological dysfunction arising from glaucoma that is associated with noticeable patient functioning defects. When these two elements are put together, we can then identify not only those who are at higher risk of developing loss that interferes with their quality of vision and quality of life but also those individuals for whom we should intervene *before* noticeable decrements occur in functioning.

HOW CAN WE BEST DELIVER GLAUCOMA CARE?

Glaucoma of all forms is a leading cause of impaired vision and blindness around the world. Even in the United States, 19% of blindness among blacks is caused by glaucoma.[1] Such vision loss and blindness has large and significant effects and costs on both the individuals affected and our society. In order to assess this burden, we need to address two questions:

1. Should we screen for glaucoma?
2. How can we ensure access to health care for those who are diagnosed as having glaucoma?

Screening for Glaucoma

All current preventive care guidelines and screening strategies uniformly state that mass glaucoma screening is not warranted and should not be conducted.[56] Using traditional means of IOP evaluation, optic disc examination, or traditional visual field testing, insufficient sensitivity, specificity, predictive values, and cost-effectiveness have been found.[56,57] One study in the United Kingdom estimated screening would be worthwhile if the value of detecting a case (in terms of savings) would exceed $850 per case, using existing resources and staff.[58] Furthermore, the open questions about the effectiveness of treatment for POAG militate against aggressive screening, because the benefits of treatment once cases are identified are as yet not completely resolved.

The recent development of the frequency-doubled perimeter (FDP), however, suggests that the test performance of the perimeter as a screening instrument may finally be sufficient for use on a population screening basis.[59] With sensitivities and specificities in excess of 95%, the posterior probabilities of a positive test result are sufficiently high as to justify its use. Together with the new definition of POAG and the finding of any visual field defect defines one as at least a moderate case of glaucoma, the FDP offers the possibility of economically feasible screening for glaucoma. To the extent that the prior probability of glaucoma is enhanced by use of a second screening technique (such as risk factor analysis), the performance of the FDP will only be more accurate.

Nevertheless, efforts to provide more accurate and reliable methods of screening still leave unanswered questions surrounding the value of treatment once the diagnosis of glaucoma has been made. No screening strategy would be cost-effective if no effective treatment existed for cases so identified. Thus, the final endorsement for glaucoma screening necessarily awaits the results of the ongoing randomized, controlled trials with a no-treatment arm to confirm the findings of the CNTGSG results.

Access to Care

Care Patterns by Ophthalmologists

Assuming that treatment is found to be effective, significant issues still exist about whether people receive appropriate care for glaucoma. Although the survey of the membership of the AAO conducted for the RAND Workforce Study suggests that the average patient with POAG should be seen four times per year,[9] data from the Medicare Provider (Part B) files indicate that only a minority of patients with any eye condition are seen at least this many times per year.[60]

Furthermore, although patients cared for in an academic setting appear to receive care in accordance with the recommendations of the AAO PPP,[61] patients receiving care in the community setting often receive care not in line with the recommendations of the PPP for POAG.[62] Thus, for all patients, significant attention needs to be paid to how care is provided.

Differential Access by Groups

This concern is even more troubling relative to care provided to minorities and the poor in the United States. Data clearly indicate that black Americans do not access the health care system in proportion to the rates of glaucoma that have been detected on the basis of population studies. Although black Americans undergo glaucoma surgery twice as often as white Americans, this rate is still 50% less than what would be expected.[63] Similarly, the homeless and the poor do not access health care in a manner similar to those in better socioeconomic situations.[64] Finally, blacks and the elderly do not have glaucoma treatment initiated at rates that might otherwise be expected.[65] The problem does not appear to be the care provided by physicians once patients enter the care system, unlike the situation with many other areas of medical care. Nevertheless, the lack of expected access raises important questions for providers to address.[66] Why is this the case?

Traditional approaches to this issue have cited the lack of income and the lack of sufficient insurance coverage for the groups just cited. Yet, even among Medicare beneficiaries, where these influences are far less, one sees the same patterns of care.[66] As such, additional factors or obstacles to care need to be examined. One important new finding is that black Americans trust the health care system and health care providers much less than white Americans.[67] The result of such lower trust may be a decrease in the likelihood of seeking care or of complying with provider recommendations once care is sought. Thus, access may be decreased on the basis of the patient's conscious decisions and behaviors.

Second, loss of vision may be seen culturally as part of the aging process, so that loss of vision in one eye is not cause for alarm. Similarly, there may be other cultural barriers to receiving care for a chronic condition.[68] Although this may appear to be an educational issue on the surface, there may be hidden subtexts that severely diminish the returns from traditional educational efforts. For example, among Latino women with diabetes, the cultural norms of their gender roles severely hamper their ability to care for themselves, both in terms of diet and in their being able to attend regular medical follow-up.[68] Such scenarios also are likely to be present for minorities relative to glaucoma care. Thus, it is clear that a wider set of factors needs to be evaluated in enhancing access to care.

CONCLUSION

When we examine the population prevalence of POAG and PACG, we can easily see that these estimates are strongly dependent on how one defines each condition and the quality of the screening and examination technique employed.[69,70] Nevertheless, it is clear that many patients who might benefit from treatment are not currently receiving it. Yet, several outstanding questions remain.

First, is treatment effective in altering the natural history of POAG? We know that treatment does alter the natural history of PACG favorably, and we have evidence that it also does so for POAG (though not yet definitive evidence). Second, can we identify those at greatest risk for the most rapid progression of damage to vision? We know that visual field loss has a measurable effect on vision-related quality of life, so targeting those at greatest risk for developing such field loss prior to its onset clearly would be beneficial. Third, can we enhance the likelihood that those who do have glaucoma will receive adequate care? This obligation involves not only increasing access to those at greatest risk of developing severe glaucoma but also optimizing the quality of care that all patients with glaucoma receive. Each of these tasks is a major undertaking that will challenge our profession and ourselves.

REFERENCES

1. American Academy of Ophthalmology. *Preferred practice pattern: primary open-angle glaucoma.* San Francisco, Calif: American Academy of Ophthalmology; 1992.
2. Guzman G, Javitt J, Glick H, Tielsch J, McDonald R. Glaucoma in the United States population: the economic burden of illness. *Invest Ophthalmol Vis Sci.* 1992;33(suppl):759.
3. Lee P. Economic concerns in glaucoma management in the 21st century. *J Glaucoma.* 1993;2:148-151.
4. American Academy of Ophthalmology. *Preferred practice pattern: primary open-angle glaucoma.* San Francisco, Calif: American Academy of Ophthalmology; 1996.
5. Caprioli J. Clinical evaluation of the optic nerve in glaucoma. *Trans Am Ophthalmol Soc.* 1994;92:589-641.
6. Quigley JA, Addicks EM, Green WR. Optic nerve damage in human glaucoma. III: quantitative correlation of nerve fiber loss and visual field defect in glaucoma, ischemic neuropathy, papilledema, and toxic neuropathy. *Arch Ophthalmol.* 1982;100:135-146.
7. Herndon LW, Choudhri SA, Cox T, et al. Central corneal thickness in normal, glaucomatous, and ocular hypertensive eyes. *Arch Ophthalmol.* 1997;115:1137-1141.
8. Sommer A, Tielsch JM, Katz J, et al. Relationship between intraocular pressure and primary open angle glaucoma among white and black Americans. *The Baltimore Eye Survey. Arch Ophthalmol.* 1991;109:1090-1095.
9. Lee PP, Jackson CJ, Relles DA. *Estimating Eye Care Provider Supply and Workforce Requirements.* Santa Monica, Calif: RAND, MR-516-AAO; 1995.
10. Lichter PR. Variability of expert observers in evaluating the optic disc. *Trans Am Ophthalmol Soc.* 1977;74:532-572.
11. Varma R, Steinmann WC, Scott IU. Expert agreement in evaluating the optic disc for glaucoma. *Ophthalmology.* 1992;99:215-221.
12. Klein BE, Klein R, Sponsel WE, et al. Prevalence of glaucoma. The Beaver Dam Eye Study. *Ophthalmology.* 1992;99:1499-1504.
13. Tielsch JM, Sommer A, Katz J, et al. Racial variations in the prevalence of primary open-angle glaucoma. The Baltimore Eye Survey. *JAMA.* 1991;266:369-374.
14. Mitchell P, Smith W, Attebo K, Healey PR. Prevalence of open-angle glaucoma in Australia. The Blue Mountains Eye Study. *Ophthalmology.* 1996;103:1661-1669.
15. Dielemans I, Vingerling JR, Wolfs RC, et al. The prevalence of open-angle glaucoma in a population-based study in the Netherlands. The Rotterdam Study. *Ophthalmology.* 1994;101:1851-1855.
16. Mason RP, Kosoko O, Wilson MR, et al. National survey of the prevalence and risk factors of glaucoma in St. Lucia, West Indies. Part I. Prevalence findings. *Ophthalmology.* 1989;96:1363-1368.
17. Quigley HA. Medical progress: open-angle glaucoma (review article). *N Engl J Med.* 1993;328:1097-1106.
18. Leske MC, Connell AM, Schachat AP, Hyman L. The Barbados Eye Study. Prevalence of open angle glaucoma. *Ophthalmology.* 1994;112:821-829.
19. Congdon N, Wang F, Tielsch JM. Issues in the epidemiology and population-based screening of primary angle-closure glaucoma. *Surv Ophthalmol.* 1992;36:411-423.
20. Congdon NG, Youlin Q, Quigley H, et al. Biometry and primary angle-closure glaucoma among Chinese, white, and black populations. *Ophthalmology.* 1997;104:1489-1495.
21. Wen L-Y, Myopic choroidal degenerations. In: Tso MOM, ed. *Retinal Diseases: Biomedical Foundations and Clinical Management.* New York, NY: JB Lippincott Co; 1988;242-246.
22. Arkell SM, Lightman DA, Sommer A, et al. The prevalence of glaucoma among Eskimos of northwest Alaska. *Arch Ophthalmol.* 1987;105:482-485.

23. Tielsch JM, Katz J, Quigley HA, Javitt JC, Sommer A. Diabetes, intraocular pressure, and primary open-angle glaucoma in the Baltimore Eye Survey. *Ophthalmology.* 1995;102:48-53.

24. Mitchell P, Smith W, Chey T, Healey PR. Open-angle glaucoma and diabetes: the Blue Mountains Eye Study, Australia. *Ophthalmology.* 1997;104:712-728.

25. Dielemans I, de Jong PT, Stolk R, et al. Primary open-angle glaucoma, intraocular pressure, and diabetes mellitus in the general elderly population. The Rotterdam Study. *Ophthalmology.* 1996;103:1271-1275.

26. Klein BE, Klein R, Jensen SC. Open-angle glaucoma and older-onset diabetes. The Beaver Dam Eye Study. *Ophthalmology.* 1994;101:1173-1177.

27. Hollows FC, Graham PA. Intra-ocular pressure, glaucoma, and glaucoma suspects in a defined population. *Br J Ophthalmol.* 1996;50:570-586.

28. Davanger M. Low-pressure glaucoma and the concept of the IOP tolerance distribution curve. *Acta Ophthalmol.* 1989;67:256-260.

29. Davanger M, Ringvold A, Blika S. The frequency distribution of the glaucoma tolerance limit. *Acta Ophthalmol.* 1991;69:782-775.

30. Davanger M, Ringvold A, Blika S. The probability of having glaucoma at different IOP levels. *Acta Ophthalmol.* 1991; 69:565-568.

31. Comparison of glaucomatous progression between untreated patients with normal-tension glaucoma and patients with therapeutically reduced intraocular pressures. Collaborative Normal-Tension Glaucoma Study Group. *Am J Ophthalmol.* 1998;126(4):487-497.

32. The effectiveness of intraocular pressure reduction in the treatment of normal-tension glaucoma. Collaborative Normal-Tension Glaucoma Study Group. *Am J Ophthalmol.* 1998;126(4):498-505.

33. Erie JC, Hodge DO, Bray DT. The incidence of primary angle-closure glaucoma in Olmsted County, Minnesota. *Arch Ophthalmol.* 1997;115:177-181.

34. Kass MA, Kolker AE, Becker B. Prognostic factors in glaucomatous visual field loss. *Arch Ophthalmol.* 1976;94:1274-1276.

35. Quigley HA, Tielsch J, Katz J, et al. Rate of progression in open-angle glaucoma estimated from cross-sectional prevalence of visual field damage. *Am J Ophthalmol.* 1996;122:355-363.

36. Mao LK, Stewart WC, Shields MB. Correlation between intraocular pressure control and progressive glaucomatous damage in primary open-angle glaucoma. *Am J Ophthalmol.* 1991;111:51-55.

37. Hattenhauer MG, Johnson DH, Ing HH, et al. The probability of blindness from open-angle glaucoma. *Ophthalmology.* 1998;105(11):2099-2104.

38. Hart WM. The epidemiology of primary open-angle glaucoma and ocular hypertension. In: Ritch R, Shields MB, Krupin T, eds. *The Glaucomas.* Baltimore, Md: CV Mosby Co; 1989;790-791.

39. Leske MC. The epidemiology of open-angle glaucoma: a review. *Am J Epidemiology.* 1983;118:166-191.

40. Ritch R, Lowe RF, Reyes A. Therapeutic overview of angle-closure glaucoma. In: Ritch R, Shields MB, Krupin T, eds. *The Glaucomas.* Baltimore, Md: CV Mosby Co; 1989;860.

41. Sample PA, Bosworth CF, Weinreb RN. Short-wavelength automated perimetry and motion automated perimetry in patients with glaucoma. *Arch Ophthalmol.* 1997;115:1129-1133.

42. Joint National Committee on Prevention, Detection, Evaluation and Treatment of High Blood Pressure. The sixth report of the Joint National Committee on Prevention, Detection, Evaluation and Treatment of High Blood Pressure. *Arch Int Med.* 1997;157:2413-2446.

43. Zeimer RC, Wilensky JT, Gieser DK, Viana MA. Association between intraocular pressure peaks and progression of visual field loss. *Ophthalmology.* 1991;98:64-69.

44. Sacca SC, Rolando M, Marletta A, et al. Fluctuations of intraocular pressure during the day in open-angle, normal-tension glaucoma and normal subjects. *Ophthalmologica.* 1998;212(2):115-119.

45. Tielsch JM, Katz J, Sommer A, Quigley HA, Javitt JC. Hypertension, perfusion pressure, and primary open-angle glaucoma. *Arch Ophthalmol.* 1995;113:216-221.

46. Hayreh SS, Zimmerman MB, Podhajsky P, Alward WLM. Nocturnal arterial hypotension and its role in optic nerve head and ocular ischemic disorders. *Am J Ophthalmol.* 1994;117:603-624.

47. Tinetti ME, Sppechley M, Ginter SF. Risk factors for falls among elderly persons living in the community. *N Engl J Med.* 1988;319:1701-1707.

48. Mangione CM, Lee PP, Hays RD. Measurement of visual functioning and health-related quality of life in eye disease and cataract surgery. In: Spilker B, ed. *Quality of Life and Pharmacoeconomics in Clinical Trials.* 2nd ed. (pp. 1045-1051). Philadelphia, Pa: Lippincott-Raven Publishers; 1996.

49. Kington R, Rogowski R, Lillard L, Lee PP. Functional associations of "trouble seeing." *J Gen Int Med.* 1997;12:125-128.

50. Lee PP, Spritzer K, Hays R. The impact of blurred vision on functioning and well-being. *Ophthalmology.* 1997;104:390-396.

51. Fryback DG, Dasbach EJ, Klein R, et al. The Beaver Dam Health Outcomes Study: initial catalog of health-state quality factors. *Med Decis Making.* 1993;13:90-102.

52. Parrish RK. Visual impairment, visual functioning, and quality of life assessments in patients with glaucoma. *Trans Am Ophthalmol Soc.* 1996;94:919-1028.

53. Javitt JC, Brenner MH, Curbow B, et al. Vision change and quality of life in the elderly: response to cataract surgery and treatment of other chronic ocular conditions. *Arch Ophthalmol.* 1993;111:680-685.

54. Steinberg EP, Tielsch JM, Schein OD, et al. The VF-14: an index of functional impairment in patients with cataract. *Arch Ophthalmol.* 1994;112:630-638.

55. Gutierrez P, Wilson MR, Johnson C, et al. Influence of glaucomatous visual field loss on health-related quality of life. *Arch Ophthalmol.* 1997;115:777-784.

56. Canadian Task Force on the Periodic Health examination. Periodic health examination, 1995, update: 3. Screening for visual problems among elderly patients. *Can Med Assoc J.* 1995;152(8):1211-1222.

57. Tielsch JM, Katz J, Singh K, et al. A population-based evaluation of glaucoma screening: the Baltimore Eye Survey. *Am J Epidemiol.* 1991;134:1102-1110.

58. Tuck MW, Crick RP. The cost-effectiveness of various modes of screening for primary open angle glaucoma. *Ophthalmic Epidemiol.* 1997;4:3-17.

59. Sponsel WE, Ritch R, Stamper R, et al. Prevent Blindness America Visual Field Screening Study. *Am J Ophthalmol.* 1995;120:699-708.

60. Ellwein LB, Friedlin V, McBean AM, Lee PP. Use of eye-care services among the 1991 Medicare population. *Ophthalmology.* 1996;103:1732-1743.

61. Albrecht K, Lee PP. Conformance with Preferred Practice Patterns in glaucoma care. *Ophthalmology.* 1994;101:1668-1671.

62. Hertzog LH, Albrecht KG, LaBree L, Lee PP. Glaucoma care and conformance with preferred practice patterns: examination of the private, community-based ophthalmologist. *Ophthalmology.* 1996;103:1009-1013.

63. Javitt JC, McBean AM, Nicholson GA, et al. Undertreatment of glaucoma among black Americans. *N Engl J Med.* 1991;325:1418-1422.

64. Ho JH, Change RJ, Wheeler NC, Lee DA. Ophthalmic disorders among the homeless and nonhomeless in Los Angeles. *J Am Optom Assoc.* 1997;68:567-573.

65. Glynn RJ, Gurwitz JH, Bohn RL, et al. Old age and race as determinants of initiation of glaucoma therapy. *Am J Epidemiol.* 1993;138:395-406.

66. Wang F, Javitt JC, Tielsch JM. Racial variations in treatment for glaucoma and cataract among Medicare recipients. *Ophthalmic Epdiemiol.* 1997;4(2):89-100.

67. Corbie-Smith G, Thomas SB, Duncan T, et al. Racial differences in perceptions of physicians and research: results of a national telephone survey. *J Gen Int Med.* 1998;13(supp):63.

68. Van Boemel GB, Lee PP. Adherence to traditional female sex role as a hidden barrier in preventable eye disease: a case history. *J Vis Impair & Blindness.* In press.

69. Bathija R, Gupta N, Zangwill L, Weinreb RN. Changing definition of glaucoma. *J Glaucoma.* 1998;7:165-169.

70. Kahn HA, Milton RC. Alternative definitions of open-angle glaucoma. Effect on prevalence and associations in the Framingham eye study. *Arch Ophthalmol.* 1980;98:2172-2177.

71. Wensor MD, McCarty CA, Sttanislavsky YL, Livingston PM, Taylor HR. The prevalence of glaucoma in the Melbourne Visual Impairment Project. *Ophthalmology.* 1998;105:733-739.

72. Bonomi L, Marchini G, Marraffa M, et al. Prevalence of glaucoma and intraocular pressure distribution in a defined population. The Egna-Neumarkt Study. *Ophthalmology.* 1998;105:209-215.

73. Cedrone C, Culaasso F, Cesareo M, et al. Prevalence of glaucoma in Ponza, Italy: a comparison with other studies. *Ophthalmic Epidemiol.* 1997;4:59-72.

74. Foster PJ, Baasanhu J, Alsbirk PH, et al. Glaucoma in Mongolia. A population-based survey in Hovsgol province, northern Mongolia. *Arch Ophthalmol.* 1996;114:1235-1241.

Chapter Two

GENETICS IN GLAUCOMA

Mansoor Sarfarazi, PhD
Ivaylo Stoilov, MD

INTRODUCTION

The glaucomas are a group of eye conditions with a broad range of clinical presentations, definitions, diagnoses, variable ages of manifestation and modes of inheritance, and different molecular etiologies. The genetic study of glaucoma has further been complicated because the nature of this phenotype can be primary or secondary to other ocular and/or non-ocular conditions. During the past few years, significant progress has been made in identifying the chromosomal locations of a number of primary and secondary forms of glaucoma. A number of functional genes underlying the molecular etiology of these genetic loci also have been cloned, and causative mutations have been identified in familial as well as sporadic cases. For the primary forms of glaucoma, as of this writing, two loci for congenital glaucoma/buphthalmos ([PCG]; GLC3A & B), one locus for juvenile-onset open-angle glaucoma ([JOAG]; GLC1A), and five loci for adult-onset chronic open-angle glaucoma ([COAG]; GLC1B to GLC1F) have been reported. Of

these, only the GLC3A (ie, CYP1B1) and GLC1A (ie, TIGR/MYOC) genes have been cloned and mutations are widely shown in different ethnic populations. For the secondary forms of glaucoma, more than 10 different loci have been described, of which the genes for only three have been cloned and shown to be directly causative of their respective ocular conditions.

This chapter assumes a working knowledge of terms frequently encountered in the field of genetics. The chapter emphasizes the molecular genetics of primary forms of glaucoma, but a brief description of all other ocular conditions for which the glaucoma manifests itself as a secondary phenotype also will be provided.

PCG/BUPHTHALMOS

The severe congenital form of glaucoma has an onset in the neonatal or infantile period, manifested by symptoms of increased intraocular pressure (IOP) and corneal edema such as excessive tearing, photophobia, and an enlargement of the globe (buphthalmos). The disease has an aggressive course, requiring filtration surgery for alleviation of the high IOP.[1] The term *primary congenital glaucoma*, or PCG, is reserved for cases where the only anatomic defect observed is isolated trabeculodysgenesis. This particular form is classified as isolated congenital glaucoma according to the Shaffer and Weiss classification, and as isolated trabeculodysgenesis according to the anatomic classification of developmental glaucomas presented by Hoskins et al.[2,3]

Etiology and Pathogenesis of PCG

Studies of the affected eyes from individuals with PCG have found evidence for maldevelopment of the anterior chamber angle of the eye.[4] By gonioscopy, the peripheral iris is seen to be inserted more anteriorly than normal, and the trabecular meshwork seems to have a shiny surface. Under microscopic examination, the iris and the ciliary body occupy a position in relation to the trabecular meshwork equivalent to the seventh or eighth month of fetal development. The trabecular beams are thickened, and there is an absence of vacuoles in the endothelial lining of Schlemm's canal. The hypotheses proposed to explain this abnormal morphology include a membrane covering the anterior chamber angle and blocking the aqueous humor outflow, abnormal cleavage of the mesoderm during embryonal development, developmental arrest of the anterior chamber angle structures derived from neural crest cells, and inhibited posterior migration of the ciliary body and iris root.[4-7] It has been suggested that these pathogenic mechanisms are triggered by genetic and environmental etiologic factors acting individually or in a multifactorial fashion. While it has been difficult to clarify the importance and the exact nature of environmental causes, the role played by genetic factors in the etiology and pathogenesis of PCG is supported by numerous genetic and epidemiological studies.

Genetics of PCG

The highest reported incidence of PCG of 1:1250 was observed among the Slovakian Roms. In Europe, incidences from 1:5000 (Switzerland) to 1:22,000 (Slovakia) were reported with 1:10,000 being the average number.[8-10] The disease is familial in 10% to 40% of cases with the transmission being that of an autosomal recessive with variable penetrance (40% to 100%). Parental consanguinity also is reported in many familial cases. There is a high rate of concordance among monozygotic twins and discordance among dizygotic ones.[8-11] Some authors have questioned the autosomal-recessive mode of inheritance.[12,13] Their arguments were based on the observation of unequal sex distribution among the affected individuals, with boys being affected nearly twice as frequently as girls, as well as a lower than expected number of affected siblings in the familial cases. Additionally, several pedigrees were reported in which the disease was transmitted in successive generations suggesting autosomal-dominant inheritance.[11] Molecular genetic studies conducted during the past 5 years have shed some light on these questions raised by the classical geneticists.

Genetic Linkage Studies in PCG Families

In 1995, we applied the methods of genetic linkage analysis to a panel of 17 families segregating PCG in an autosomal-recessive fashion. All families originated from Turkey. In 11 families, genetic linkage was detected between the disease phenotype and genetic markers from chromosomal region 2p21.[14] Haplotype analysis and homozygosity mapping enabled us to map the disease gene within 2.5 cM interval flanked by DNA markers D2S2186 and D2S1346. This locus was designated GLC3A. Inspection of the haplotypes and heterogeneity analysis indicated that six families were not linked to locus GLC3A. Subsequent studies found that in four of these families the disease phenotype is linked to genetic markers spanning a region of about 3 cM on chromosome 1p36.[15] This genetic interval was defined by two groups of tightly linked markers—D1S1597/D1S485/D1S228 and D1S1176/D1S507/D1S407. This second locus associated with PCG was designated GLC3B. Two families were not linked to both loci indicating the existence of at least one more PCG locus. The association between locus GLC3A and PCG was subsequently confirmed in a large panel of families from Saudi Arabia and Slovakian Roms.[16,17] All families reported in these two studies were linked to locus GLC3A, thus establishing it as a major locus for this condition.

The genetic linkage studies made two important contributions to our understanding of PCG. First, the

Table 2-1

PCG Mutations in the CYP1B1 Gene

Exon	Mutation	Location	Ethnicity	Reference
II	Trp-57 Cys	Hinge region	Hisp	20
II	Gly-61 Glu	Hinge region	T, SA	16,20
II	4306insT		T	20
II	Glu-281 stop		T	20
II	4668insC		T	18
III	Large del.		T	18
III	7901del13		T	18
III	Gly-365 Trp	J-helix	US	20
III	Asp-374 Asn		SA	16
III	Pro-379 Leu	K-helix	T	20
III	Glu-387 Lys	K-helix	Hisp, Roms, Fr Can	19,20
III	Arg-390 His	K-helix	Pk	20
III	8037dup10		US, UK, T	20
III	Pro-437 Leu	Meander	T	20
III	8182delG		Hisp	20
III	Arg-469 Trp	Heme-binding	UK, T, SA	16,20
III	8240dup27		T	20

The origin of the analyzed families is indicated as Fr Can=French Canadian, Hisp=Hispanic, Pk=Pakistani, Roms=Slovakian, SA=Saudi Arabian, T=Turkish, UK=British, US=American.
Numbering of the aminoacid residues and nucleotides is according to the genomic sequence of CYP1B1 gene (GeneBank U56438).

detection of a strong linkage between the disease phenotype and discrete chromosomal region was new evidence that mutations in a single gene may be sufficient for disease to develop. Second, the identification of two different genetic loci associated with PCG was the first direct confirmation of genetic heterogeneity for this phenotype.

Causative Mutations in the Cytochrome P4501B1 (CYP1B1) Gene

The identification of genetic loci associated with PCG made it possible to initiate a search for the actual disease gene. The first gene to be directly implicated in the pathogenesis of PCG was cytochrome P4501B1 (CYP1B1).[18] This gene was mapped to chromosome 2p21 by in situ hybridization. Higher resolution mapping placed this gene within the GLC3A candidate region. Sequence analysis of CYP1B1 coding regions resulted in the identification of three DNA mutations which segregated with disease phenotype in five families previously linked to locus GLC3A. These mutations were not present in the normal population.

This initial study was followed by the publication of a detailed molecular analysis of three panels of PCG families from Turkey, Saudi Arabia, and Slovakian Roms.[16,19,20] The major findings detailed in these four reports could be summarized as follows.

- A total of 73 families were analyzed. From these, 70 had more than one affected individual and three had only one affected child.
- Screening for mutations within the CYP1B1 coding regions resulted in the identification of 23 DNA changes. Seventeen of these changes were characterized as disease-causing mutations (Table 2-1) and six were found to be a naturally occurring polymorphism.
- In all familial cases, the mutant alleles co-segregated with the disease phenotype in an autosomal-recessive fashion (Figure 2-1a). In the three families with only one affected individual, the parents were found to be normal carriers with the affected child being homozygote or compound heterozygote for the mutant alleles carried by his or her parents (Figure 2-1b). Both sexes were equally represented among the affected individuals.
- Parent-child transmission was present in five families (Figure 2-1c). Molecular analysis found that in all instances the affected parent was a homozygote for mutant allele, while the other parent was a normal carrier. Therefore, these are examples of pseudodominant inheritance of an autosomal-recessive trait.
- The penetrance was 100% in the Turkish and Rom families. Evidence for reduced penetrance (80%) was found in the Saudi Arabian families where 18 apparently unaffected individuals had haplotypes and mutations identical to those of their affected siblings. Two of these individuals were subsequently diagnosed with congenital glaucoma.
- Evidence for founder effect was present in the Rom population of Slovakia, where all affected individuals were homozygotes for Glu387(Lys mutation and all shared an identical haplotype for the six intragenic markers.

- In addition to the Turkish, Saudi Arabian, and Rom families, CYP1B1 mutations segregating in an autosomal-recessive manner with PCG phenotype were observed in families from various ethnic origin: German-American, French-Canadian, Hispanic, British, and Pakistani.

Therefore, molecular genetic analysis has confirmed the existence of a hereditary form of PCG, inherited as an autosomal-recessive trait with high penetrance (80% to 100%) and caused by mutations in the CYP1B1 gene. This appears to be the major familial form of PCG. There also is evidence for sporadic cases of PCG being a result of marriages between two normal carriers of CYP1B1 mutations. At this moment, there is no sufficient data to confirm or reject the existence of dominant or multifactorial forms of the disease.

Human Cytochrome P4501B1 (CYP1B1)

Cytochrome P450 enzymes are a family of monomeric mixed function mono-oxygenases, responsible for the phase I metabolism of a wide range of substrates.[21] Identification of CYP1B1 as the gene mutated in PCG is the first example in which mutations in a member of the cytochrome P450 superfamily are shown to result in a developmental defect. The existence of a link between members of the cytochrome P450 superfamily and the processes of growth and differentiation has been proposed in the early 1990s.[22] It was hypothesized that in addition to the metabolism of xenobiotics, the P450s are responsible for controlling the steady state levels of small bio-organic molecules that act as a ligand in various signal transduction pathways. It, therefore, is plausible to expect that CYP1B1 participates in the metabolism of biologically active molecule(s) essential for normal development of the anterior chamber angle of the eye. CYP1B1 is expressed in the anterior uveal tract of the eye—ciliary body, nonpigmented ciliary epithelium, iris, and trabecular meshwork.[18,20] These structures have highly specialized functions including accommodation, regulation of outflow facility, and formation of aqueous humor. CYP1B1 may influence these processes by participating in the metabolism of regulatory molecules like steroids and derivatives of arachidonic acid. Such molecules could be synthesized locally or delivered via the bloodstream. It has been shown that CYP1B1 can catalyze the 4-hydroxi-

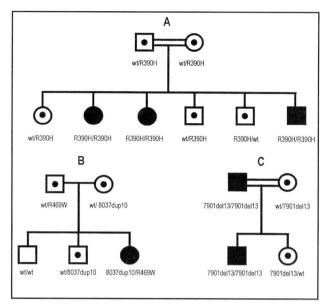

Figure 2-1. Pedigrees of PCG illustrating the classic features of (A) an autosomal-recessive inheritance, (B) isolated case, and (C) pseudo-dominant transmission.

lation of 17β-estradiol.[23] Unfortunately, it remains unclear if hydroxyestrogens play any physiological role in the development of the anterior chamber angle of the eye.

Molecular modeling experiments have provided some clues regarding the mechanism by which the mutations found in PCG individuals may interfere with the normal function of CYP1B1 molecule. Eight of the reported mutations were predicted to introduce premature stop codons or frameshifts in the CYP1B1 open reading frame. These mutations would eliminate at least the hem-binding region of CYP1B1, which is essential for the normal function of every P450 molecule. It is expected, therefore, that these mutations would result in functional null alleles. Alternatively, these mutations may interfere with RNA metabolism by the nonsense-mediated mRNA-decay mechanism. The remaining nine mutations were missence. They were found to affect highly conserved residues located in the hinge region and/or conserved core structures of CYP1B1.[20] These structures are shared by the P450 molecules and are responsible for proper protein folding and hem-binding. In vitro mutagenesis experiments have demonstrated that mutations in these regions have deleterious effects on the ability of P450 to adopt a normal conformation, bind hem, and metabolize substrates.[24,25]

PRIMARY OPEN-ANGLE GLAUCOMA (POAG)

POAG is a group of ocular conditions with variable severity and phenotypic expressively.[26] For example, it may be manifested by IOP measurements ranging between 10 to over 50 mmHg, and age of onset varying from 5 to over 80 years. Additionally, phenotypically similar findings may be secondary to other ocular conditions.[26] The pedigree structure of the majority of families used in genetic linkage analysis clearly suggests that inheritance is autosomal dominant with an incomplete penetrance.[27-30] POAG has been divided arbitrarily into the two groups of "juvenile" and "adult" with an overlapping clinical presentation and a sliding scale age of onset.[26,31] Clinical diagnosis of both groups is based on the presentation of the visual field loss and glaucomatous changes of the optic nerve, which usually are accompanied by increased IOP. Nevertheless, the juvenile-onset phenotype is more severe and often presents with significantly higher IOPs (ie, >40 to 50 mmHg). This phenotype usually does not respond to medical treatment and often requires multiple surgical interventions to achieve IOP control.[32-34]

Juvenile-Onset Primary Open-Angle Glaucoma (JOAG)

In 1993, a locus for this condition was mapped to a 1q21-q31 region and named GLC1A.[35] (Note: Use of GLC1 symbol for all types of POAG has been approved by the HUGO Nomenclature Committee; The letter A, B, C, etc will be assigned to each newly identified locus.) This initial report soon was followed by reports in many other families from North America,[36,37] Ireland, United Kingdom, Germany, France,[38] Denmark,[39] and Canada.[40] Nevertheless, a number of other Swedish,[39] African-American,[41] and French[42] JOAG families have been described that do not map to this region of chromosome 1q.

A number of larger families linked to the GLC1A locus included subjects with variable age of onset as both juvenile- and adult-onset-affected patients were present within the same family.[40,42] The presence of these "mixed" affected subjects within the same pedigree implied that either a single gene is involved in the etiology of both types of glaucoma, or a modifying gene has altered the phenotype in these late-onset affected subjects. Nevertheless, the clinical features in the majority of the affected individuals reported so far are very similar and resemble typical JOAG. Despite the existing variability in the exact age of detection, the majority of the patients were diagnosed with glaucoma in childhood to early adulthood (average age: 18 years). The IOP typically was very high, often in the range of 40 to 50 mmHg. Medical treatment initially was effective, but surgery eventually was required to control the progress of glaucoma.

Causative Mutations in the TIGR/MYOC Gene

A combination of linkage analysis, radiation hybrids mapping of known and unknown (ie, ESTs) genes, together with construction of YAC and PAC contigs of the GLC1A locus[43-46] provided a complete physical map of about 4 to 5 Mb that was expected to contain the causative JOAG gene. In January 1997, this research led to the identification and publication of TIGR or myocilin (MYOC) as the causative gene for JOAG.[47] Initially, three mutations were described in a group of 10 familial (JOAG and POAG) and three isolated cases, as well as in one normal subject.[47] In September 1997, this initial observation was confirmed by identification of a new mutation in a previously well-documented Edinburgh JOAG family that spanned over six generations.[48] In November 1997, additional mutations were reported in French[49] and Japanese[50] families. Soon after, more mutations were noted in North American,[51-55] British,[56] French,[57] German,[58] Spanish,[59,60] North Korean,[61] Canadian,[62] and Italian families.[63] At least 30 mutations in 65 families so far have been described in the TIGR/MYOC gene for both JOAG and POAG types of glaucoma. Identification of these mutations has opened up a new possibility that the TIGR gene may not only be involved in the juvenile-onset type of POAG, but also in a certain portion of adult-onset POAG cases. A comprehensive list of these mutations is provided in Table 2-2. The majority of reported mutations are missense and clustered in exon III of the TIGR/MYOC gene with exception of only two. One is a previously mentioned Gln368STOP mutation that is the most commonly reported so far,[47,51,52] and another is a deletion of three base pairs in the exon III that was reported in four families from a small southern Italian village.[63] As all individuals of these four families carried a common haplotype, this mutation most likely result-

Table 2-2

List of Reported Mutations in the TIGR/MYOC Gene

Number	Mutation	Family	Age of Onset	Population	References
1	Gln19His	1	Not specified	Not specified	51
2	Arg82Cys	1	Not specified	Not specified	51
3	Gly246Arg	1	Juvenile	French	49
4	Gly252Arg	1	Juvenile	N. American	55
5	Trp286Arg	1	Not specified	Not specified	51
6	Thr293Lys	1	Not specified	Not specified	51
7	Glu323Lys	1	Juvenile	Panamanian	55
8	Pro334Ser	2	Not specified	Korean	61
9	Gln337Arg	1	Juvenile	Scottish	48
10	Pro361Ser	1	Not specified	Not specified	51
11	Gly364Val	2	Juvenile/Adult	Not specified	47,51
12	Gly367Arg	1	Adult	Japanese	50
		1	Juvenile	German	58
		1	Adult	Irish	60
13	Gln368Stop	15	Adult	N. American	47,51
		3	Adult	N. American	52
14	Pro370Leu	2	Juvenile	French	49
		1	Juvenile	German	58
		1	Juvenile	Japanese	50
		1	Juvenile	English	56
		1	Juvenile	N. American	55
15	Thr377Met	2	Adult	N. American	53
		1	Juvenile/Adult	Not specified	51
16	Asp380Ala	1	Juvenile	Spanish	59
		1	Juvenile	Canadian	56
		1	Not specified	Not specified	51
17	1177GACA->T	1	Juvenile	Italian	63
18	396INS397	1	Juvenile	Not specified	51
19	Arg422His	1	Not specified	Not specified	51
20	Lys423Glu	1	Juvenile/Adult	Canadian	62
21	Val426Phe	1	Juvenile	Spanish	60
		1	Juvenile	N. American	55
22	Tyr437His	2	Juvenile	N. American	47,51
23	Ala445Val	1	Not specified	Not specified	51
24	Agr470Cys	1	Not specified	Not specified	51
25	Ile477Ser	1	Juvenile/Adult	French	49
26	Ile477Asn	1	Juvenile	N. American	54
		1	Not specified	Not specified	51
27	Asn480Lys	3	Juvenile/Adult	French	49
28	Ile499Phe	1	Juvenile/Adult	French	49
29	Lys500Arg	1	Not specified	Not specified	51
30	Ser502Pro	1	Juvenile	English	56
Total		**65**			

ed from a founder effect with a common ancestral mutation.[63]

Several investigators have documented a number of recurrent/spontaneous mutations, but the predominantly reported observation is the Gln368STOP mutation.[47,51,52] This mutation truncates the TIGR protein by 136 amino acids prematurely, and it has almost exclusively been observed in families with later onset and with moderately raised IOPs. Interestingly, this mutation seems to have spontaneously arisen in our group of subjects, as the closely flanking markers within the inherited haplotype of different families do not share a single common allelic composition (unpublished observation). As shown in Table 2-2, most missense mutations lead to an early and more severe form of JOAG phenotype. Nevertheless, a few other mutations can produce both early- or late-onset forms of this condition. Although the exact biochemical pathways through which the TIGR gene functions have not been identified as of yet, co-exhibition of early- and late-onset phenotypes due to the same mutation is indicative that other unknown modifying genes also may play an important role in the etiology of this condition. Alternatively, because different phenotypic expressions of the same mutation have been observed mainly in extensively large families, the basis for this variation may be non-genetics. Additionally, it may be attributed to some unknown environmental factors and/or other living conditions of these otherwise distantly related affected subjects.

One other interesting occurrence has been observed in a very large French-Canadian pedigree in which four subjects born to two affected parents inherited two copies of the affected haplotype from their parents, but all are clinically normal for glaucoma.[62] TIGR screening of this family has identified a Lys423Glu mutation in all of the affected-bearing haplotypes, in which all phenotypically affected subjects were heterozygote for this mutation, but the abovementioned normal subjects were homozygote for the same mutation.[62] The authors indicated that homoallelic complementation of the affected haplotypes is a likely mechanism to account for these normal homozygous subjects. Furthermore, the authors speculated that this observation appears to be the first mutation that caused an autosomal-dominant heterozygote-specific disease phenotype in man.

It is also worthy to note that several other families have been indicated as segregating with a group of

GLC1A flanking DNA markers on 1q, but no mutations have ever been identified when the coding regions of the TIGR/MYOC gene[56,64] were screened. Although there are no accurate data on the exact size of many of these pedigrees, it is equally likely that either a mutation in the promoter of the TIGR/MYOC gene or, alternatively, mutations in another neighboring gene are responsible for the JOAG phenotype in these families. Although it already has been demonstrated that a number of TIGR promoter mutations are overpresented in the POAG cases when compared to the controls,[65] there is no indication as yet that other genes within the GLC1A region also may partially participate in the etiology of JOAG or POAG.

In order to illustrate the power of mutation screening of the TIGR/MYOC gene in families with JOAG (or POAG), an example pedigree has been provided in Figure 2-2. This is one of our typical JOAG families that previously has been shown to have a Ser502Pro mutation in the TIGR gene.[56] As illustrated, this mutation can be easily documented by screening the family with single strand conformational polymorphism (SSCP) assay. The letter "M" on the left side of this picture shows the presence of this mutation, while the letter "W" is indicative of the wild type band. Note that not only all the affected subjects carry this mutant allele (ie, upper band) but also two additional healthy subjects have inherited it as well. These two subjects (persons IV:6 and IV:9) are still in their mid 20s and, thus, are at very high risk of developing glaucoma. Therefore, detection of a given mutation in one such family can be used to identify and clinically monitor healthy subjects at a very regular interval (ie, every 3 to 4 months) if they have been proven to carry the mutation. Likewise, all other healthy subjects who are free of such a mutation can be monitored much less frequently, depending on their age and the type of glaucoma phenotype.

Human TIGR or MYOC Gene

The TIGR gene was originally identified and isolated by induction of primary cultured cells of trabecular meshwork tissue with glucocorticoids.[66] The responding protein named TIGR subsequently was shown to be present not only in the trabecular meshwork but also in the ciliary body,[67] retina,[68] and almost all other ocular tissues. This gene also is expressed in many other non-ocular tissues.[66] The TIGR gene encodes for a polypeptide that is 504 amino acids long. The gene is over 20 kb long and consists of three exons (604, 126, and 782 bp, respectively) that are separated by two large introns. At the C-terminus part of this protein, there is a domain with 40% identity with olfactomedin, a major component of the extracellular matrix of the olfactory neuroepithelium. Interestingly, this region contains almost all of the known TIGR mutations (see Table 2-2) and has been suggested as possibly being involved in the cell binding activity of this protein.[66] Therefore, mutations in this region may interfere with uptake or metabolism of the protein leading to its accumulation, obstruction of aqueous outflow, and increased IOPs.

In summary, mutations in the TIGR/MYOC have been established to play a significant role in the etiology of most JOAG as well as a limited number of COAG families. Nevertheless, at minimum, screening of this gene in the steroid-induced forms of glaucoma has not identified any causative mutations in this gene.[61]

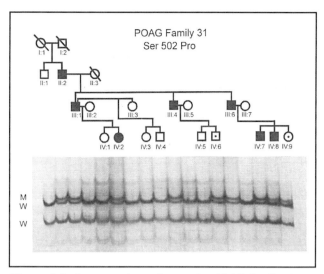

Figure 2-2. An example pedigree of a JOAG family showing a Ser502Pro mutation in the TIGR/MYOC gene. The two identified gene carriers (persons IV:6 and IV:9) are shown with a "dot" inside their respective symbol. The SSCP analysis of this family for this particular mutation is illustrated below this kindred. Letter "M" donates the mutatnt allele, while "W" shows the normal and wild type allele.

Adult-Onset COAG

This insidious type of POAG accounts for the majority (ie, 70%) of glaucoma cases in white populations. Its prevalence has been found to be four or more times higher in those of African extraction.[69-71] Diagnosis of this condition is based on characteristic glaucomatous optic nerve damage, characteristic visual field loss, and increased IOPs.[31,71,72] Most COAG patients do not manifest the disease before the age of 40. Unfortunately, many patients have the disease for some time before the diagnosis is made because COAG is asymptomatic until very late in the disease.

Inheritance of COAG

The late onset and painless nature of this condition has complicated the diagnosis and proper treatment of COAG. As a consequence, it has been difficult to determine the exact mode of inheritance for this condition, because the majority of the patients are either isolated cases or, by the time of first presentation, no accurate clinical information or systematic ophthalmic examination would be possible on the previous generations. Therefore, autosomal-dominant, autosomal-recessive, X-linked, and even multifactorial modes of inheritance have been suggested.[73-75] In the majority of COAG families that have been systematically studied, however, the autosomal-dominant mode of inheritance with a reduced penetrance has been suggested.[76-82]

In addition to the GLC1A locus on the long arm of chromosome 1, for which a subgroup of COAG families are also shown to be due to the same TIGR/MYOC mutations, a number of other chromosomal locations already have been identified for families with only the COAG phenotype. A total of five additional loci (GLC1B to GLC1F) have been identified for other COAG families that are briefly described below.

The GLC1B Locus on the 2cen-q13 Region

In 1996, we presented clinical, two-point linkage and haplotype transmission data that assigned the first locus (GLC1B) for adult-onset POAG to the 2cen-q13 region.[78] Six British families previously excluded from the GLC1A locus (and 215 other DNA markers) were found to be linked to a group of STRP markers located on 2p11-2q13. Further analysis extended this initial linkage data and identified another 12 British families that segregated with this region of chromosome 2. The newly generated linkage data, however, did not help to reduce the critical region of the GLC1B locus any further.

The phenotype of glaucoma patients linked to 2cen-q13 generally is less severe as compared to the GLC1A-linked families. The mean age of onset/diagnosis in these families was 53 years, and 33% of the affected subjects in these families had IOPs of <22 mmHg. The remaining 67% had moderate to high pressures that varied between 22 to 40 mmHg. With the exception of one family that showed very high IOP values, the remaining families had IOPs between 22 to 34 mmHg suggesting that the GLC1B locus on chromosome 2q is responsible for families with moderate tension COAG. Furthermore, other large families with IOP values consistently below 22 mmHg (ie, classic low-tension glaucoma) did not segregate with this region of chromosome 2, thereby suggesting that IOP values are not a significant predeterminant factor for linkage of other COAG families to the GLC1B locus. Of the 52 affected subjects in the GLC1B-linked families, a total of 22 (42%) had ocular surgery to control their pressures.

We also have excluded another 22 COAG families that do not show any linkage to the 2cen-q13 region and, therefore, provided evidence for genetic heterogeneity of this group of conditions. The families linked to the GLC1B-locus may represent a distinct entity with further genetic heterogeneity. So far, a number of potential candidate genes from this region of chromosome 2 have been screened for mutation, but as yet, no definite causative mutations have been identified in any of the genes studied. A comprehensive physical map of this region recently has been constructed. This map eventually will help to identify a putative gene involved in the etiology of this group of GLC1B-linked families.

Recently, one additional large French-Canadian family comprising 132 individuals spanning over three living generations has been mapped to the same region of the GLC1B locus. All the affected members of this family have IOP>22 mmHg with variable age of onset ranging between 38 to 58 years of age.[83] This single large family has provided statistically significant evidence for linkage to this location, and reduced the expected size of the region that harbors the putative GLC1B gene.

The GLC1C Locus on the 3q21-q24 Region

The second locus (GLC1C) for adult-onset COAG maps to the 3q21-24 region in a single American family.[79] Nine living affected, seven possibly affected, and another four healthy members of this pedigree share a common affected-bearing haplotype. Another nine offspring of affected subjects, who showed no sign of COAG, also inherited a normal haplotype from their respective parents. The patients in this study presented with a phenotype that is characteristic of the common form of glaucoma including onset after the age of 35, high IOPs, compromised disc/cup ratio, and visual field loss. Three of the 10 affected individuals (30%) have had to resort to surgery to control their pressures. No additional families, as yet, have been shown to be linked to the GLC1C locus, despite the fact that over 70 COAG families already have been tested for linkage to this region of chromosome 3 (our unpublished observation).

The clinical presentation of affected subjects segregating for GLC1B or GLC1C loci are very similar. The average age of onset in the affected subjects is 53 and 55 years for the GLC1B and GLC1C, respectively. Ocular surgery was required in 42% of GLC1B-linked patients as compared to 30% of the GLC1C-linked affected subjects. The IOP values presented for the GLC1C-linked affected subjects are not directly comparable to those reported for the GLC1B-linked families, however, because these values (ie, 18 to 32 mmHg) are presented for individuals after medical treatment was initiated and/or diagnosis was made. There are no other differences between the clinical presentation of the GLC1B- and GLC1C-linked affected subjects.

The GLC1D Locus on the 8q23 Region

Recently, we studied a four-generation American family with adult-onset POAG in which the disease did not map to the two previously described loci of GLC1B and GLC1C.[80] The phenotype in this family appears to be variable, with onset of visual field loss in middle age, followed by modest elevation of IOP and progression of the disease in older individuals. A total of 20 subjects in three successive generations, including eight affected subjects and one glaucoma suspect, were used to establish linkage to the 8q23 region. This localization delineated the third locus that was being identified COAG. Haplotype transmission data identified two recombination events that placed the gene in a 6.3-cM region flanked by D8S1830 and D8S592. Eight affected subjects and three glaucoma suspects inherited the disease-bearing haplotype. The genetic heterogeneity of adult-onset glaucoma has been demonstrated further by the multiplicity of chromosomal loci associated with this disease. As yet, no other large families have been shown to be linked to the GLC1D locus, a number of smaller COAG families have been segregating for this region of chromosome 8q (our unpublished data). Nevertheless, because the sizes of these families are not sufficient to prove linkage by themselves, testing of additional large families in this region must be carried out before the contribution of this locus to the overall clinical presentation of the COAG phenotype can be determined fully.

The GLC1E Locus on the 10p15-p14 Region

In early 1998, by using a very large British family with a classical form of normal-tension open-angle glaucoma (NTG or LTG), we were able to identify a new locus on the 10p15-p14 region.[81] Although this was the fourth COAG locus identified, it represented the first locus for the LTG phenotype. The clinical manifestation in most of the affected subjects of this family represents a classical NTG with cupping of the optic nerve head and visual field loss, in the absence of increased IOP. Inspection of 15 affected members of this family revealed a lower mean age at detection of 43 years (range: 23 to 65 years) in 12 subjects. These individuals were classified as NTG compared with three others defined as COAG, with an average age of 48 years (range: 38 to 62 years). The average IOP for family members with NTG was 17.58 mmHg (range: 14 to 21 mmHg) untreated and 14 mmHg (range: 6 to 17 mmHg) treated, whereas in the COAG members average IOP was 23 mmHg (range: 21 to 25 mmHg) untreated and 13 mmHg (range: 10 to 18 mmHg) treated, with a diurnal variation of 5 to 6 mmHg. The cup/disc ratios averaged 0.78 (range: 0.60 to 0.95) in patients with NTG and 0.80 (range: 0.50 to 0.90) in the COAG patients. Although some ocular

and systemic findings such as myopia, systemic hypertension, vascular disease, and migraine are reported to be unusually common in NTG patients,[84] we could not prove any association between these and the NTG phenotype in the family investigated. There is clearly much clinical overlap between COAG and NTG, if indeed it is basically justifiable to separate POAG into these two components. Genetic determination of families such as the one identified in this kindred, together with DNA genotyping, almost certainly will lead to more coherence in the subclassification of POAG.

Of the 42 individuals genotyped in this pedigree, 39 subjects (16 affected) inherited a haplotype compatible with their prior clinical designation, whereas the remaining three were young, clinically healthy, normal subjects who were at risk of developing this condition. Two critical recombination events in the affected subjects positioned the GLC1E locus to a region of approximately 21 cM, flanked by D10S1729 and D10S1664. An additional recombination in a 59-year-old unaffected female suggests, however, that this locus resides between D10S585 (or D10S1172) and D10S1664, within a genetic distance of 5 to 11 cM. The latter minimum region must be taken cautiously, however, because incomplete penetrance has previously been documented for this group of ocular conditions. A maximum LOD score of 10.00 at a recombination fraction of 0=0.00 was obtained with D10S1216. When only the affected meioses of this kindred were analyzed, LOD scores remained statistically significant, ranging from 3.16 (D10S527) to 3.57 (D10S506). Although this was the first locus being described for a classical form of LTG, no other families with a similar clinical presentation have, as yet, been tested for this region of chromosome 10. Therefore, the accurate percentage that this locus contributes to the overall phenotype of LTG has not as yet been determined.

The kindred that was used to identify the GLC1E locus is illustrated in Figure 2-3. Although we have not as yet identified a causative gene in this family, the linkage information obtained so far has provided sufficient evidence for subdividing the healthy subjects into two categories of very low to very high risk. In particular, there are five normal subjects in the fourth generations that share the same affected haplotype (ie, gene carriers shown with a dot inside their symbol) and, therefore, are at very high risk of developing LTG. All the other

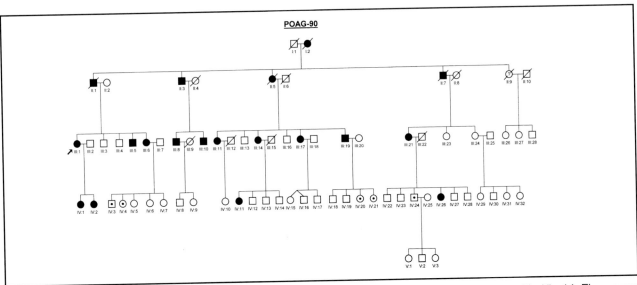

Figure 2-3. Pedigree structure of a LTG family that was originally used to map the GLC1E locus to 10p15-p14. Five young and unaffected subjects identified as carrying the common affected haplotype are presented with a "dot" inside their respective symbol. These individuals are, therefore, at much higher risk of developing LTG later in life. All other normal subjects have inherited the normal haplotype from their respective affected parents and, therefore, at are lower risk of developing LTG.

healthy subjects of this family inherited the normal haplotype-bearing from their affected parent and, therefore, are at very low risk. Nevertheless, one cannot infer that these individuals are at a lower risk of developing other types of glaucoma when they are compared to a general population.

The GLC1F Locus on the 7q35-q36 Region

A single large family with at least four consecutive affected generations has been used to map a new locus to the 7q35-q36 region.[82] This family consisted of 12 affected subjects, 10 of whom were alive and participated in the study. Eleven additional family members also were included; two of these were later found to be gene carriers. The phenotype in this family is characterized by a mean age of 53 years (range: 22 to 70 years) with moderately elevated IOPs ranging from 22 to 38 mmHg. The GLC1F locus is flanked by two microsatellite markers of D7S2442 and D7S482, within a region of about 5.3 cM. This locus maps very close to a previously reported region for the pigment dispersion syndrome (PDS) and, therefore, it remains to be determined whether these two loci are allelic.

In summary, genetic linkage studies of COAG families have indicated clearly that this form of glau-coma is very heterogeneous and, thus, a large number of loci are expected to be involved in the etiology of this condition. What already has been observed for retinitis pigmentosa (RP), in which more than 30 loci were identified in the syndromic and non-syndromic RP types,[85] may also be the case for glaucoma phenotypes.

SECONDARY FORMS OF GLAUCOMA

Although secondary glaucoma may potentially be part of many different systemic and non-systemic syndromes, only two well-known ocular conditions, namely pseudoexfoliation (PEX) syndrome and PDS, are frequently reported to produce a secondary glaucoma phenotype.

PEX Syndrome

Grayish flakes that coat the surfaces of the anterior segment of the eye characterize PEX syndrome. The deposits can be found on the lens capsule, the ciliary processes, the zonules, and the pupillary margin.[86] This disorder was first described in 1917 by Lindberg[87] and has now been accepted as being a systemic disorder.[88] Exfoliation material was shown to occur in the conjunctiva, in the wall of vessels, in the dermis of skin, and it is consistently associated with connective tissue components. Other extraocular locations in which the material has been found include heart, meninges, lungs, skin, liver, and gallbladder. There is increased cardiovascular morbidity and mortality. Therefore, identification of the PEX gene is much more interesting, as its expression does not affect only the eye, but also many other systems in the body.

Although this condition has long been associated with Scandinavia, PEX syndrome occurs in virtually every population of the world, except in Eskimos.[89] It also is frequent in American Indians, Greeks, and in the African Bantu. In Finland and elsewhere in Scandinavia, it may have a frequency as high as 20% in individuals over the age of 80. Although the prevalence of the PEX syndrome varies considerably worldwide, in many countries it appears as a common late-onset disorder that is frequently associated with open-angle glaucoma, cataract, and increased complications during cataract surgery.

Familial occurrence of PEX syndrome often has been described, but as yet, no clear hereditary pattern has been prospectively proposed for this condition. Although male preponderance has been reported, many other reports have given an equal sex distribution. Autosomal-dominant inheritance with reduced penetrance was suggested as the most likely mode of inheritance of this phenotype.[90] The advanced age of onset and asymptomatic course of the disease have always been the two main obstacles for determining the segregation pattern and/or identifying the responsible PEX gene. Nevertheless, with the availability of new molecular genetic techniques, it has been possible to provisionally identify two separate, but as yet unconfirmed, chromosomal locations for this condition.

The first provisional locus was mapped to the 2q35-q37 region that includes a region of about 21 cM.[91] The second provisional locus has been placed on the 2p13-p11 region.[92] Although some of the families mapping to the 2q35-q37 region have definitely been excluded from the 2p13-p11 region,[91] the converse data have not been available at the time of this writing. It is very important to note that linkage of the PEX phenotype to both of these two loci is still provisional. This conclusion mainly is due to the fact that the size of families used in these studies is small and not a single large family has been identified that could conclusively show linkage to one of these two locations. The only way of proving which of these two locations may possibly play a significant role in the etiology of this condition is to pool the genetic linkage data from many affected subjects in many reasonably sized PEX families. A large number of affected subjects are currently being screened for a possible linkage to one or both of these two locations.

PDS and Pigmentary Glaucoma

Pigmentary glaucoma is a form of open-angle glaucoma that usually manifests itself within the second or third decade of life. Disruption and loss of iris pigment epithelium, deposition of the dispersed pigment granules in the anterior chamber, iris transillumination, and dense trabecular pigmentation are characteristic features of the PDS condition. In 1997, the first locus (PDS1) for this condition was mapped to 7q35-q36 region in a group of four families, one of which had 16 affected subjects in four generations.[93] More recently, a second locus (PDS2) for this condition has been mapped to 18q11-q21 region in another family that consists of at least nine affected subjects.[94] Identification of two separate loci for this condition is another example of genetic heterogeneity in this group of eye conditions. Nevertheless, the ability to do a genetic analysis using these two linked loci can help to identify asymptomatic individuals and minimize, delay, or control the development of this condition.

OCULAR CONDITIONS ASSOCIATED WITH GLAUCOMA

Presentation of the glaucoma phenotype is not limited to its pure primary or secondary forms. Frequently, this condition has been seen to co-segregate with various ocular and non-ocular conditions. Although the list of these conditions is quite extensive, only a brief description of those ocular phenotypes that have recently been subjected to a more detailed molecular study will be given.

Rieger Syndrome (RS)

Two separate genetic loci have been identified on the 4q25-q26[95] and 13q14[96] regions. This phenotype exhibits a variety of ocular conditions that include malformation of the anterior chamber, microcornea with opacity, hypoplasia and/or coloboma of the iris, and glaucoma. Other features such as hypodontia, broad nasal root with telecanthus, maxillary hypoplasia with protruding lower lip, and umbilical hernia also are associated with this phenotype.

The gene on chromosome 4q already has been cloned. This is a bicoid-related homeobox transcription factor gene (known as RIEG1 or PITX2), and mutations in this gene are not only associated with the RS phenotype[97] but also with an autosomal-dominant form of iris hypoplasia[98] as well as the iridogoniodysgenesis syndrome type 2, which is a type of iris hypoplasia with an early-onset glaucoma.[99]

The second RS locus on chromosome 13q14 has been identified in a single family with 11 affected subjects, nine of whom showed evidence of glaucoma. Although the clinical presentation of this family is very similar to those reported for the 4q-linked families, the redundancy of the periumbilical skin was absent in the affected members of this kindred. The responsible gene for this form of RS has not been identified as yet.

Anomalies of the Anterior Segment Development at the 6p25 Region

In 1996, a locus was mapped to the 6p25 region in two families segregating for iridogoniodysgenesis anomaly (IGDA).[100] The IGDA phenotype is inherited an autosomal dominant condition with clinical presentation that includes abnormal iridocorneal angle differentiation (or goniodysgenesis), iris hypoplasia, elevated IOP, and juvenile glaucoma. This region of chromosome 6 involves many other ocular conditions, including congenital glaucoma,[101] POAG with iris hypoplasia,[102] Rieger and Axenfeld anomalies, and other ocular conditions that are generally associated with the anterior segment development. Therefore, clustering of these eye anomalies either represents a group of allelic disorders or alternatively exemplifies a cluster of tightly linked genes at the 6p25 region.

Recently, a gene from this region has been cloned and shown to be mutated in a number of eye anomalies that exhibit a spectrum of glaucoma phenotypes.[101,103] This is a forkhead-like transcription factor (FKHL7) gene that was independently isolated by two different groups.[101,103] FKHL7 mutations have been reported in a group of distinct families segregating for Rieger anomaly, Axenfeld anomaly, and iris hypoplasia. Nevertheless, mutations in this gene have not been

found in the original IGDA families that were used to identify this location on 6p25.[103] Furthermore, another large family with a combination of POAG and iris hyperplasia has been excluded as having mutation in the FKHL7 gene.[104] Contrary to this observation, additional novel mutations have been identified in families with only Axenfeld or Rieger anomaly.[103,105] Therefore, it is likely that mutations in the FKHL7 are predominantly associated with the Axenfeld-Rieger anomaly and contribute very little to other eye abnormalities that are associated with this region of chromosome 6. This fact, in turn, indicates that additional eye-related genes must reside on 6p25 and contribute to development of the remaining ocular phenotypes mapping to this region.

Glaucoma and Nail-Patella Syndrome (NPS)

NPS is one the phenotypes that have been studied for over 100 years. The co-segregation of this phenotype with the ABO blood group on 9q34 was the first example of a genetic linkage that was identified in man. It was not until very recently, however, that the first association of this phenotype with open-angle glaucoma was demonstrated in two families.[106] So far, co-segregation of open-angle glaucoma with NPS has been identified in nine out of 29 (31%) families that have systematically been investigated for these two phenotypes. It has recently been shown that three mutations in the LIM homeobox transcription factor 1, beta (LMX1B) are responsible for the NPS phenotype.[107,108] Additional mutations have also been shown in four families segregating for both NPS and open-angle glaucoma.[106] The onset of glaucoma in the first family was between 18 to 41 years (mean: 32 years), in the second from birth to 54 (mean: 24 years), in the third from 40 to 77 (mean: 56 years), and in the fourth family between 40 to 50 (mean: 45 years). Therefore, the four mutations identified in the NPS families included glaucoma phenotypes that ranged from congenital to very late-onset POAG form.

In another study, 41 NPS families were screened for the LMX1B gene and 25 mutations have been identified in a total of 37 families.[109] Six families with the mutation had open-angle glaucoma reported in one or more members. Of these, mutations in the open-angle glaucoma members of four families were reported, and the open-angle glaucoma members of the remaining two families were not available for screening. This study included open-angle glaucoma members in another two families for whom mutations have yet to be identified. Moreover, one of the same mutations reported in an earlier family with both NPS and open-angle glaucoma[108] also was seen in another family[109] that only exhibited the NPS but not the open-angle glaucoma phenotype. Therefore, this observation together with the reported finding of anterior segment ocular abnormalities in mice with targeted disruption of the LMX1B gene[109] are two strong indications that glaucoma is a genuine pleiotropic effect of the NPS gene.

REFERENCES

1. De Luise V, Anderson DR. Primary infantile glaucoma (congenital glaucoma). *Surv Ophthalmol.* 1983;28:1-19.
2. Hoskins DH Jr, Shaffer RN, Hetherington J. Anatomical classification of the developmental glaucomas. *Arch Ophthalmol.* 1984;102:1331-1336.
3. Shaffer RN, Weiss DI. *Congenital and Pediatric Glaucomas.* St Louis: Mosby;1970.
4. Anderson DR. The development of the trabecular meshwork and its abnormality in primary infantile glaucoma. *Tr Am Ophthalmol Soc.* 1981;79:458-485.
5. Allen L, Burion HM, Braley AE. A new concept of development of anterior chamber angle: its relationship to developmental glaucoma and other structural anomalies. *Arch Ophthalmol.* 1955;53:783-798.
6. Barkan O. Pathogenesis of congenital glaucoma. *Am J Ophthalmol.* 1955;40:1-11.
7. Kupfer C, Kaiser-Kupfer M. Observations on the development of the anterior chamber angle with reference to the pathogenesis of congenital glaucomas. *Am J Ophthalmol.* 1979;88:424-426.
8. Francois J. Congenital glaucoma and its inheritance. *Ophthalmologica.* 1972;181:61-73.
9. Francois J. *Heredity in Ophthalmology.* St Louis, Mo: CV Mosby; 1961:218-225.
10. Gencik A. Epidemiology and genetics of primary congenital glaucoma in Slovakia. Description of a form of primary congenital glaucoma in gypsies with autosomal recessive inheritance and complete penetrance. *Dev Ophthalmol.* 1989;16:75-115.
11. Duke-Elder S. Congenital deformities. In: Duke-Elder S, ed. *System of Ophthalmology.* St Louis, Mo: CV Mosby;1969:548-565.
12. Demenias F, Bonaiti C, Briard ML, Feingold J, Frezal J. Congenital glaucoma: genetic models. *Hum Genet.* 1979;46:305-317.
13. Jay MR, Rice NSC. Genetic implications of congenital glaucoma. *Metab Ophthalmol.* 1978;2:257-258.
14. Sarfarazi M, Akarsu AN, Hossain A, et al. Assignment of a locus (GLC3A) for primary congenital glaucoma (Buphthalmos) to 2p21 and evidence for genetic heterogeneity. *Genomics.* 1995;30:171-177.
15. Akarsu AN, Turacli ME, Aktan GS, et al. A second locus (GLC3B) for primary congenital glaucoma (Buphthalmos) maps to the 1p36 region. *Hum Mol Gen.* 1996;5:1199-1203.
16. Bejjani BA, Lewis RA, Tomey KF, et al. Mutations in CYP1B1, the gene for cytochrome P4501B1, are the predominant cause of primary congenital glaucoma in Saudi Arabia. *Am J Hum Genet.* 1998;62:325-333.
17. Plasilova M, Ferakova E, Kadasi L, et al. Linkage of autosomal recessive primary congenital glaucoma to the GLC3A locus in Roms (Gypsies) from Slovakia. *Hum Hered.* 1998;48:30-33.
18. Stoilov I, Akarsu AN, Sarfarazi M. Identification of three different truncating mutations in the cytochrome P4501B1 (CYP1B1) gene as the principal cause of primary congenital glaucoma (Buphthalmos) in families linked to the GLC3A locus on chromosome 2p21. *Hum Mol Gen.* 1997;6:641-647.
19. Plasilova M, Stoilov I, Sarfarazi M, Kadasi L, Ferakova E, Ferak V. Identification of single ancestral CYP1B1 mutation in Slovak gypsies (Roms) affected with primary congenital glaucoma. *J Med Genet.* 1999;36(4):290-294..
20. Stoilov I, Akarsu AN, Alozie I, et al. Sequence analysis and homology modeling suggest that primary congenital glaucoma on 2p21 results from mutations disrupting either the hinge region or the conserved core structures of cytochrome P4501B1. *Am J Hum Genet.* 1998;62:573-584.
21. Nelson DR, Kamataki T, Waxman DJ, et al. The P450 superfamily: update on new sequences, gene mapping, accession numbers, early trivial names of enzymes, and nomenclature. *DNA Cell Biol.* 1993;12:1-51.
22. Nebert DW. Proposed role of drug-metabolizing enzymes: regulation of steady state levels of the ligands that effect growth, homeostasis, differentiation, and neuroendocrine functions. *Mol Endocrinol.* 1991;5:1203-1214.
23. Hayes CL, Spink DC, Spink BC, Cao JQ, Walker NJ, Sutter TR. 17 β-Estradiol hydroxylation catalyzed by cytochrome P4501B1. *Proc Natl Acad Sci USA.* 1997;93:9776-9781.
24. Chen CD, Kemper B. Different structural requirements at specific proline rich residue positions in the conserved proline-rich region of cytochrome P4502C2. *J Biol Chem.* 1996;271:28607-28611.
25. Yamazaki S, Sato K, Suhara K, Sakaguchi M, Michara K, Omura T. Importance of the proline-rich region following signal-anchor sequence in the formation of correct conformation of microsomal cytochrome P-450s. *J Biochem.* 1993;114:652-657.
26. Shields M, Ritch R, Krupin T. Classification of the glaucomas. In: Ritch R, Shields BM, Krupin T, eds. *The Glaucomas.* Vol 2. St Louis, Mo: Mosby;1996:717-725.
27. Lichter PR. Genetic clues to glaucoma's secrets. The Jackson memorial lecture Part 2. *Am J Ophthalmol.* 1994;117:706-727.
28. Johnson AT, Alward W, Sheffield V, Stone E. (1996) Genetics and glaucoma. In: Ritch R, Shields BM, Krupin T, eds. *The Glaucomas.* Vol 2. St Louis, Mo: Mosby;1996:39-54.
29. Raymond V. Molecular genetics of glaucomas: mapping of the first five "GLC" loci. *Am J Hum Genet.* 1997;60:272-277.
30. Sarfarazi M. Recent advances in molecular genetics of glaucomas. *Hum Mol Genet.* 1997;6(10):1667-1677.

31. Quigley HA. Open angle glaucoma. *N Engl J Med.* 1993; 328:10971106.
32. Ellis OH. The etiology, symptomatology and treatment of juvenile glaucoma. *Am J Ophthalmol.* 1948;31:1589-1596.
33. Goldwin R, Waltman SR, Becker B. Primary open angle glaucoma in adolescents and young adults. *Arch Ophthalmol.* 1970;84:579-582.
34. Johnson AT, Drack AV, Kwitek AE, Cannon RL, Stone EM, Alward WLM. Clinical features and linkage analysis of a family with autosomal dominant juvenile glaucoma. *Ophthalmology.* 1993;100:524-529.
35. Sheffield VC, Stone EM, Alward WLM, et al. Genetic linkage of familial open angle glaucoma to chromosome 1q21q31. *Nature Genet.* 1993;4:4750.
36. Richards JE, Lichter PR, Boehnke M, et al. Mapping of a gene for autosomal dominant juvenile onset open angle glaucoma to chromosome 1q. *Am J Hum Genet.* 1994;54:62-70.
37. Wiggs JL, Haines JL, Paglinauan C, Fine A, Sporn C, Lou D. Genetic linkage of autosomal dominant juvenile glaucoma to 1q21q31 in three affected pedigrees. *Genomics.* 1994;21:99-303.
38. Meyer A, Valtot F, Bechetoille A, et al. Linkage between juvenile glaucoma and chromosome 1q in two French families. *Comp Rend Acad Sci (Paris).* 1994;317:565-570.
39. Graff C, Urbak SF, Jerndal T, Wadelius C. Confirmation of linkage to 1q21-31 in a Danish autosomal dominant juvenile-onset glaucoma family and evidence of genetic heterogeneity. *Hum Genet.* 1995;96:285-289.
40. Morissette J, Cote G, Anctil JL, et al. A common gene for juvenile and adult onset primary open angle glaucomas confined on chromosome 1q. *Am J Hum Gent.* 1995;56:1431-1442.
41. Wiggs JL, Del Bono EA, Schuman JS, et al. Clinical features of five pedigrees genetically linked to the juvenile glaucoma locus on chromosome 1q21q31. *Ophthalmology.* 1995;2:1782-1789.
42. Meyer A, Bechetoille A, Valtot F, et al. Age dependent penetrance and mapping of the locus for juvenile and early-onset open-angle glaucoma on chromosome 1q (GLC1A) in a French family. *Hum Genet.* 1996;98:567-571.
43. Sunden S, Alward WLM, Nichols BE, et al. Fine mapping of the autosomal dominant juvenile open-angle glaucoma (GLC1A) region and evaluation of the candidate genes. *Genome Res.* 1996;6:862-869.
44. Clepet C, Dauwerse HJG, Desmaze C, Ommen GJB, Weissenbach J, Morissette J. A 10cM YAC contig spanning GLC1A, the primary open-angle glaucoma locus at 1q23-q25. *Eur J Hum Genet.* 1996;4:250-259.
45. Belmouden A, Adam M, Dupont de Dinechin S, et al. Recombinational and physical mapping of the locus for primary open-angle glaucoma (GLC1A) on chromosome 1q23-q25. *Genomics.* 1997;39:348-358.
46. Williams H, Scott D, McDonald L, Vaudin M, Kenwrick S, Wooster R. Construction of PAC contig of human chromosome 1q22-q25 including the GLC1A candidate region. *Eur Soc Hum Genet Meeting.* 1997;Abstract 195.
47. Stone EM, Fingert JH, Alward WLM, et al. Identification of a gene that causes primary open angle glaucoma. *Science.* 1997;275:668-670.
48. Stoilova D, Child A, Brice G, Crick RP, Fleck BW, Sarfarazi M. Identification of a new 'TIGR' mutation in a family with juvenile-onset primary open angle glaucoma. *Ophthalmic Genet.* 1997;18(3):109-118.
49. Adam MF, Belmouden A, Binisti P, et al. Recurrent mutations in a single exon encoding the evolutionarily conserved olfactomedin-homology domain of TIGR in familial open-angle glaucoma. *Hum Mol Genet.* 1997;6(12):2091-2097.
50. Suzuki Y, Shirato S, Taniguchi F, Ohara K, Nishimaki K, Ohta S. Mutations in the TIGR gene in familial primary open-angle glaucoma in Japan. *Am J Hum Genet.* 1997;61(5):1202-1204.
51. Alward WL, Fingert JH, Coote MA, et al. Clinical features associated with mutations in the chromosome 1 open-angle glaucoma gene. *N Engl J Med.* 1998;338(15):1022-1027.
52. Allingham RR, Wiggs JL, De La Paz MA, et al. Gln368STOP myocilin mutation in families with late-onset primary open-angle glaucoma. *Invest Ophthalmol Vis Sci.* 1998;39(12):2288-2295.
53. Wiggs JL, Allingham RR, Vollrath D, et al. Frequence of mutations in TIGR/myocilin in families with juvenile and adult primary open-angle glaucoma. *Invest Ophthalmol Vis Sci.* 1998;39(4):S31. Abstract 129.
54. Richards JE, Ritch R, Lichter PR, et al. Novel trabecular meshwork inducible glucocorticoid response mutation in an eight-generation juvenile-onset primary open-angle glaucoma pedigree. *Ophthalmology.* 1998;105(9):1698-1707.
55. Rozsa FW, Shimizu S, Lichter PR, et al. GLC1A mutations point to regions of potential functional importance on the TIGR/MYOC protein. *Mol Vis.* 1998;4:20.
56. Stoilova D, Child A, Brice G, et al. Novel TIGR/MYOC mutations in families with juvenile onset primary open angle glaucoma. *J Med Genet.* 1998;35(12):989-992.
57. Brezin AP, Bechetoille A, Hamard P, et al. Genetic heterogeneity of primary open angle glaucoma and ocular hypertension: linkage to GLC1A associated with an increased risk of severe glaucomatous optic neuropathy. *J Med Genet.* 1997;34:546-552.
58. Michels-Rautenstrauss KG, Mardin CY, Budde WM, et al. Juvenile open angle glaucoma: fine mapping of the TIGR gene to 1q24.3-q25.2 and mutation analysis. *Hum Genet.* 1998;102(1):103-106.
59. Kennan AM, Mansergh FC, Fingert JH, et al. A novel Asp380Ala mutation in the GLC1A/myocilin gene in a family with juvenile onset primary open angle glaucoma. *J Med Genet.* 1998;35(11):957-960.
60. Mansergh FC, Kenna PF, Ayuso C, Kiang AS, Humphries P, Farrar GJ. Novel mutations in the TIGR gene in early and late onset open angle glaucoma. *Hum Mutat.* 1998;11(3):244-251.
61. Kee C, Ahn BH. TIGR gene in primary open-angle glaucoma and steroid-induced glaucoma. *Korean J Ophthalmol.* 1997;11(2):75-78.
62. Morissette J, Clepet C, Moisan S, et al. Homozygotes carrying an autosomal dominant TIGR mutation do not manifest glaucoma. *Nat Genet.* 1998;19(4):319-321.

63. Angius A, De Gioia E, Loi A, et al. A novel mutation in the GLC1A gene causes juvenile open-angle glaucoma in 4 families from the Italian region of Puglia. *Arch Ophthalmol.* 1998;116(6):793-797.

64. Wiggs JL, Allingham RR, Vollrath D, et al. Prevalence of mutations in TIGR/myocilin in patients with adult and juvenile primary open-angle glaucoma. *Am J Hum Genet.* 1998;63(5):1549-1552.

65. Chen H, Chen P, Do T, et al. Identification of a TIGR promoter sequence variant, TIGR.mt1, in a POAG pedigree and estimation of its frequency in adult POAG. *Invest Ophthalmol Vis Sci.* 1998;39(4):S3156. Abstract 3156.

66. Polansky J, Fauss D, Chen P, et al. Cellular pharmacology and molecular biology of the trabecular meshwork inducible glucocorticoid response gene product. *Ophthalmologica.* 1997;211:126-139.

67. Ortego J, Escribano J, Coca-Prados M. Cloning and characterization of subtracted cDNAs from a human ciliary body library encoding TIGR, a protein involved in juvenile open angle glaucoma with homology to myosin and olfactomedin. *FEBS Lett.* 1997;413(2):349-353.

68. Kubota R, Noda S, Wang Y, et al. A novel myosin-like protein (myocilin) expressed in the connecting cilium of the photoreceptor: molecular cloning, tissue expression, and chromosomal mapping. *Genomics.* 1997;41:360-369.

69. Quigley HA, Vitale S. Models of open angle glaucoma prevalence and incidence in the United States. *Invest Ophthalmol Vis Sci,* 1997;38:83-91.

70. Quigley HA. The number of people with glaucoma worldwide. *Br J Ophthalmol.* 1996;80:389-393.

71. Wilson R, Matrone J. Epidemiology of chronic open angle glaucoma. In: Ritch R, Shields BM, Krupin T, eds. *The Glaucomas.* Vol 2. St Louis, Mo: Mosby; 1996;753-768.

72. Crick RP, Reynolds PM, Daubs JG. Epidemiological aspects of primary open angle glaucoma. *Glaucoma.* 1983;5:4-14.

73. Francois J. Genetics and primary open-angle glaucoma. *Am J Ophthalmol.* 1966;61:652-665.

74. Jay B, Peterson G. The genetics of simple glaucoma. *Trans Ophthalmol Soc UK.* 1970;90:161-171.

75. Netland PA, Wiggs JL, Dreyer EB. Inheritance of glaucoma and genetic counseling of glaucoma patients. *Int Ophthalmol Clin.* 1993;33:101-120.

76. Avramopolus D, Kitsos G, Economou-Petersen E, et al. Exclusion of one pedigree affected by adult onset primary open angle glaucoma from linkage to the juvenile glaucoma locus on chromosome 1q21-q31. *J Med Genet.* 1996;3:1043-1044.

77. Richards JE, Lichter PR, Herman S, et al. Probable exclusion of GLC1A as a candidate gene in a family with middle-age-onset primary open-angle glaucoma. *Ophthalmology.* 1996;103:1035-1040.

78. Stoilova D, Child A, Trifan OC, Crick RP, Coakes RL, Sarfarazi M. Localization of a locus (GLC1B) for adult-onset primary open angle glaucoma to the 2cen-q13 region. *Genomics.* 1996;36:142-150.

79. Wirtz MK, Samples JR, Kramer PL, et al. Mapping a gene for adult-onset primary open angle glaucoma to chromosome 3q. *Am J Hum Genet.* 1997;60:296-304.

80. Trifan OC, Traboulsi EI, Stoilova D, et al. A third locus (GLC1D) for adult-onset primary open-angle glaucoma maps to the 8q23 region. *Am J Ophthalmol.* 1998;126:17-28.

81. Sarfarazi M, Child A, Stoilova D, et al. Localization of the fourth locus (GLC1E) for adult-onset primary open-angle glaucoma to the 10p15-p14 region. *Am J Hum Genet.* 1998;62:641-652.

82. Wirtz MK, Samples JR, Kramer PL, Yount J, Rust K, Acott TS. Identification of a new adult-onset primary-open angle glaucoma locus – GLC1F. *Arch Ophthalmol.* 1999;117(2):237-241.

83. Faucher M, Dubois S, Cote G, Anctil JL, Morissette J, Raymond V. Mapping of a gene for adult-onset primary open-angle glaucoma to the GLC1B locus at chromosome 2cen-q13 in a French-Canadian family. *Invest Ophthalmol Vis Sci.* 1999. Abstract.

84. Werner EB. Normal-tension glaucoma. In: Ritch R, Shields BM, Krupin T, eds. *The Glaucomas.* Vol 2. St Louis, Mo: Mosby;1996;768-797.

85. Dry JA, Li T. Molecular genetics of retinitis pigmentosa. *Hum Mol Genet.* 1995;4:1739-1743.

86. Johnson DH. The exfoliation syndrome—a continuing challenge. In: Albert DM, Jakobiec FA, eds. *Principles and Practice of Ophthalmology.* Philadelphia, Pa: Saunders; 1995.

87. Lindberg JG. Clinical studies of the depigmentation of the pupillary margin and transillumination of the iris in cases of senile cataract and also in normal eyes of the aged. Diss. Heslingfors University, 1917.

88. Amari F, Nagata S, Umihira J, Nohora M, Usuda N, Sevaga K. Lectin electron microscopy histochemistry of the pseudoexfoliative material in the skin. *Invest Ophthalmol Vis Sci.* 1994;35:3962-3966.

89. McKusik VA. *Mendelian Inheritance in Man.* Baltimore, Md: The John Hopkins University Press.

90. Wiggs JL. Genetics of glaucoma. *Ophthalmol North Am.* 1995;8(2):203-215.

91. Sotirova V, Irkec M, Caudill M, Orhan M, Akarsu A, Sarfarzi M. Ascertainment and molecular genetic study of families with pseudoexfoliation syndrome (PEX). *Invest Ophthalmol Vis Sci.* 1998;39(4):S32. Abstract 139.

92. Wiggs JL, Andersen JS, Stefansson E, et al. A genomic screen suggests a locus on chromosome 2p16 for pseudoexfoliation syndrome. *Am J Hum Genet.* 1998;63(4):A314. Abstract 1818.

93. Anderson J, Pralea A, Del Bono EA, et al. A gene responsible for the pigment dispersion syndrome maps to chromosome 7q35-q36. *Arch Ophthalmol.* 1997;115:384-388.

94. Andersen JS, Parrish R, Greenfield D, Del Bono EA, Haines JL, Wiggs JL. A second locus for the pigment dispersion syndrome and pigmentary glaucoma maps 18q11-q21. *Am J Hum Genet.* 1998;63(4):A279. Abstract 1611.

95. Murray JC, Bennett SR, Kwitek AE, et al. Linkage of Rieger syndrome to the region of the epidermal growth factor gene on chromosome 4. *Nat Genet.* 1992;2:46-49.

96. Phillips JC, Del Bono EA, Haines JL, et al. A second locus for Rieger syndrome maps to chromosome 13q14. *Am J Hum Genet.* 1996;59:613-619.

97. Semina EV, Reiter R, Leysens NJ, et al. Cloning and characterization of a novel bicoid-related homeobox transcription factor gene, RIEG, involved in Rieger syndrome. *Nature Genet.* 1996;14:392-399.

98. Alward WL, Semina EV, Kalenak JW, et al. Autosomal dominant iris hypoplasia is caused by a mutation in the Rieger syndrome (RIEG/PITX2) gene. *Am J Ophthalmol.* 1998;125(1): 98-100.

99. Kulak SC, Kozlowski K, Semina EV, Pearce WG, Walter MA. Mutation in the RIEG1 gene in patients with iridogoniodysgenesis syndrome. *Hum Mol Genet.* 1998;7(7):1113-1117.

100. Mears AJ, Mirzayans F, Gould DB, Pearce WG, Walter MA. Autosomal dominant iridogoniodysgenesis anomaly maps to 6p25. *Am J Hum Genet.* 1996;59:1321-1327.

101. Nishimura DY, Swiderski RE, Alward WL, et al. The forkhead transcription factor gene FKHL7 is responsible for glaucoma phenotypes which map to 6p25. *Nat Genet.* 1998;19(2):140-147.

102. Jordan T, Ebenezer N, Manners R, McGill J, Bhattacharya S. Familial glaucoma iridogoniodysplasia maps to a 6p25 region implicated in primary congenital glaucoma and iridogoniodysgenesis anomaly. *Am J Hum Genet.* 1997;61(4):882-888.

103. Mears AJ, Jordan T, Mirzayans F, et al. Mutations of the forkhead/winged-helix gene, FKHL7, in patients with Axenfeld-Rieger anomaly. *Am J Hum Genet.* 1998;63(5):1316-1328.

104. Raymond V, Dubois S, Mears AJ, et al. Absence of mutations in the coding region of the FREAC3/FKHL7 gene in a large open-angle glaucoma family showing linkage to the IRID locus at 6p25. *Am J Hum Genet.* 1998;63(4):A305. Abstract 1765.

105. Caudill M, Barsoum-Homsy M, Chevrette L, et al. Mutation screening of the forkhead transcription factor FKHL7 in families with Axenfeld-Reiger anomaly. *Am J Hum Genet.* 1998;63(4):A99. Abstract 545.

106. Lichter PR, Richards JE, Downs CA, Stringham HM, Boehnke M, Farley FA. Cosegregation of open-angle glaucoma and the nail-patella syndrome. *Am J Ophthalmol.* 1997;124(4):506-515.

107. Dreyer SD, Zhou L, Machado MA, et al. Cloning, characterization, and chromosomal assignment of the human ortholog of murine Zfp-37, a candidate gene for Nager syndrome. *Mamm Genome.* 1998;9(6):458-462.

108. Vollrath D, Jaramillo-Babb VL, Clough MV, et al. Loss-of-function mutations in the LIM-homeodomain gene, LMX1B, in nail-patella syndrome. *Hum Mol Genet.* 1998;7(7):1091-1098.

109. McIntosh I, Dreyer SD, Clough MV, et al. Mutation analysis of LMX1B gene in nail-patella syndrome patients. *Am J Hum Genet.* 1998;63(6):1651-1658.

Chapter Three

ANATOMY AND PATHOPHYSIOLOGY OF AQUEOUS PRODUCTION AND OUTFLOW

Thomas F. Freddo, OD, PhD

The mechanisms that underlie aqueous production and drainage are complex. To understand the glaucomas, the basic anatomy and physiology of aqueous humor production and drainage must first must be mastered. The following is an overview and introduction to these subjects and is not meant to be comprehensive.

AQUEOUS HUMOR

Aqueous humor is a clear nutritive fluid that supports most of the metabolic demands of the avascular tissues of the eye. Aqueous is derived from a filtrate of plasma and secreted by the bi-layered ciliary epithelium into the posterior chamber of the eye at a rate of approximately 2.5 to 3.0 μL/min. Given that the combined volumes of the anterior (250 μL) and posterior (50 μL) chambers of the eye total 300 μL, it is simple to calculate that the entire volume of the aqueous humor is replaced approximately every 100 minutes.

Numerous studies have compared the relative concentrations of the various constituents in plasma and aqueous humor. These are summarized in Table 3-1. Although many similarities exist between the aqueous and plasma, several significant differences are found as well. As one important example, aqueous humor has a substantially higher concentration of ascorbate, which is widely assumed to be present as an antioxidant and scavenger of superoxide radicals.[1]

Free amino acid levels vary with respect to their relative concentrations in plasma. Certain of these, including arginine, isoleucine, leucine, methionine, phenylalanine, serine, threonine, tyrosine, and valine, are in higher concentration in the aqueous than in plasma, suggesting that active transport mechanisms are involved.[2,3]

The protein concentration of aqueous humor, as sampled from the anterior chamber, is less than 1% of that found in plasma (ratio of aqueous/plasma = 0.024/7 gm/dL). Recent improvements in protein chemistry methods have permitted a more complete analysis of this protein spectrum.[4,5] Although the blood-derived proteins present in aqueous generally reflect their relative concentrations in plasma, there are some clear exceptions. Among these are certain proteins found in higher concentration in aqueous than in plasma, including transferrin, an iron-scavenging protein.[6] Still other proteins are locally produced within the tissues of the eye and serve an array of recently identified regulatory functions. Foremost among these proteins are growth factors, the most intensively studied of which is TGF-β. TGF-β has been shown to play an array of important roles in the unique immunoregulatory processes of the anterior chamber.[7] A most provocative finding has been preliminary data suggesting that TGF-β_2 may be elevated in the aqueous humor of patients with primary open-angle glaucoma (POAG).[8] The significance of this finding remains to be fully explored, but it speaks to the importance of further inquiry into the mechanisms of these important classes of proteins in aqueous humor.

Other recent evidence suggests that the amount of plasma-derived protein present in the aqueous humor of the anterior chamber is supplemented just prior to its entry into the outflow pathway. Using fluorophotometry and, more recently, magnetic resonance imaging with contrast materials (Figure 3-1), it has been demonstrated that an anterior diffusional protein pathway exists in the normal eye that moves protein from a depot in the ciliary body stroma, through the uninterrupted stromal pathway to the root of the iris, bypassing the posterior chamber.[9-11]

In the absence of an epithelium on the anterior iris surface, this additional protein enters the aqueous humor. Proteins entering the anterior chamber in this fashion are prevented from returning to the posterior chamber by tight junctions joining the posterior epithelial cells of the iris.[12] Additional protein likely enters the adjacent outflow pathways that lead to Schlemm's canal (Figure 3-2). The question of whether any of these additional proteins are factors in aqueous outflow resistance is only beginning to be examined.[13] There is some evidence to support the theory that certain of the proteins added to aqueous humor, particularly those of low molecular weight and known as "fines," may play a role in generating normal outflow resistance as they are carried by aqueous flow into the trabecular meshwork.[14,15]

Table 3-1

Constituents of Human Aqueous Humor*

Constituent (µmol/mL)	Anterior Chamber Aqueous	Plasma
Ascorbate	1.06	0.04
Bicarbonate	22.0	26.0
Calcium	2.5	4.9
Chloride	131.0	107.0
Glucose	2.8	5.9
Lactate	4.5	1.9
Magnesium	1.2	1.2
Phosphate	0.6	1.1
Potassium	22.0	26.0
Sodium	152.0	148.0
Urea	6.1	7.3
Protein (gm/dL)	0.024	7.0
pH	7.21	7.4

*Adapted from Krupin and Civan[27]

AQUEOUS CIRCULATION

Aqueous humor is secreted by the ciliary epithelium into the posterior chamber. To enter the anterior chamber, aqueous must pass through the pupil. Changes in the anatomical relationship between the pupillary margin and anterior capsule of the lens can reduce the flow of aqueous humor into the anterior chamber (relative pupillary block). Similarly, inflammation-induced adhesions of the pupillary margin to the anterior surface of the lens (posterior synechiae) can obstruct aqueous flow.

Upon entering the anterior chamber, aqueous circulates in a convection current driven by the temperature difference between the warmer iris and the cooler cornea. Rising posteriorly and falling anteriorly, the aqueous humor finally leaves the eye via one of two principal outflow pathways described later. Because the aqueous humor is normally free of particulates, this circulation is difficult to appreciate. However, when particulates are present, such as uveal pigment in pigment dispersion syndrome or inflammatory cells in anterior uveitis, one can often observe that the par-

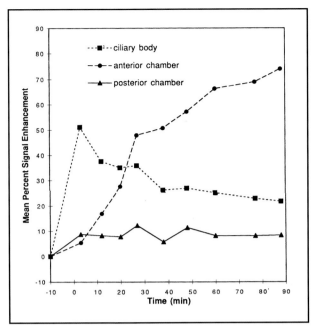

Figure 3-1. Mean percent signal enhancement from magnetic resonance images of the ciliary body and anterior and posterior chambers of the normal rabbit eye following intravenous administration of gadolinium-DTP. Enhancement occurs rapidly in the ciliary body and more slowly in the anterior chamber. Note that virtually no enhancement occurs in the posterior chamber during the 90 minute time course. Reprinted with permission from Kolodny N, Freddo T, Lawrence B, et al. Contrast-enhanced magnetic resonance imaging confirmation of an anterior protein pathway in normal rabbit eyes. *Invest Ophthalmol Vis Sci.* 1996;37(8):1602-1607. Copyright by Association for Research in Vision and Ophthalmology.

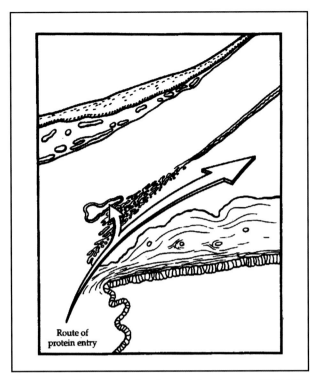

Figure 3-2. Predominant pathway taken by non-transported, plasma-derived proteins entering the aqueous humor. Reprinted with permission from Morrison JC, Freddo TF. Anatomy, microcirculation, and ultrastructure of the ciliary body. In: Ritch R, Shields MB, Krupin T, eds. *The Glaucomas.* 2nd ed. St Louis, Mo: CV Mosby Co; 1996.

ticulates in the posterior portion of the anterior chamber are rising while those just posterior to the cornea are falling. As the aqueous falls along the inward curvature of the inferior cornea, particulates such as pigment tend to sediment out and are phagocytosed by the corneal endothelium. If sufficient pigment is released, a vertically oriented line of pigment gradually becomes evident decorating the inferior half of the central cornea (Krukenberg's spindle).

AQUEOUS FORMATION

Aqueous humor formation is most easily described as a two-step process, realizing that these two steps are not independent. The first step is elaboration of a filtrate of plasma from the ciliary body microvasculature into the ciliary body stroma, and the second is forma-

tion of aqueous humor from this filtrate by the ciliary epithelium and its secretion into the posterior chamber.

The Ciliary Body

Aqueous humor is produced exclusively by the ciliary body, the intermediate portion of the uvea, which extends from the root of the iris posteriorly to the choroid. Aqueous humor production by the ciliary epithelium is but one of three principal functions ascribed to the ciliary body. The second function is enhancement of aqueous outflow through the connections of its longitudinal bundle of smooth muscle pulling the scleral spur posteriorly (described later). Finally, the third function is to provide the active, energy-requiring component of accommodation through contraction of the circular bundle of the ciliary muscle.

Gross Anatomy

The ciliary body is grossly subdivided into two regions. The anterior-most of these begins at the iris root and is termed the *pars plicata*. The pars plicata is named for the numerous fin-like ciliary processes that project into the posterior chamber (Figure 3-3).

Continuing from the posterior margin of the ciliary processes, the ciliary body has a flat inner surface. This flat portion, which extends to the anterior choroid, is termed the *pars plana*. The zonular fibers that support the crystalline lens originate within the epithelial layers covering the inner surface of the posterior pars plana, running forward along its inner surface as a continuous mat. Upon reaching the pars plicata, the zonular fibers are channeled into the valleys between adjacent ciliary processes before making their insertions onto the anterior and posterior edges of the equatorial lens capsule. Thus, under normal circumstances only the ridges of the pars plicata region remain exposed in the posterior chamber.

Histology

The inner surface of the ciliary body is covered by two layers of epithelial cells. The layer closest to the posterior chamber contains no melanin pigment granules and is termed the *non-pigmented ciliary epithelium* (Figure 3-4). This layer is continuous anteriorly with the posterior pigmented epithelium of the iris and posteriorly with the sensory retina at the ora serrata.

The epithelial layer closest to the ciliary body stroma does contain melanin pigment granules and is termed the *pigmented ciliary epithelium*. This layer is continuous with the anterior myoepithelium of the iris anteriorly and with the retinal pigmented epithelium at the ora serrata. It is the basal surface of these cells that face the ciliary body stroma. Despite their appearance, these two cell layers do not constitute a compound or stratified epithelium. They actually represent two simple epithelia arranged with their apical surfaces in apposition. This unique arrangement is the result of invagination of the neuroectoderm of the optic cup during embryologic development.

The ciliary body stroma is a loose, areolar connective tissue continuous with the iris stroma anteriorly and with the choroid at the ora serrata (see Figure 3-4). The ciliary body stroma in the pars plana region is a thin layer between the pigmented ciliary epithelium and the smooth muscle fibers of the ciliary muscle, which lie against the sclera. In the pars plicata region, this thin strip of stroma continues anteriorly to become continuous with the iris stroma at the iris root. The stroma also extends into the core of each of the ciliary processes, carrying with it its vascular supply.

The microvascular pattern of the ciliary body has only recently been documented with the advent of

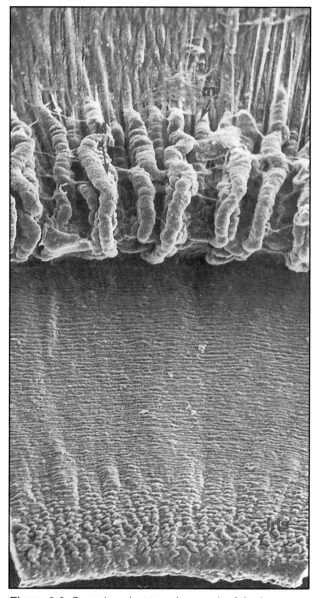

Figure 3-3. Scanning electron micrograph of the inner surface of the iris and ciliary body with the lens and some zonules removed. Major (M) and minor (m) ciliary processes are evident in the pars plicata region of the ciliary body (x16).

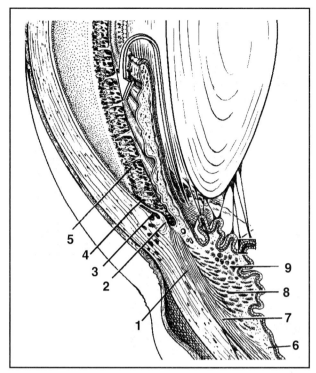

Figure 3-4. Sketch demonstrating the relationships between the ocular tissues of the anterior segment and denoting the pathway of aqueous flow. Two layers of epithelial cells line the inner surface of the ciliary body. The layer closest to the posterior chamber is the non-pigmented ciliary epithelium, while the layer closest to the ciliary body stroma is the pigmented ciliary epithelium. (1) Supraciliary space, (2) Scleral spur, (3) Canal of Schlemm, (4) Schwalbe's line, (5) Trabecular meshwork, (6) Ciliary body stroma of pars plana region, (7) Longitudinal bundle of the ciliary muscle, (8) Radial bundle of the ciliary muscle, (9) Circular bundle of the ciliary muscle. Modified from Freddo T. Ocular anatomy and physiology related to aqueous production and outflow. In: Lewis T, Fingeret M, eds. *Primary Care of the Glaucomas.* Stamford, Conn: Appleton and Lange; 1993.

vascular casting methods. Elegant scanning electron micrographs by Morrison et al now document that each of the ciliary processes actually has a dual vascular supply (Figure 3-5a).[16] Emanating from the discontinuous major circle of the iris, each process receives an anterior and posterior arteriole. The posterior arteriole, smaller in diameter, provides the vascular supply for the ciliary muscle, and gives rise to non-fenestrated capillaries that do not normally leak plasma proteins. By contrast, the tip of each ciliary process is served by one of a series of larger anterior arterioles, which give rise to a more robust vascular system of large fenestrated capillaries. The direction

of blood flow in both sets of arterioles is from anterior to posterior, toward a network of choroidal veins (Figure 3-5b).

Elaboration of a Plasma Filtrate from the Microvasculature of the Ciliary Body

The physiological process whereby fluid is forced across a membrane by pressure is termed *filtration*. The amount of filtrate crossing a particular membrane depends upon the pressure difference across the membrane and the surface area over which filtration can occur. The composition of the filtrate (eg, water, ions, proteins) is determined largely by the size of the pores in the membrane (ie, by the permeability of the blood vessel wall). A filtrate of plasma is produced across the walls of the microvasculature within the ciliary processes. Evidence suggests that blood flow in the ciliary body is regionalized and that these various regions respond differently to agents such as epinephrine.[17] Adrenergic nerve endings are associated with the ciliary body microvasculature, which prompt a reduction in blood flow following sympathetic stimulation.[18,19] This reduction in blood flow likely reduces filtrate production.

Unlike the capillaries of the ciliary muscle, which are non-fenestrated, the capillaries derived from the anterior arterioles are fenestrated (Figure 3-6). These capillaries also lack continuous tight junctions and are freely permeable not only to solute and ions but to plasma proteins as well.

In the rabbit, the concentration of plasma protein in the ciliary body stroma reaches nearly 75% of that in the bloodstream, contributing a significant oncotic pressure. The ions, fluid, and small molecules of the plasma filtrate also leave the fenestrated microvasculature driven by the hydrostatic pressure within the capillaries of the ciliary processes.[20] This hydrostatic pressure is dependent upon neuroregulatory and/or humoral influences that serve to control the amount of filtrate available in the ciliary body stroma.

The hydrostatic pressure within the microvasculature is opposed by the interstitial fluid pressure of the ciliary body stroma. The interstitial fluid pressure increases with intraocular pressure (IOP).[20] Thus, moderate elevations of IOP can actually suppress aqueous inflow indirectly leading to a decrease in IOP. The dynamics of this relationship are actually more complex, and the effect is insufficient to serve as a

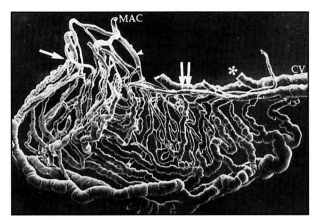

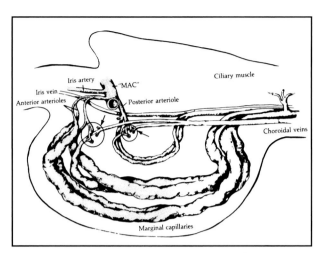

Figure 3-5a. A cast of the microvasculature within a single ciliary process. The major arterial circle (MAC) gives rise to an anterior (arrow) and posterior (arrowhead) arteriole. Double arrow denotes the choroidal vein. Drainage from the ciliary muscle to choroidal veins has been removed at the asterisk (x110). Reprinted with permission from Morrison JC, Van Buskirk EM, Freddo TF. Anatomy, microcirculation, and ultrastructure of the ciliary body. In: Ritch R, Shields MB, Krupin T, eds. *The Glaucomas.* 2nd ed. St Louis, Mo: CV Mosby Co; 1996.

Figure 3-5b. Diagrammatic representation of the vascular cast shown in Figure 3-5a. Reprinted with permission from Morrison JC, Van Buskirk EM, Freddo TF. Anatomy, microcirculation, and ultrastructure of the ciliary body. In: Ritch R, Shields MB, Krupin T, eds. *The Glaucomas.* 2nd ed. St Louis, Mo: CV Mosby Co; 1996.

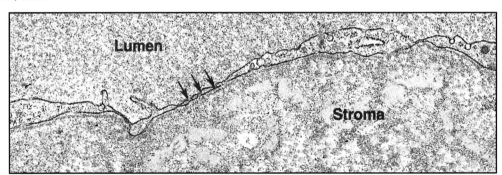

Figure 3-6. Transmission electron micrograph demonstrates that granular horseradish reaction product, mimicking the distribution of plasma proteins, leaks through fenestrations (arrows) from a capillary in the ciliary body stroma into the surrounding stroma (x40,800). Reprinted with permission from Morrison JC, Van Buskirk EM, Freddo TF. Anatomy, microcirculation, and ultrastructure of the ciliary body. In: Ritch R, Shields MB and Krupin T, eds. *The Glaucomas.* 2nd ed. St Louis, Mo: CV Mosby Co; 1996.

protective mechanism against the elevated pressure that characterizes POAG.

Nonetheless, there is an important clinical consequence of the relationship between IOP and inflow, but this effect manifests itself as an effect on the measurement of aqueous outflow. Certain methods for measuring outflow facility, such as tonography and constant pressure perfusion techniques, rely upon artificially elevating the IOP and then calculating the outflow facility from the rate of decrease in the elevated pressure over time.[21,22] Because reduction in aqueous production contributes a fraction of this fall in IOP, the resulting outflow facility is proportionally increased. The proportion of total outflow facility resulting from the pressure-induced reduction in aqueous production is termed *pseudofacility*. The percent of total outflow represented by pseudofacility appears to vary markedly among species. Although early estimates suggested that pseudofacility might account for as much as 20% of total outflow in humans,[23] methodological refinements have reduced this estimate to only about 5% to 10% of the total human outflow.[24]

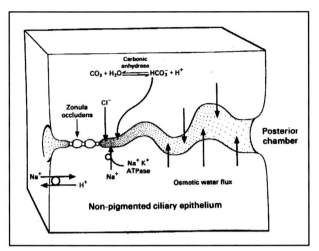

Figure 3-7. Simplified, schematic overview of major ion movement in the non-pigmented ciliary epithelium in aqueous humor production. Modified from Freddo T. Ocular anatomy and physiology related to aqueous production and outflow. In: Lewis T, Fingeret M, eds. *Primary Care of the Glaucomas*. Stamford, Conn: Appleton and Lange; 1993.

Formation and Secretion of Aqueous Humor from the Plasma Filtrate by the Ciliary Epithelium

The formation of aqueous humor by the ciliary epithelium is dependent primarily upon two forces: hydrostatic pressure and the magnitude of the oncotic pressure gradient across the ciliary epithelium. A diurnal fluctuation in the rate of aqueous production is known to occur. Flow rates are highest just after awakening and reach their lowest during sleep.[25] The magnitude of this effect is significant (approximately a 50% decrease), emphasizing the importance of recording time of day when taking tonometric measurements of IOP.

One of the most commonly cited models for the process of aqueous secretion is the modified Diamond-Bossert model for standing gradient osmotic flow.[20,26] An extremely simplified version is presented in Figure 3-7. A more detailed discussion of the numerous ion channels and ports that have recently been documented in various ciliary body preparations is available elsewhere.[27]

To produce aqueous, the ions that leave the microvasculature in the ciliary processes must enter the ciliary epithelial cells. Recent evidence suggests that sodium, potassium, and chloride ions are actively transported from the plasma filtrate in the ciliary body stroma into the pigmented ciliary epithelial cells by a resident $Na^+/K^+/2Cl^-$ exchanger (symport).[28,29] Once inside the pigmented ciliary epithelial cells, these ions move to the non-pigmented ciliary epithelial cells via gap junctions that unite both cell layers into a functional syncytium through both electrotonic and metabolic coupling.[30] From the non-pigmented epithelial cells, Na^+, Cl^- and HCO_3^- ions are pumped into the intercellular clefts between adjacent non-pigmented ciliary epithelial cells. The presence of these solutes creates a standing osmotic gradient that draws water into the cleft. The tight junctions joining the apico-lateral surfaces of the non-pigmented cells, restrict aqueous flow at the apical end of the cleft, directing it toward the posterior chamber.

The tight junctions of the ciliary epithelium[31] and those of the iris vascular endothelium[32] serve to limit diffusion of macromolecules into the aqueous humor, thus constituting the anatomical equivalents of the blood-aqueous barrier. Compromises in the integrity of this barrier caused by such provocations as anterior uveitis[33-35] or paracentesis[36] permit macromolecules to stream into the aqueous. This added protein scatters light and is clinically referred to as *flare*. Compromise of these junctions also reduces the oncotic pressure gradient from the ciliary body stroma into the posterior chamber, thus leading to a variable reduction in aqueous production. This decrease does not always lead to a reduction in IOP because significant elevation of aqueous humor serum protein concentration can obstruct aqueous outflow,[37] thus compensating for the reduction in inflow.

Evidence Supporting the Model

Evidence for the dependency of aqueous secretion upon oxidative metabolism comes from numerous studies demonstrating that metabolic inhibitors, reduction of oxygen tension, and hypothermia all reduce the rate of aqueous production.[38-40]

Na^+/K^+ ATPase

Sodium potassium ATPase is the enzyme that drives the Na^+/K^+ exchange pump. A currently accepted model of this pump (Post-Albers) proposes that the enzyme switches successively between two conformations within the cell membrane.[41,42] The conformation presented to the cytoplasmic surface exhibits a high affinity for sodium but a low affinity for potassium. The affinities of the alternate conformation, presented to the extracellular surface under normal conditions, are opposite. By successively switching from one conformation to the other, in a cyclical fashion, three sodium ions are extruded and two potassium ions are imported per ATP molecule. The exchange is thus not electrically neutral and results in a net outward movement of positive charge.

Evidence that such a system is central to the process of aqueous secretion comes from studies that have localized sodium potassium ATPase activity to the non-pigmented ciliary epithelium[43] and others documenting that inhibition of this enzyme with ouabain reduces aqueous secretion.[39]

Carbonic Anhydrase

The enzyme carbonic anhydrase also plays a central but as yet incompletely understood role in the process of aqueous secretion by generating bicarbonate ions. Within the ciliary epithelium, this enzyme has been histochemically localized solely to the non-pigmented layer at the tips of the ciliary processes.[44] The valleys between the major ciliary processes, normally covered by bundles of zonular fibers, do not exhibit staining for carbonic anhydrase.

The basic reaction catalyzed by the enzyme is quite straightforward, accelerating the hydration of carbon dioxide to carbonic acid, which dissociates into hydrogen and bicarbonate ions according to the following equation:

$$H_2O + CO_2 <\!\!-\!\!> H_2CO_3 <\!\!-\!\!> HCO_3^- + H^+$$

The roles of the ionic products of this reaction in the overall process of aqueous humor secretion remain uncertain. Indeed, the role of bicarbonate ion in aqueous production may vary by species. One function of bicarbonate ion in aqueous is to alter pH. Rabbit aqueous humor, high in bicarbonate, is alkaline relative to plasma, whereas human aqueous humor, low in bicarbonate, is acidic relative to plasma (see Table 3-1).

Inhibition of carbonic anhydrase decreases not only the entry of bicarbonate ions into the posterior chamber, but also the entry of sodium ions.[45] Whether a direct linkage between sodium and bicarbonate transport exists remains, however, unclear. One theory regarding the role played by bicarbonate ions in aqueous humor production maintains that HCO_3^- is transported in parallel with Na^+, primarily to offset the net outward movement of cations by the Na^+/K^+ ATPase pump. Another states that HCO_3^- movement may serve to alter pH in order to optimize Na^+/K^+ ATPase activity. Still other theories include facilitation of chloride transport[46] and/or alteration of the transepithelial voltage difference.[47]

Regardless of the mechanisms, the importance of this enzyme to aqueous secretion is amply illustrated by the clinical utility of carbonic anhydrase inhibitors (CAIs), such as acetazolamide[45] and the more recently available topical derivative, in the treatment of glaucoma.[48,49]

Receptor Systems Related to Aqueous Production

An array of receptors have been identified in the ciliary body of various species, including those for natriuretic peptides and others.[50] Moreover, a host of additional neuropeptides (eg, vasoactive intestinal peptide, neuropeptide Y, opioids, substance P) have been identified within the tissues of the ocular anterior segment. Uncovering possible roles for these agents in aqueous dynamics is at a very early stage. Also of interest is a proposed role for various nitrovasodilators in control of IOP, possibly mediated via nitric oxide.[51,52]

Beta Adrenergic Receptors

The most thoroughly examined of the receptor systems relating to aqueous production is that of the β-adrenergic receptor, which appears to have its effects primarily through the adenylyl-cyclase enzyme-receptor complex. Beta-adrenergic receptors have been localized to the ciliary epithelium.[53] Stimulation of these receptors initiates a signal transduction cascade beginning with activation of a regulatory intramembranous G-protein. In the case of β-adrenergic stimulation, the G-protein activates the second messenger adenylyl cyclase, which has also been localized to the ciliary body.[54,55] This, in turn, leads to elevation of cyclic-AMP levels resulting in phosphorylation of protein kinase-A (Figure 3-8).

What is currently unclear is the mechanism through which these events lead to the ultimate effect on aqueous humor inflow.[56] The literature in this area is remarkably contradictory, even disregarding the added complexities that arise in trying to compare data obtained from different species.[57,58] Regardless of the molecular mechanisms at work, it does seem clear

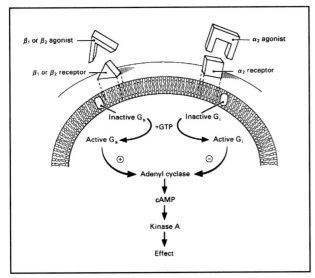

Figure 3-8. Schematic outline of major steps in signal transduction pathways following binding of β_1, β_2, and α_2 receptors. Reprinted with permission from Freddo T. Ocular anatomy and physiology related to aqueous production and outflow. In: Lewis T, Fingeret M, eds. *Primary Care of the Glaucomas*. Stamford, Conn: Appleton and Lange; 1993.

that β-antagonists such as timolol maleate lead to reductions in both aqueous inflow and IOP.[59] Equally well-established, if not well-explained, is the belief that neither β-agonists nor β-antagonists demonstrate an outflow-mediated effect on IOP, despite the presence of β-receptors on cells within the trabecular outflow pathways.[56]

Alpha Adrenergic Receptors

Alpha$_2$ adrenergic receptors also are present in the ciliary body.[60] Like β-receptors, they are coupled through G-proteins to adenylyl cyclase, but in a negative fashion that serves to block the elevations of cyclic-AMP levels induced by β-agonists (see Figure 3-8).[56] If this is the actual mechanism, it remains paradoxical that both α-adrenergic agonists and antagonists have been reported to lower IOP.[61] They appear to act through suppression of aqueous inflow without an apparent effect on outflow facility,[62] although effects mediated via reductions in episcleral venous pressure and ciliary body vascular flow also have been reported.[63] Initially approved only for use prophylactically to prevent acute elevations of IOP that often follow argon laser trabeculoplasty,[64,65] apraclonidine and the more recent and promising brimonidine now

are available for management of glaucoma, and add useful alternatives to our armamentarium, at least on the inflow side of the equation.

AQUEOUS OUTFLOW

The outflow of aqueous humor occurs predominately through two pathways: trabecular outflow, which is pressure-dependent, and uveoscleral outflow, which is pressure-independent.

The Trabecular Meshwork

The trabecular meshwork is a wedge-shaped band of tissue encircling and bridging the anterior chamber angle (Figure 3-9). The apex of this wedge is attached to Schwalbe's line, the peripheral edge of Descemet's membrane of the cornea. Expanding as it moves posteriorly from its point of origin, the trabecular meshwork attaches to the respective stromas of the ciliary body and the peripheral iris. Indeed, thin strands of pigmented tissue often rise from the peripheral iris to meet the trabecular meshwork. These are called iris processes (see Figures 3-9 through 3-10b).

Projecting into the base of this wedge is a shelf-like projection of sclera termed the *scleral spur* (see Figures 3-9 through 3-10b). Attached to the posterior surface of the scleral spur are the smooth muscle fibers of the longitudinal bundle of the ciliary muscle. When these fibers contract, they pull the spur posteriorly. In doing so, the layers of the corneoscleral meshwork attached to the anterior surface of the spur are spread apart. Tendons of ciliary muscle fibers also likely change the configuration of the juxtacanalicular region of the meshwork by acting through the cribriform plexus or through contractile cells that have been identified within the scleral spur of the human eye.[66] It is generally assumed that opening the meshwork in this fashion facilitates aqueous drainage and represents the most likely basis for the use of miotics in increasing aqueous outflow to reduce IOP in glaucoma.

A portion of the meshwork lies wholly within a recess in the sclera termed the *internal scleral sulcus*. The limits of this sulcus are defined by an imaginary line drawn on a sagittal section of the meshwork from Schwalbe's line to the anterior tip of the scleral spur (see Figure 3-9). Within the confines of the sulcus are the corneoscleral and juxtacanalicular (cribriform) regions of the meshwork and the Canal of Schlemm.

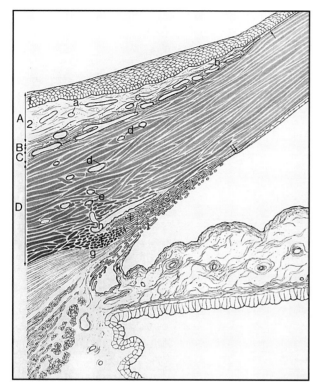

Figure 3-9. Drawing of the limbal region. The limbal con-junctiva (A) is formed by an epithelium (1) and an areolar connective tissue stroma (2). Tenon's capsule (B) forms an ill-defined layer of connective tissue over the episclera (C). The limbal corneosclera occupies area D. (a) Conjunctival vessels, (b) corneal arcades, single arrow, terminus of Bowman's layer. The trabecular meshwork (i) originates from Schwalbe's line (double arrows), broadening from its apex to become continuous with the iris and ciliary body (j). An iris process is evident (k). The scleral spur (f) projects into the meshwork forming a point of attachment for the fibers of the longitudinal bundle of the ciliary muscle (g). Aqueous flows into Schlemm's canal (h) and from there into a deep scleral plexus (e), intrascleral plexus (d), and finally, the episcleral vessels (c). Reprinted with permission from Hogan M, Alvarado J, Weddell J. *Histology of the Human Eye*. Philadelphia, Pa: WB Saunders; 1971.

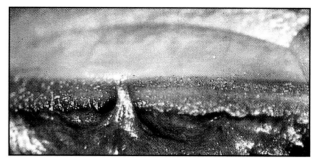

Figure 3-10a. Macroscopic photograph of angle structures viewed from the same perspective as in gonioscopy. Schlemm's canal is filled with blood in this specimen show-ing its relationship to the other structures. Reprinted with permission from Freddo T. Ocular anatomy and physiology related to aqueous production and outflow. In: Lewis T, Fingeret M, eds. *Primary Care of the Glaucomas*. Stamford, Conn: Appleton and Lange; 1993.

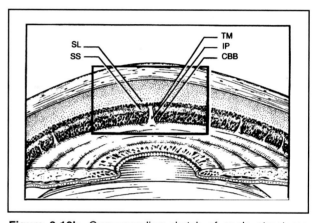

Figure 3-10b. Corresponding sketch of angle structures viewed from the same perspective as in gonioscopy. (SL) Schwalbe's line, (SS) scleral spur, (TM) trabecular mesh-work, (IP) iris process, (CBB) ciliary body band. Reprinted with permission from Freddo T. Ocular anatomy and physi-ology related to aqueous production and outflow. In: Lewis T, Fingeret M, eds. *Primary Care of the Glaucomas*. Stamford, Conn: Appleton and Lange; 1993.

The portion of the meshwork that is not confined within the sulcus, and which is most readily viewed gonioscopically, is termed the *uveal meshwork*.

For any clinician intent upon managing glaucoma, understanding the relationship between the views of the meshwork obtained from sagittal sections and those obtained gonioscopically is essential. Compare the diagrammatic representation of the angle struc-tures seen in a sagittal section (see Figure 3-9) with the appearance of these same structures viewed *en face* (see Figures 3-10a and 3-10b). Because the Canal of Schlemm is filled with blood in Figure 3-10a, the

relationship between the canal and the other angle structures also is evident. These views should each be compared with the goniophotograph of a normal, open angle seen in Figures 3-11a and 3-11b.

The principal landmarks evident in such a view of an open anterior chamber angle include, from superi-or to inferior:
- Schwalbe's line (ie, the peripheral terminus of Descemet's membrane)
- The trabecular meshwork
- The scleral spur
- The ciliary body band

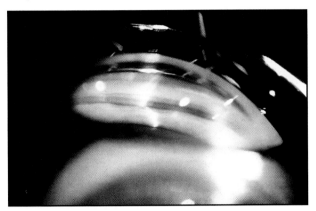

Figure 3-11a. Goniophotograph of a normal, open angle representing a view analogous to that shown in Figures 3-10a and 3-10b. Note that trabecular meshwork can be divided into an upper lighter band (anterior) and a lower darker band (posterior) seen just above the scleral spur. Courtesy of Rodney Gutner, OD, New England College of Optometry.

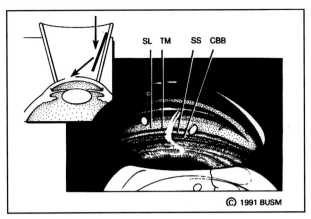

Figure 3-11b. (SL) Schwalbe's line, (SS) scleral spur, (CBB) ciliary body band. Reprinted with permission from Freddo T. Ocular anatomy and physiology related to aqueous production and outflow. In: Lewis T, Fingeret M, eds. *Primary Care of the Glaucomas.* Stamford, Conn: Appleton and Lange; 1993.

The portion labeled trabecular meshwork can be further subdivided into a minimally pigmented anterior meshwork and a more heavily pigmented posterior meshwork. In sagittal sections, the anterior portion of the meshwork corresponds to the portion of the meshwork that has no Schlemm's canal external to it. As a result, this portion of the meshwork sees little aqueous flow and thus its trabecular endothelial cells phagocytose relatively little pigment. It is this anterior, low-flow portion of the meshwork that is ideally targeted in argon laser trabeculoplasty.

The Uveal and Corneoscleral Meshwork

The tissue of the trabecular meshwork delimits a series of progressively smaller spaces for aqueous flow. The uveal meshwork is composed of intersecting beams (Figure 3-12). In section, these beams are seen to be composed of a non-vascularized core of collagens and elastin, surrounded by a basement membrane and a single layer of thin endothelial cells (Figure 3-13). The corneoscleral meshwork has essentially the same composition but the openings available for aqueous flow are reduced such that the appearance is more aptly described as a perforated sheet.

For many years, it had been widely assumed that a gel of hyaluronic acid fills the flow spaces of the trabecular meshwork, contributing to the resistance of aqueous outflow that generates normal IOP. Indeed, it

also was assumed that a progressive increase in such a gel might likely be the cause of the increased resistance that characterizes POAG. Results of more recent histochemical studies, however, do not support this view. Using a biotinylated hyaluronan-binding protein, hyaluronate was found mainly in the juxtacanalicular region, surrounding Schlemm's canal and in collector channels (Figure 3-14a). And contrary to what had been widely presumed some years ago, hyaluronate levels in the meshwork, in fact, decrease with age and decrease even further in glaucomatous eyes when compared to age-matched controls (Figures 3-14b and c).[67,68]

The endothelial cells of the trabecular meshwork are known to be phagocytic.[69,70] They are capable of ingesting both endogenous materials such as pigment[71,72] and exogenous particulates such as latex microspheres,[73] presumably for the purpose of keeping the trabecular outflow channels free of potentially obstructive debris. It appears that this phagocytic capacity may be at some long-term cost to the meshwork, however, because phagocytosis appears to prompt endothelial cells to detach from their beams and migrate out of the eye.[70]

Unfortunately, trabecular endothelial cells, like corneal endothelial cells, have a limited capacity for cell division.[74] Thus, as with the corneal endothelium, a progressive, age-related reduction in the number of trabecular endothelial cells has been observed.[75,76] Whether this cell loss is a major factor leading to the development of glaucoma remains to be established.[77]

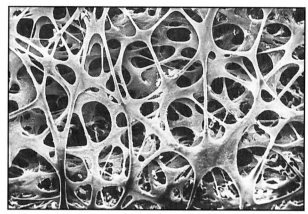

Figure 3-12. Scanning electron micrograph of the face of the uveal meshwork showing intersecting trabecular beams (x504). Reprinted with permission from Freddo TF, Patterson M, Scott D, et al. Influence of Mercurial sulfhydryl agents on aqueous outflow pathways in enucleated eyes. *Invest Ophthalmol Vis Sci.* 1984;25(3):278-285. Copyright by Association for Research in Vision and Ophthalmology.

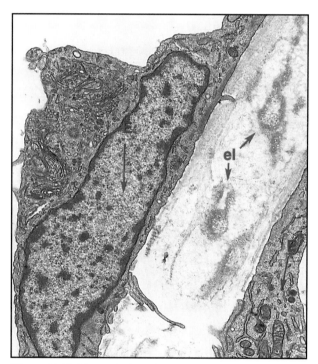

Figure 3-13. Transmission electron micrograph of a trabecular beam surrounded by a single layer of endothelial cells (E) and containing an avascular core of collagen and elastin (el).

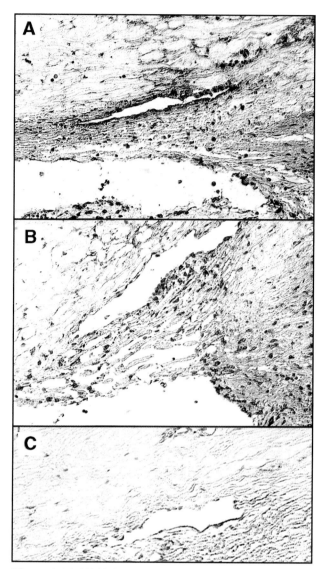

Figure 3-14. (A) Light micrograph of non-glaucomatous 47-year-old human trabecular meshwork. Red stain denotes location of hyaluronate, primarily in the region of the meshwork closest to Schlemm's canal. (B) Light micrograph of a non-glaucomatous 79-year-old human trabecular meshwork shows age-related decrease in hyaluronate staining. (C) Light micrograph of a glaucomatous 79-year-old human meshwork shows even less staining for hyaluronate.

Although their mitotic activity is limited, trabecular endothelial cells should not be thought of as inert. These cells are capable of producing a range of substances that likely play critical roles in regulating the extracellular matrix of the meshwork thereby influencing outflow, particularly in the juxtacanalicular region. Two groups of compounds produced by the meshwork that are likely involved in regulation of outflow are the matrix metalloproteinases (MMPs) and their inhibitors (tissue inhibitors of metalloproteinases [TIMPs]).[78] MMPs are zinc-dependent, calcium-stabilized, endopeptidases used by an array of connective tissues to initiate and regulate turnover of extracellular matrix. MMPs, including interstitial collagenase, Gelatinase A and B, and Stromelysin are all made in the trabecular meshwork and degrade ECM.[78] TIMPs, also made by the meshwork, serve to limit MMP activity. An array of modulators influence the balance between these two forces including growth factors, cytokines, and exogenously applied agents such as dexamethasone. Whether an imbalance in these forces represents a contributing or initiating event in the development of glaucoma remains to be established.

Most recently, a novel protein, induced by exposure of trabecular cell cultures to glucocorticoids has been identified, along with its gene. This protein, called TIGR (trabecular meshwork inducible glucocorticoid response [myocilin]) is an olfactomedin-related glycoprotein that increases in amount in response to glucocorticoid exposure.[79,80] In normal human eyes, TIGR is immunohistochemically localized to the inner uveal meshwork region and the anterior portion of the meshwork. In most glaucomatous eyes examined, TIGR staining was observed to be more intense and more widely distributed.[81] TIGR is presently under intense investigation as playing a possible role in steroid-induced glaucoma and possibly even POAG itself.

The Cribriform or Juxtacanalicular Meshwork

The tissue found in the region of the meshwork lying between the innermost corneoscleral trabecular beam and the inner wall of Schlemm's canal does not have a beam configuration. Instead, an open connective tissue matrix is found, which contains fibroblast-like cells that lack a basal lamina Figure 3-15.[82] The region of the meshwork occupied by these cells, and the extracellular matrix with which these cells are associated, represents the cribriform or juxtacanalicular region of the trabecular meshwork.

Running through this matrix is a plexus of elastin-containing fibers that are connected at one end to tendons from the longitudinal bundle of the ciliary muscle. At the other end, these fibers are connected to the basal surface of the endothelial cells that line the inner wall of Schlemm's canal. This anatomical system, called the *cribriform plexus*,[82] has the potential to effect alter-

ations in the permeability of this region. Such changes are likely of clinical importance, for it is the cribriform region of the aqueous outflow system that is generally held to represent the principal site of aqueous outflow resistance.[83] Underscoring the physiological importance of these various anatomical connections is the work of Kaufman and Bárány, who first demonstrated that surgical disinsertion of the ciliary muscle eliminates the outflow-enhancing effects of pilocarpine.[84]

The "Open" Spaces of the Trabecular Meshwork

In photomicrographs of trabecular meshwork prepared using conventional methods of tissue preparation, it appears that there is ample "open-space" even in an early to moderate stage of POAG. Nevertheless, calculations of outflow resistance in the juxtacanalicular meshwork, using a mathematical model that assumed the "open" spaces seen in conventional electron micrographs to be real, have been shown to fall two orders of magnitude short of generally accepted values for outflow resistance.[85] This fact has led some to seek alternate methods of tissue preparation that may better preserve the complex extracellular matrix presumed to reside in the JCT region. Using a recently developed method known as Quick-Freeze/Deep-Etch, it is now possible to obtain an electron microscopic view of the JCT region that does not require the series of chemical extractions employed using conventional methods. The resulting new view demonstrates a substantially more complex matrix present in the JCT region than could previously be demonstrated (Figures 3-16a and 3-16b). Preliminary morphometric and modeling studies suggest that this new view of the JCT region correlates much better with fluid dynamic predictions,[86] supporting previous work by others concluding that the JCT region is the principal site of resistance, at least in the normal eye.[87]

The Canal of Schlemm

The Canal of Schlemm is a continuous, circumferentially oriented channel, situated deep within the internal scleral sulcus. The lumen of the canal has direct connections to the venous system of the eye. Despite this connection, blood usually is not seen in the canal unless IOP falls below that of episcleral venous pressure.

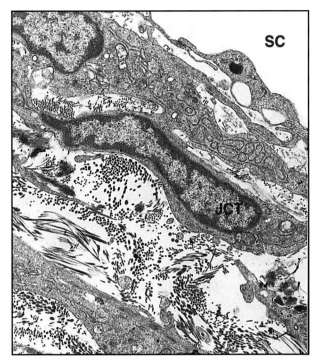

Figure 3-15. Transmission electron micrograph demonstrating the appearance of cells in the juxtacanalicular (JCT) region of the trabecular meshwork. These cells lack a basal lamina and are enmeshed within a connective tissue matrix that includes fibrillar collagen. These cells commonly extend paddle-like processes (arrows) to reach the endothelial cells lining Schlemm's canal (SC). Courtesy of Haiyan Gong, MD, PhD, Boston University. Reprinted with permission from Freddo T. Ocular anatomy and physiology related to aqueous production and outflow. In: Lewis T, Fingeret M, eds. *Primary Care of the Glaucomas.* Stamford, Conn: Appleton and Lange; 1993.

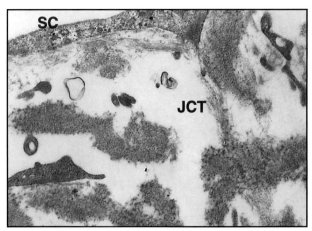

Figure 3-16a. Transmission electron micrograph of conventionally prepared normal human trabecular meshwork shows ample "open-space" in the juxtacanalicular (JCT) region beneath Schlemm's canal (SC) (X40,400).

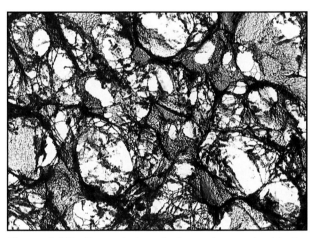

Figure 3-16b. Transmission electron micrograph of juxtacanalicular region of normal human trabecular meshwork at the same magnification as in Figure 3-16a, but prepared using quick-freeze/deep-etch, shows much less "open-space." Courtesy of Haiyan Gong, MD, PhD, Boston University.

The canal usually appears slit-like and, at several points around the circumference of the eye, it divides into two parallel channels that rejoin after a short distance. The outer wall of Schlemm's canal directly abuts the sclera. The inner wall of Schlemm's canal faces the juxtacanalicular region of the meshwork.

When subjected to pressure, as exists in vivo, the inner wall of Schlemm's canal exhibits unusual structures termed *giant vacuoles* (Figure 3-17). The formation of these vacuoles is pressure-dependent but not energy dependent. As IOP is increased (within physiological limits), the size of vacuoles in the inner wall of Schlemm's canal also increases.[88] Conversely, when IOP is reduced, as in paracentesis, vacuoles also are reduced.[36,89]

Giant vacuoles rarely are found if the tissue has not been fixed under conditions of active flow. As odd as these vacuoles appear, similar vacuoles are present in the arachnoid villi of the meninges, surrounding the brain, where they are believed to play a role in the resorption of cerebrospinal fluid.[88,90,91]

Very small openings called *pores* are found both in vacuoles and in non-vacuole-containing areas of the inner wall.[92] Pores are presumed to represent the actual flow pathways used by aqueous to traverse the inner wall of Schlemm's canal. Two types of pores have recently been examined: so-called intracellular pores and "border" or intercellular pores.[93] The significance of these two classes of pores remains to be established, but only one of them, the border pore, corre-

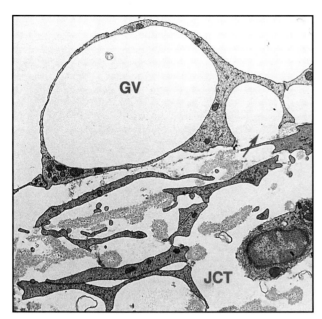

Figure 3-17. Transmission electron micrograph demonstrates a giant vacuole (GV) in the inner wall of Schlemm's canal (SC). Another vacuole is seen in the process of formation (arrow) (JCT) (X6,500). Reprinted with permission from Freddo T. Ocular anatomy and physiology related to aqueous production and outflow. In: Lewis T, Fingeret M, eds. *Primary Care of the Glaucomas.* Stamford, Conn: Appleton and Lange; 1993.

lates with perfusion pressure.[93] Border pores occur along the intercellular cleft between adjacent endothelial cells. Ultrastructural studies, using the technique of freeze-fracture electron microscopy, have demonstrated that the endothelial cells of the inner wall are joined by two types of intercellular junctions, gap junctions and discontinuous tight junctions in monkey[94] and normal human eyes.[95] More recent studies also have documented that the complexity of the junctions between inner wall cells decreases with increasing pressure.[96] Taken together, these data raise the prospect that border pores could represent focal areas where the number of tight junctional strands has been reduced to zero, thus creating a temporary, focal opening between endothelial cells.

From Schlemm's Canal to the Episclera

Upon reaching the lumen of Schlemm's canal, aqueous humor flows by one of two pathways to join the venous blood of the episcleral vessels. As a consequence, elevations of episcleral venous pressure (eg, carotid-cavernous sinus fistula) can give rise to signif-

icant elevations of IOP. The most commonly used pathway from Schlemm's canal to the episcleral vasculature is via a complex system of tortuous pathways that obliquely traverse the thickness of the sclera. These are outlined in the right-hand side of Figure 3-18. Within Schlemm's canal, aqueous flows circumferentially toward one of approximately 30 external collector channels. From the external collector channels, aqueous flows successively through a deep scleral plexus and an intrascleral venous plexus prior to reaching the episcleral veins. During this tortuous passage, aqueous and blood are mixed.

A smaller volume of aqueous humor bypasses the complex pathway outlined above by entering aqueous veins (of Ascher).[97] Few in number, the aqueous veins lead from either the outer wall of Schlemm's canal or an external collector channel, directly to the episclera (see Figure 3-18, left side). Absent the tortuous pathway taken by most of the aqueous, the blood and aqueous have not mixed by the time they reach the episclera. As a consequence, aqueous veins are readily identified by biomicroscopy as blood vessels appearing only half filled with blood.[97]

Current estimates are that less than 20% of total resistance resides in the portion of the outflow pathway beyond Schlemm's canal; however, the recently identified presence of contractile elements within the walls of the external collector channels in human eyes has spurred renewed interest in these issues.[98]

Uveoscleral Outflow

A smaller but nonetheless important fraction of total aqueous outflow leaves the eye in a pressure-independent fashion via a pathway beginning at the face of the ciliary body band and, ultimately, through the sclera (uveoscleral) or the scleral emissaria provided for the vortex veins (uveo-vortex).[99] The amount of total outflow represented by uveoscleral flow at normal IOP varies significantly among species. The pathway can be followed using tracer molecules and appears to pass within the connective tissue septae that separate the fascicles of smooth muscle fibers in the ciliary muscle (Figure 3-19). Contraction of this muscle reduces the available space for uveoscleral flow. Thus, it is not surprising that pilocarpine reduces uveoscleral outflow.[100] Current estimates are that in the normal human eye, uveoscleral flow accounts for less than 10% of the total.[100]

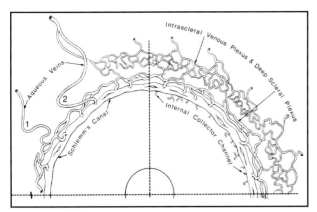

Figure 3-18. Diagrammatic representation of the distal portion of the aqueous outflow pathways from Schlemm's canal to the episcleral vessels. External collector channels arising from the outer wall of Schlemm's canal (upper right) lead to deep and intrascleral plexi and then to the episcleral vessels. Aqueous veins (upper left) arising from either external collector channels or the outer wall of Schlemm's canal, bypass this more convoluted pathway. Modified from Hogan M, Alvarado J, Weddell J. *Histology of the Human Eye*. Philadelphia, Pa: WB Saunders; 1971.

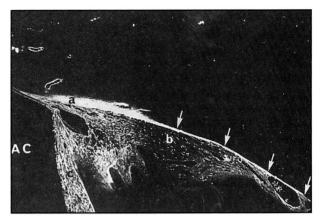

Figure 3-19. Light micrograph demonstrates the distribution of fluoresceinated dextran after intracameral perfusion. The tracer has moved from the anterior chamber (AC) posteriorly through the angle tissues (a) including the connective tissue septae of the ciliary muscle (b) to the supraciliary and suprachoroidal spaces (arrows). Note the tracer enters the iris stroma (c) but does not cross the iris into the posterior chamber (X38.5). Reprinted with permission from Tripathi RC. Uveoscleral drainage of aqueous humor. *Exp Eye Res*. 1977;25(suppl):305.

In recent years, however, the uveoscleral pathway has been the subject of increased interest with the discovery that several prostaglandin analogs are capable of augmenting uveoscleral outflow, possibly by solubilizing elements of the intramuscular connective tissue matrix of the ciliary body.[101] One of these, Latanoprost (Xalatan) has become available commercially. Two interesting discoveries have emerged as clinical use of this medication has increased. First, prolonged use stimulates melanin pigment production in the uvea leading to a progressive darkening of iris color.[102] Most surprising, however, has been developing empirical evidence that pilocarpine and Xalatan are additive in reducing IOP.[103,104] Since pilocarpine has been shown to profoundly reduce uveoscleral outflow, this surprising eventuality clearly demonstrates that our knowledge of the anatomy and physiology of uveoscleral outflow is incomplete and further study is warranted.

Fluid Mechanics of Trabecular Outflow

From the previous discussion, it is clear that an array of basic factors, some known and some yet to be elucidated, all contribute to the measured IOP at any point in time. Accounting for each of them in attempting to understand aqueous humor dynamics is exceedingly difficult. A general appreciation for how the major factors involved in this process interact is, however, very useful. These major factors include the measured IOP, the pressure in the venous system of the episclera, the flow rate of aqueous humor, and a factor that represents the ability of aqueous to leave the eye. This latter factor is referred to as facility of outflow, which is the inverse of outflow resistance. These factors were first incorporated into simplified mathematical constructs by Goldmann as follows:

$$\Delta P = IOP - \text{episcleral venous pressure}$$

and

facility of trabecular outflow = aqueous flow rate/ΔP

where IOP and episcleral venous pressure are measured in mmHg and aqueous flow is in μL/min at steady state. These equations assume that trabecular outflow occurs in an entirely passive manner as a bulk flow down a pressure gradient. They also assume that all outflow is trabecular. Under steady-state conditions, episcleral pressure is a negligible variable, and the facility of outflow through the trabecular meshwork is predominant. Under these circumstances the equations can be simplified as follows:

$$F_{in} = F_{out} = C_{trab}(\Delta P) + F_u$$

Kaufman has provided an illustrative example of this modified equation using measured values for the normal human eye.[105]

$F_{in} = F_{out} = 2.5 \ \mu L/min$

$C_{trab} = 0.3 \ \mu L/min/mmHg$

$IOP = 16 \ mmHg$

episcleral venous pressure = 9 mmHg

$\Delta P = (16 - 9) = 7$

$F_u = 0.4 \ \mu L/min$

Substitution of these values into the equation

$F_{in} = F_{out} = C_{trab}(\Delta P) + F_u$

gives the following:

$2.5 = 0.3(7) + 0.4$

In an overview such as this, certain oversimplifications and omissions are inevitable. Naturally, ample resources are available to the reader interested in developing an in-depth understanding of the numerous aspects of aqueous humor dynamics touched upon here. The reader should be encouraged to pursue these additional resources to supplement the rudimentary understanding provided herein.

REFERENCES

1. Varma SD, Kumar S, Richards RS. Light-induced damage to ocular lens cation pump: prevention by vitamin C. *Proc Nat Acad Sci USA.* 1979;76:3504.

2. Reddy DVN, Rosenberg C, Kinsey VE. Steady-state distribution of free amino acids in the aqueous humors, vitreous body, and plasma of the rabbit. *Exp Eye Res.* 1961;1:175.

3. Riley MV. The chemistry of aqueous humor. In: Anderson RE, ed. *Biochemistry of the Eye.* San Francisco, Calif: American Academy of Ophthalmology;1983.

4. Russell P, Epstein DL. Protein analysis of monkey aqueous humor. *Curr Eye Res.* 1992;11:1239.

5. Tripathi RC, Millard CB, Tripathi BJ. Protein composition of human aqueous humor: SDS-PAGE analysis of surgical and post-mortem samples. *Exp Eye Res.* 1989;48:117.

6. Tripathi RC, Borisuth NS, Tripathi BJ, Gotsis SS. Quantitative and qualitative analyses of transferrin in aqueous humor from patients with primary and secondary glaucomas. *Invest Ophthalmol Vis Sci.* 1992;33:2866.

7. Cousins SW, McCabe MM, Danielpour D, Streilein JW. Identification of transforming growth factor-beta as an immunosuppressive factor in aqueous humor. *Invest Ophthalmol Vis Sci.* 1991;32:2201.

8. Tripathi RC, Li J, Chan WF, Tripathi BJ. Aqueous humor in glaucomatous eyes contains an increased level of TGF-beta$_2$. *Exp Eye Res.* 1994;59:723.

9. Barsotti, MF, Bartels SP, Freddo TF, Kamm RD. The source of protein in the aqueous humor of the normal monkey eye. *Invest Ophthalmol Vis Sci.* 1992;33:581.

10. Freddo TF, Bartels SP, Barsotti MF, Kamm RD. The source of proteins in the aqueous humor of the normal rabbit. *Invest Ophthalmol Vis Sci.* 1990;31:125.

11. Kolodny N, Freddo T, Lawrence B, Suarez C, Bartels SP. Contrast-enhanced MRI confirmation of an anterior protein pathway in the normal rabbit eye. *Invest Ophthalmol Vis Sci.* 1996;37:1602.

12. Freddo T. Intercellular junctions of the iris epithelia in Macaca mulatta. *Invest Ophthalmol Vis Sci.* 1984;25:1094.

13. Sit AJ, Gong H, Ritter N, Freddo TF, Kamm RD, Johnson M. The role of soluble proteins in generating aqueous outflow resistance in the bovine and human eye. *Exp Eye Res.* 1997;64:813.

14. Doss EW, Ward KA, Koretz JF. Investigation of the "fines" hypothesis of primary open-angle glaucoma: the possible role of alpha-crystallin. *Ophthalmol Res.* 1998;30:142.

15. Russell P, Koretz J, Epstein DL. Is primary open angle glaucoma caused by small proteins? *Med Hypoth.* 1993;41:455.

16. Morrison J, VanBuskirk EM. Ciliary process microvasculature of the primate eye. *Am J Ophthalmol.* 1984;97:372.

17. Funk R, Rohen JW. Intraocular microendoscopy of the ciliary-process vasculature in albino rabbits: effects of vasoactive agents. *Exp Eye Res.* 1987;45:597.

18. Bill A. Autonomic nervous control of uveal blood flow. *Acta Physiol (Scand).* 1962;56:70.

19. Bill A. The protective role of ocular sympathetic vasomotor nerves in acute arterial hypertension. Proceedings of the Ninth European Conference in Microcirculation, Antwerp, Belgium. *Bibl Anat.* 1977;16:30.

20. Cole DF. Secretion of aqueous humor. *Exp Eye Res.* 1977;25(suppl):161.

21. Bill A, Bárány EH. Gross facility, facility of conventional routes, and pseudofacility of aqueous humor outflow in the cynomolgus monkeys: the reduction in aqueous humor formation rate caused by moderate increments in intraocular pressure. *Arch Ophthalmol.* 1966;75:665.

22. Brubaker RF. The measurement of pseudofacility and true facility by constant pressure perfusion in the normal rhesus monkey eye. *Invest Ophthalmol.* 1970;9:42.

23. Kupfer C, Sanderson P. Determination of pseudofacility in the eye of man. *Arch Ophthalmol.* 1968;80:194.

24. Kaufman PL, Bill A, Bárány EH. Formation and drainage of aqueous humor following total iris removal and ciliary muscle disinsertion in the cynomolgus monkey. *Invest Ophthalmol Vis Sci.* 1977;16:226.

25. Reiss GR, et al. Aqueous humor flow during sleep. *Invest Ophthalmol Vis Sci.* 1984;25:776.

26. Diamond J, Bossert WH. Standing gradient osmotic flow: a mechanism for coupling of water and solute transport in epithelia. *J Gen Physiol.* 1967;50:2061.

27. Krupin T, Civan M. Physiologic basis of aqueous humor formation. In: Ritch R, Shields MB, Krupin T, eds. *The Glaucomas.* 2nd ed. St Louis, Mo: CV Mosby Co;1996.

28. Edelman JL, Sachs G, Adorante JS. Ion transport asymmetry and functional coupling in bovine pigmented and nonpigmented ciliary epithelial cells. *Am J Physiol.* 1994;266:C1210.

29. Xu JC, et al. Molecular cloning and functional expression of the bumetanide-sensitive Na-K-Cl co-transporter. *Proc Nat Acad Sci USA.* 1994;91:2201.

30. Green K, Bountra C, Georgiou C, House R. An electrophysiological study of rabbit ciliary epithelium. *Invest Ophthalmol Vis Sci.* 1985;26:371.

31. Raviola G, Raviola E. Intercellular junctions in the ciliary epithelium. *Invest Ophthalmol Vis Sci.* 1978;17:958.

32. Freddo T, Raviola, G. Freeze-fracture analysis of the interendothelial junctions in blood vessels of the iris in Macaca mulatta. *Invest Ophthalmol Vis Sci.* 1982;23:154.

33. Freddo T. Intercellular junctions of the ciliary epithelium in anterior uveitis. *Invest Ophthalmol Vis Sci.* 1987;28:320.

34. Freddo TF, Sacks-Wilner R. Interendothelial junctions of the iris vasculature in anterior uveitis. *Invest Ophthalmol Vis Sci.* 1989;30:1104.

35. Freddo TF, Bartels SP, Barsotti MF. Morphological correlations with fluorophotometric data from monkey eyes with anterior uveitis. *Invest Ophthalmol Vis Sci.* 1992;33:1642.

36. Raviola G. Effects of paracentesis on the blood-aqueous barrier. An electron microscope study on Macaca mulatta using horseradish peroxidase as a tracer. *Invest Ophthalmol Vis Sci.* 1974;13:828.

37. Epstein DL, Hashimoto JM, Grant WM. Serum obstruction of aqueous outflow in enucleated eyes. *Am J Ophthalmol.* 1978;86:101.

38. Bartels SP. Aqueous humor formation: fluid production by a sodium pump. In: Ritch R, Shields MB, Krupin T, eds. *The Glaucomas.* 1st ed. St Louis, Mo: CV Mosby Co;1989.

39. Becker B. Ouabain and aqueous humor dynamics in the rabbit eye. *Invest Ophthalmol.* 1963;2:325.

40. Becker B. Hypothermia and aqueous humor dynamics of the rabbit eye. *Trans Am Ophthalmol Soc.* 1960;58:337.

41. Glynn IM. Annual review prize lecture: all hands to the sodium pump. *J Physiol (London).* 1993;462:1.

42. Horisberger JD. *The Na,K-ATPase: Structure-Function Relationship.* Austin, Texas: RG Landes;1994.

43. Flügel C, Lütjen-Drecoll E. Presence and distribution of Na+/K+ -ATPase in the ciliary epithelium of the rabbit. *Histochemistry.* 1988;88:613.

44. Lütjen-Drecoll E, Lönnerholm G, Eichorn M. Carbonic anhydrase distribution in the human and monkey eye by light and electron microscopy. *Graefe's Arch Clin Exp Ophthalmol.* 1983;220:285.

45. Maren TH. The rates of movement of sodium, chloride and bicarbonate from plasma to posterior chamber: effect of acetazolamide and relation to the treatment of glaucoma. *Invest Ophthalmol.* 1976;15:356.

46. Weiderholt M, Helbig H, Korbmacher C. Ion transport across the ciliary epithelium: lessons from cultured cell and proposed role of the carbonic anhydrase. In: Botre F, Gross G, Storey BT, eds. *Carbonic Anhydrase.* New York, NY: VCH;1991.

47. Coca-Prados M, et al. PKC-sensitive Cl- channels associated with ciliary epithelial homologue of pl(sb cln). *Am J Physiol.* 1995;37:C572.

48. Lippa EA, et al. Dose-response and duration of action of dorzolamide, a topical carbonic anhydrase inhibitor. *Arch Ophthalmol.* 1992;110:495.

49. Podos SM, Serle JB. Topically active carbonic anhydrase inhibitors for glaucoma. *Arch Ophthalmol.* 1991;109:38.

50. Korenfeld MS, Becker B. Atrial natriuretic peptide: effects on intraocular pressure, cGMP, and aqueous flow. *Invest Ophthalmol Vis Sci.* 1989;30:2385.

51. Nathanson JA. Nitrovasodilators as a new class of ocular hypotensive agents. *J Pharmacol Exp Therap.* 1992;260:956.

52. Nathanson JA. Nitric oxide and nitrovasodilators in the eye: implications for ocular physiology and glaucoma. *J Glaucoma.* 1993;2:206.

53. Lavah M, Melamed E, Dofna Z, Atlas D. Localization of β-receptors in the anterior segment of the eye by a fluorescent analog of propranolol. *Invest Ophthalmol Vis Sci.* 1978;17:645.

54. Nathanson JA. Adrenergic regulation of intraocular pressure: identification of β-adrenergic stimulated adenylate cyclase in ciliary process epithelium. *Proc Natl Acad Sci USA.* 1980;77:7421.

55. Tsukahara S, Maizawa N. Cytochemical localization of adenyl cyclase in the rabbit ciliary body. *Exp Eye Res.* 1978;26:99.

56. Mittag T. Adrenergic and dopaminergic drugs in glaucoma. In: Ritch R, Shields MB, Krupin T, eds. *The Glaucomas.* 2nd ed. St Louis, Mo: CV Mosby Co;1996.

57. Bill A. Effects of norepinephrine, isoproterenol, and sympathetic stimulation on aqueous humor dynamics in vervet monkeys. *Exp Eye Res.* 1970;10:31.

58. Brubaker RF Gaasterland D. The effect of isoproterenol on aqueous humor formation in humans. *Invest Ophthalmol Vis Sci.* 1984;25:357.

59. Coakes RL, Brubaker RS. The mechanism of timolol in lowering intraocular pressure. *Arch Ophthalmol.* 1978;96:2045.

60. Mittag TW, Tormay A, Severin C, Podos SM. Alpha adrenergic antagonists: correlation of the effect on intraocular pressure and on α₂-adrenergic receptor binding specificity in the rabbit eye. *Exp Eye Res.* 1985;40:591.

61. Mittag TW. Ocular effects of selective alpha-adrenergic agents: a new drug paradox? *Ann Ophthalmol.* 1983;15:201.

62. Gharagozolo NZ, Relf SJ, Brubaker RF. Aqueous flow is reduced by the α₂-adrenergic agonist, apraclonidine hydrochloride, (ALO 2145). *Ophthalmology.* 1988;95:1217.

63. Abrahms DA, et al. A limited comparison of apraclonidine's dose response in subjects with normal and increased intraocular pressure. *Am J Ophthalmol.* 1989;108:230.

64. Brown RH, et al. ALO 2145 reduces the IOP elevation after anterior segment surgery. *Ophthalmology.* 1988;95:378.

65. Robin AL, et al. Effect of ALO-2145 on intraocular pressure following argon laser trabeculoplasty. *Arch Ophthalmol.* 1987;105:646.

66. Tamm E, Flügel C, Stefani FH, Rohen JW. Contractile cells in the human scleral spur. *Exp Eye Res.* 1992;54:531.

67. Gong H, Freddo TF. Hyaluronic acid in the normal and glaucomatous human outflow pathway. *Invest Ophthalmol Vis Sci.* 1994;35(suppl):2083.

68. Knepper PA, et al. GAG profile of human TM in primary open-angle glaucoma. *Invest Ophthalmol Vis Sci.* 1989;30:224.

69. Grierson I, Lee WR. Erythrocyte phagocytosis in the human trabecular meshwork. *Br J Ophthalmol.* 1973;57:400.

70. Rohen JW, van der Zypen E. The phagocytic activity of the trabecular meshwork endothelium: an electron microscope study of the vervet (Cercopithecus æthiops). *Graefe's Arch Clin Exp Ophthalmol.* 1968;175:143.

71. Epstein DL, Freddo TF, Anderson PJ, Patterson MM, Bassett-Chu S. Experimental obstruction to aqueous outflow by pigment particles in living monkeys. *Invest Ophthalmol Vis Sci.* 1986;27:387.

72. Richardson TM, Hutchinson BT, Grant MW. The outflow tract in pigmentary glaucoma: a light and electron microscopic study. *Arch Ophthalmol.* 1977;95:1015.

73. Buller C, Johnson DH, Tschumper RC. Human trabecular meshwork phagocytosis: observations in an organ culture system. *Invest Ophthalmol Vis Sci.* 1990;31:2156.

74. Johnson DH. Do trabecular cells replicate? *Invest Ophthalmol Vis Sci.* 1986;27(suppl):210.

75. Alvarado J, Murphy C, Polansky J, Juster R. Age-related changes in trabecular meshwork cellularity. *Invest Ophthalmol Vis Sci.* 1981;21:714.

76. Grierson I, Howes RC. Age-related depletion of the cell population in the human trabecular meshwork. *Eye.* 1987;1:204.

77. Alvarado J, Murphy C, Juster R. Trabecular meshwork cellularity in primary open angle glaucoma and non-glaucomatous normals. *Ophthalmology.* 1984;91:564.

78. Alexander JP, et al. Expression of matrix metalloproteinases and inhibitor by human trabecular meshwork. *Invest Ophthalmol Vis Sci.* 1991;32:172.

79. Nguyen TD, Chen P, Huang WD, Johnson D, Polansky JR. Gene structure and properties of TIGR, an olfactomedin-related glycoprotein cloned from glucocorticoid-induced trabecular meshwork cells. *J Biol Chem.* 1998;273:6341.

80. Polansky JR, et al. Cellular pharmacology and molecular biology of the trabecular meshwork inducible glucocorticoid response gene product. *Ophthalmologica.* 1997;211:126.

81. Lütjen-Drecoll E, May CA, Polansky JR, Johnson DH, Bloemendal H, Nguyen TD. Localization of the stress proteins alpha B-crystallin and trabecular meshwork inducible glucocorticoid response protein in normal and glaucomatous trabecular meshwork. *Invest Ophthalmol Vis Sci.* 1998;39: 517.

82. Rohen JW, Futa R, Lütjen-Drecoll E. The fine structure of the cribriform meshwork in normal and glaucomatous eyes as seen in tangential sections. *Invest Ophthalmol Vis Sci.* 1981;21:574.

83. Bill A, Svedbergh B. Scanning electron microscopic studies of the trabecular meshwork and the canal of Schlemm—an attempt to localize the main resistance to outflow of aqueous humor in man. *Acta Ophthalmol.* 1972;50:295.

84. Kaufman PL, Bárány EH. Loss of acute pilocarpine effect on outflow facility following surgical disinsertion and retrodisplacement of the ciliary muscle from the scleral spur in cynomolgus monkey. *Invest Ophthalmol.* 1976;15:793.

85. Ethier CR, Kamm RD, Palaszewski BA, Johnson M, Richardson TM. Calculation of flow resistance in the juxtacanalicular meshwork. *Invest Ophthalmol Vis Sci.* 1986;27:1741.

86. Gong H, Brown K, Johnson M, Kamm RD, Freddo TF. Hydraulic conductivity of juxtacanalicular connective tissue using quick-freeze/deep-etch. *Invest Ophthalmol Vis Sci.* 1997;38(suppl):S564.

87. Meapea O, Bill A. Pressures in the juxtacanalicular tissue and Schlemm's canal in monkeys. *Exp Eye Res.* 1992;54:879.

88. Tripathi RC. The functional morphology of the outflow systems of ocular and cerebrospinal fluids. *Exp Eye Res.* 1977;25(suppl):65.

89. Grierson I, Lee WR. Pressure-induced changes in the ultrastructure of the endothelium lining Schlemm's canal. *Am J Ophthalmol.* 1975;80:863.

90. Gomez DG, Potts G. Effects of pressure on the arachnoid villus. *Exp Eye Res.* 1977;25(suppl):117.

91. Tripathi BJ, Tripathi RC. Vacuolar transcellular channels as a drainage pathway for cerebrospinal fluid. *J Physiol (Lond).* 1974;239:195.

92. Inomata H, Bill A, Smelser GK. Aqueous humor pathways through the trabecular meshwork and into Schlemm's canal in cynomolgus monkey (Macaca irus). *Am J Ophthalmol.* 1972;73:760.

93. Ethier CR, Coloma FM, Sit AJ, Johnson M. Two pore types in the inner wall endothelium of Schlemm's canal. *Invest Ophthalmol Vis Sci.* 1998;39:2041.

94. Raviola G, Raviola E. Paracellular route of aqueous outflow in the trabecular meshwork and canal of Schlemm. *Invest Ophthalmol Vis Sci.* 1981;21:52.

95. Bhatt K, Gong H, Freddo T. Freeze-fracture studies of interendothelial junctions in the angle of the human eye. *Invest Ophthalmol Vis Sci.* 1995;36:1379.

96. Ye W, Gong H, Sit A, Johnson M, Freddo TF. Interendothelial junctions in normal human Schlemm's canal respond to changes in pressure. *Invest Ophthalmol Vis Sci.* 1997;38:2460.

97. Ascher KW. Aqueous veins: physiologic importance of visible elimination of intraocular fluid. *Am J Ophthalmol.* 1942;25:1174.

98. de Kater AW, Spurr-Michaud SJ, Gipson IK. Localization of smooth muscle myosin-containing cells in the aqueous outflow pathway. *Invest Ophthalmol Vis Sci.* 1990;31:347.

99. Bill A. Further studies on the influence of the intraocular pressure on aqueous humor dynamics in cynomolgus monkeys. *Invest Ophthalmol.* 1967;6:364.

100. Bill A. Uveoscleral drainage of aqueous humor in human eyes. *Exp Eye Res.* 1971;12:275.

101. Lütjen-Drecoll E, Tamm E. Morphological study of the anterior segment of cynomolgus monkey eyes following treatment with prostaglandin $F_{2\alpha}$. *Exp Eye Res.* 1988;47:761.

102. Camras CB, et al. Latanaprost, a potent ocular hypotensive prostaglandin analog, increases pigmentation in peripherally hypopigmented irides. *Ophthalmology.* 1994;101(suppl):128.

103. Fristrom B, Nilsson SEG. Interaction of PhXA41, a new prostaglandin analogue, with pilocarpine. *Arch Ophthalmol.* 1993;111:662.

104. Villumsen J, Alm A. Effect of prostaglandin $F_{2\alpha}$ analogue PhXA41 in eyes treated with pilocarpine and timolol. *Invest Ophthalmol Vis Sci.* 1992;33(suppl):1248.

105. Kaufman PL. Pressure-dependent outflow. In: Ritch R, Shields MB, Krupin T, eds. *The Glaucomas.* 2nd ed (p. 309). St Louis: CV Mosby Co;1996.

Chapter Four

Gonioscopy: An Essential Aid in the Diagnosis and Management of Glaucoma

L. Jay Katz, MD, FACS
Jonathan S. Myers, MD
George L. Spaeth, MD, FACS

INTRODUCTION

Visualization of the internal angle anatomy within the anterior chamber is essential in:
- Establishing the health status of the eye
- Differentiating numerous diseases
- Evaluating the response to certain therapies
- Enabling the proper performance of several surgical applications

The normal angle is limited posteriorly by the insertion of the iris onto the ciliary body, and, anteriorly, by the peripheral cornea. Visualization of the angle in vivo was not described until Trantas, in 1907, indented the limbus of a keratoglobus eye bringing the angle structures directly into view.[1] This distortion of the globe is uncomfortable for the patient and provides only limited clarity. Trantas in 1918 coined the term *gonioscopy* from the Greek *gonia* (angle) and *skopein* (seeing) to refer to examination of the angle.[2]

In order to clearly examine the angle structures, certain optical difficulties have to be overcome. The angle structures cannot be seen even viewing from the side of the eye because of total internal reflection of reflected light by the cornea-air interface, as originally pointed out by Salzmann.[3-5] The cornea-air interface bends light emanating from inside the eye (Figure 4-1). The difference in the refractive density of the cornea and air combined with the corneal curvature results in light reflected from the angle structures being completely reflected back inside the eye because the critical angle (45 degrees) has been exceeded. With all the light being reflected back, the angle structures cannot be examined directly. With the advent of goniolenses, this optical problem was solved by changing the angle of curvature at the cornea-air or lens-air interface, and altering the "critical angle." This technique allows light from the angle to be viewed.

GONIOLENSES

There are two basic types of goniolenses (or gonioscopes): direct and indirect. The direct gonioscope is made of clear plastic and is dome shaped (Figure 4-2). It has a steeper external curvature than

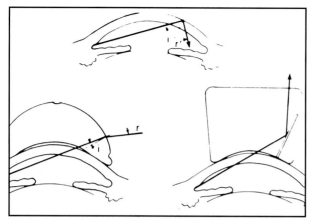

Figure 4-1. Total internal reflection of light making visibility of angle impossible (top). Domed direct goniolens (bottom left). Indirect goniolens with reflecting mirror (bottom right).

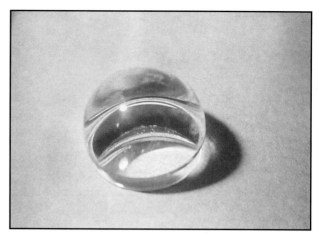

Figure 4-2. Domed direct goniolens (Koeppe).

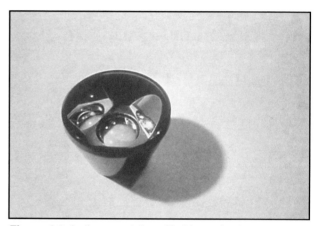

Figure 4-3. Indirect goniolens (Goldmann)—three-mirrored version.

the cornea, such that the critical angle is not exceeded. Therefore, light rays originating from the angle are allowed to escape and can be observed from the side. The indirect lens utilizes a mirror within the goniolens to redirect the exiting rays so that the angle of reflection is altered allowing the light rays to be deflected almost perpendicular to the lens-air interface (Figure 4-3).

Direct Goniolens

A prototypical diagnostic direct goniolens was introduced by Koeppe in 1920. A number of disadvantages have relegated the direct goniolens to use predominantly in the operating room. It is impractical for daily office use. The patient needs to be supine. The lens must be coupled to the cornea by balanced salt solution, or alternatively, a viscous agent (eg, methylcellulose), or a viscoelastic (eg, hyaluronate), which facilitates coupling of the lens to the corneal surface. Both a light source and adequate magnification can be provided with a portable slit-lamp or operating microscope. The observer must move around the eye in order to get a complete 360 degree view of the angle. The positive features of the direct contact lens view include:

- A wide 120 degree panoramic view from one side (Figure 4-4)
- Easy simultaneous bilateral angle comparison
- Allowance of intraoperative procedures such as goniotomy through a modified direct goniolens, such as the Barkan lens

Indirect Goniolens

There are two basic types of indirect lenses, exemplified by the Goldmann and Zeiss four-mirrored lenses. Both are conveniently used at the slit-lamp, because the mirrors of these lenses deflect the image toward the examiner nearly parallel to the visual axis.[6] The Goldmann lens has a mirror angled to view the anterior chamber angle, as well as two less sharply angled mirrors to view the retina. This goniolens affords the best optics and provides the clearest, most detailed view. Whenever careful scrutiny is required for discerning pathology of the angle, the Goldmann lens should be utilized. If angle photography or laser treatment to the angle (eg, argon laser trabeculoplasty) is to be performed, a Goldmann lens remains the preferred goniolens. Methylcellulose is used to couple the lens to the cornea. The lens must be rotated for

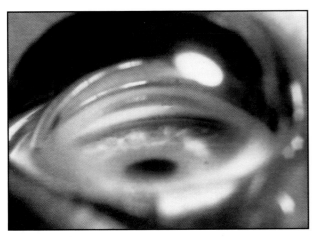

Figure 4-4. View of angle through direct goniolens.

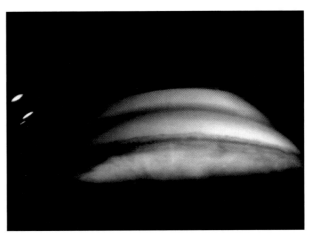

Figure 4-5a. Angle seen through Goldmann indirect goniolens.

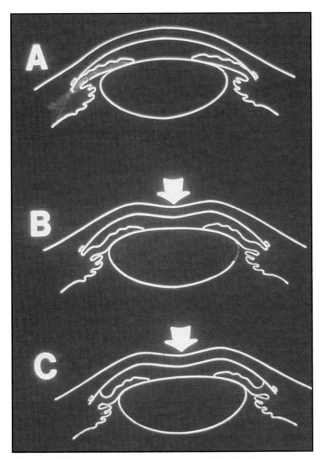

Figure 4-5b. Indentation gonioscopy. (A) Shallow anterior chamber. (B) Open angle (optically closed only). (C) Closed angle with peripheral anterior synechiae.

360 degrees and the view adjusted through the slit lamp biomicroscope in order to view the entire angle (Figures 4-5a through d). When methylcellulose is used, it makes ophthalmoscopy, fundus photography, or perimetry difficult after viewing the angle, even following copious irrigation of the eye.

The four-mirrored goniolenses, such as the Zeiss (Figures 4-6a and b), Posner, and Sussman, are the only lenses that allow dynamic indentation gonioscopy (Table 4-1).

This technique is necessary for the proper evaluation of narrow or closed angles. The portion of these gonioscopes that contact the cornea is only 9 mm wide (in comparison to the usual 12-mm Goldmann lens), which is smaller than the typical corneal diameter. Thus, when the goniolens is gently pushed against the central cornea, the central portion of the cornea is indented, displacing aqueous into the peripheral angle recess. By overly inflating the peripheral anterior chamber, the iris is pushed away from the angle, enabling the observer to ascertain the true iris insertion onto the angle (see Figure 4-5b). When pushing with the larger diameter Goldmann goniolens, the entire cornea is indented and the peripheral angle is not opened. Forbes, in 1966, underscored the utility of indentation gonioscopy in differentiating an optically closed angle from synechial angle closure.[7] With a four-mirrored lens, little or no rotation is necessary, because all four quadrants can be seen through the four mirrors. Tear fluid, not viscous coupling solution, effectively couples the lens with the cornea. The patient's own tear film usually suffices, although sometimes the use of a viscous

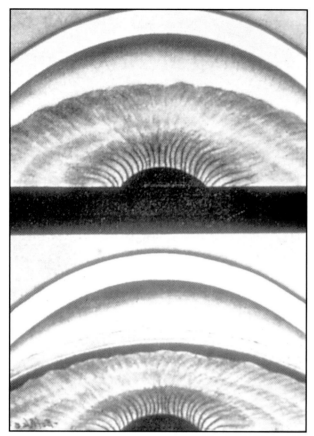

Figure 4-5c. Indentation gonioscopy. View of angle pre- and post-indentation. Open and no peripheral anterior synechiae.

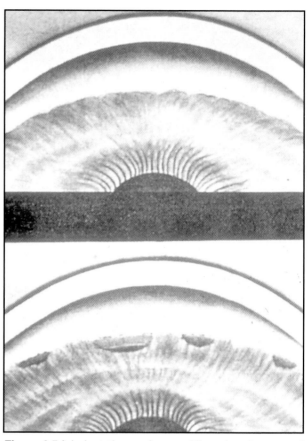

Figure 4-5d. Indentation gonioscopy. View of angle pre- and post-indentation. Partially open with peripheral anterior synechiae.

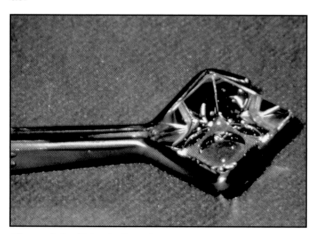

Figure 4-6a. Zeiss indirect four-mirrored goniolens.

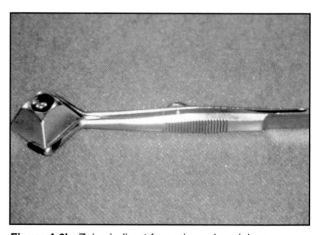

Figure 4-6b. Zeiss indirect four-mirrored goniolens.

artificial tear may be helpful, especially in patients with a history of corneal epithelial disease. Additional testing such as ophthalmoscopy, fundus photography, and perimetry can be performed without any delays following indentation gonioscopy. The negative aspects to the Zeiss four-mirrored lens include:

- The view is less clear than that achieved by other types of gonioscopy
- The technique is more difficult to master
- The potential exists for misinterpretation of the angle configuration because of artificial deepening and Descemet's folds secondary to excessive pressure

Table 4-1

Indirect Goniolenses
for Indentation Gonioscopy (Four Mirrors)

Goniolens	Material	Handle
Zeiss	Glass	Releasable-lock holder
Posner	Plastic	Fixed, built-in
Sussman	Plastic	Ring only

The correct technique for indirect gonioscopy requires that the patient's head be positioned at the proper height and that the observer be comfortable in viewing the patient through the slit lamp biomicroscope. The lateral canthus of the patient's eye should be level with the canthal mark on the slit lamp bar. After applying topical anesthesia to the globe, the contact lens is placed on the eye with the patient's gaze directed upward. The patient is then asked to look straight ahead. A small, thin beam of illumination, parallel to the viewing axis, is used to minimize light-induced miosis, which may change the angle's appearance. When viewing through the mirror, one is then looking into the angle 180 degrees opposite to the mirror (eg, looking at the mirror at 12 o'clock provides a view of the angle at 6 o'clock). If the angle is slightly narrow and the last roll of iris blocks the view of the angle, the contact lens may be minimally tilted, or preferably the patient may gaze slightly in the direction of the observing mirror. Ideally, the plane of the goniolens should always be perpendicular to the slit lamp microscope light beam. Too much angling and pushing on the cornea with a goniolens may abrade the corneal epithelium, especially in those with inherently loose epithelium (eg, anterior basement membrane dystrophy, diabetics, edematous corneas, or in recent postoperative cases). It is important to be certain that the cornea is moist before and during gonioscopy. Cleaning the goniolenses between use minimizes the potential for infectious disease transmission. Wiping the goniolens with a 70% isopropyl alcohol swab followed by air drying usually suffices. Some plastic goniolenses cannot be treated with alcohol. A 1:10 dilution of household bleach is an alternative cleansing agent.[8] Bleach needs to be thoroughly rinsed off prior to use, otherwise, significant corneal damage may result.

NORMAL ANGLE ANATOMY

Embryologically, the iris is formed by two layers of mesoderm. The anterior layer atrophies centrally giving rise to the pupil. Irregular atrophy results in iris crypts. The junction of the pupillary and ciliary zones of the iris is referred to as the frill. The iris color is determined by the amount of pigment in the anterior layer. When pigment is present only in the posterior layer, the iris is blue. When heavily pigmented in both layers, it is brown. The anterior limit of the posterior pigmented layer is the pupillary ruff.

The normal diameter of the cornea is 11 to 12.5 mm and the greatest anterior chamber depth is usually about 3.4 mm in adults. The depth is greater in myopes than in hyperopes and in men than in women. The anterior chamber shallows with age as the crystalline lens thickens with nuclear sclerosis.

In order to appreciate an abnormal clinical situation involving the angle, the normal anatomy and variability must be understood and recognized (Figure 4-7).[9,10] The whole angle itself measures approximately 1000 μm and is subdivided into several discernible layers. The insertion site of the iris on the ciliary body is approximately 1.5 mm from the limbus, or 1 to 1.5 mm from Schwalbe's line as viewed internally.

The ciliary body has a gray or light brown coloration. The width of the ciliary body varies considerably, being greatest in whites and narrowest in blacks and Asians. The ciliary body contains three muscles:
1. Longitudinal fibers
2. Oblique fibers
3. Circular fibers

The circular fibers control accommodation. The longitudinal muscle partially attaches to the trabecular meshwork. Contraction of these fibers (stimulated by accommodation or parasympathomimetic drugs such as pilocarpine) opens the trabecular meshwork and enhances aqueous outflow, thereby lowering intraocular pressure (IOP).

The scleral spur is the attachment point of the ciliary body to the sclera. It is a bone white band that remains uniform in color and width along the entire circumference of the angle, and shows little patient-to-patient variation, thus making it a useful landmark.

The trabecular meshwork, which is about 400 μm in width and is the primary site of aqueous outflow. Characteristically, it has a pigmented posterior section and a non-pigmented anterior zone. Aqueous flows only through the posterior region overlying

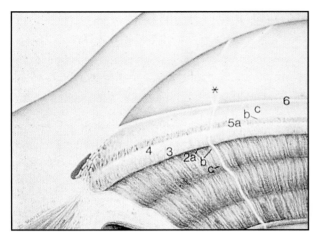

Figure 4-7. Angle anatomy. (*) Pupil, (2a-c) peripheral iris, (3) ciliary body, (4) scleral spur, (5) trabecular meshwork, (5a) pigmented, (5b) junction, (5c) non-pigmented, (6) Schwalbe's line.

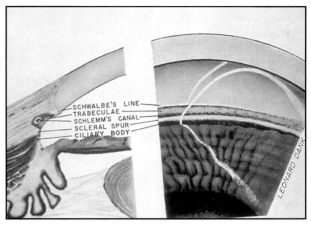

Figure 4-8. Junction of reflection off Bowman and Descemet's membranes is at Schwalbe's line.

Schlemm's canal. The trabecular meshwork has three components: The innermost layer is the uveal meshwork and has large 50 micron pores. The middle layer, the corneoscleral meshwork, has smaller pores of 10 to 20 microns. Both sections offer little resistance to aqueous outflow. The third and deepest layer is the juxtacanalicular tissue next to Schlemm's canal, which is the principal site of resistance to aqueous outflow. The meshwork pigmentation may be homogenous or quite variegated. Lacy extensions of the iris uveal meshwork onto the trabecular meshwork are termed *iris processes*.[11] When confluent, they occasionally may be confused with acquired peripheral anterior synechias. Usually the iris processes are filamentary, most dense nasally, and more prominent in young individuals with dark irides. With aging they tend to disappear.

Schwalbe's line defines the anterior boundary of the angle. It is seen as a knob-like convexity protruding into the anterior chamber. Histologically, it represents the termination of Descemet's membrane. When prominent, it is termed *posterior embryotoxin*. An optical cut through the cornea with the slit lamp beam has two reflections: from Bowman's and Descemet's membranes. They meet at Schwalbe's line (Figure 4-8). There may be a sprinkling of irregularly placed pigmentation onto Schwalbe's line, measuring about 50 to 150 μm in width.

Schlemm's canal is situated behind the posterior pigmented trabecular meshwork, and measures about 200 to 350 μm in width. Aqueous courses into 25 to 30 efferent collector channels, draining into the deep scleral plexus and episcleral venous plexus. A few collector channels empty into surface aqueous veins, especially inferonasally. This process can be visualized in 25% of patients. Compressing the aqueous veins, causing back pressure, leads to accumulation of clear aqueous within the lumen of these vessels.

Normal blood vessels frequently are seen in the angle (Figure 4-9). Three types have been identified[12]:
1. An iris radial vessel appears on the iris periphery emanating from the iris root insertion and disappears within the iris stroma. Such vessels are best seen in light blue irides.
2. The second vessel type is the short radial ciliary body vessel, which is perpendicular to the iris plane. It is a short trunk going from the ciliary body into the trabecular meshwork.
3. The largest and most conspicuous vessel is the serpentine-like circumferential ciliary body vessel. It undulates up and down going across the ciliary body occasionally dipping out of view below the iris insertion.

GRADING SYSTEMS

An orderly, systematic approach to the identification of the angle structures and anatomy (ie, configuration) helps the observer to accurately reflect upon and describe what has been seen. For example, the location and extent of peripheral anterior synechia can be drawn onto a representative circle. The pigmentation of the trabecular meshwork can be graded on a scale of 0 to 4+. It is more difficult to formulate a

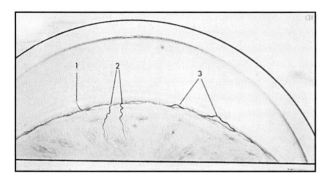

Figure 4-9. Normal blood vessels in the angle. (1) Iris radial vessel, (2) short radial ciliary body vessel, (3) circumferential ciliary body vessel.

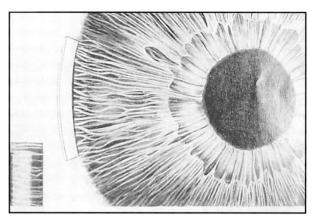

Figure 4-10. Van Herick estimation of peripheral anterior chamber depth (based on relative AC depth compared with corneal thickness).

Table 4-2		
Van Herick Grading System		
Van Herick Grade	**Peripheral Anterior Chamber Depth (Corneal Thickness)**	**Risk of Angle Closure**
1	Less than 0.25	High
2	0.25	Possible
3	0.25 to 0.5	Not likely
4	Greater than 1	Rare

three-dimensional evaluation of the peripheral angle that describes the width and shape.

Even without gonioscopy, there can be indirect clues that suggest a narrow angle may be present. A narrow anterior chamber angle may be detected by shining a pen light across the anterior chamber from the side and casting shadows on the far side of the iris in a narrow chamber. The anterior chamber depth can be measured manually by a Haag-Streit attachment to the slit lamp or by A-scan biometric ultrasonography. These techniques provide an accurate central anterior chamber depth measurement. A depth of 2.2 mm or less implies an eye at high risk for angle-closure development. The Van Herick slit lamp estimation of the peripheral anterior chamber depth also can warn of a potentially occludable angle (Figure 4-10).[13] The oculars and light beam are angled 60 degrees apart. The slit lamp beam is passed through the peripheral cornea. The width of the beam within the cornea is used as a comparative marker. If the peripheral anterior chamber depth is less than one quarter of the

corneal thickness it is estimated to be a narrow occludable angle (Table 4-2).

The measured anterior chamber depth and the Van Herick estimate technique are only indirect clues and are not substitutes for gonioscopy. Gonioscopy is the only reliable method to confirm and evaluate a narrow angle. A number of distinguished physicians have devised classification systems of the angle. The Shaffer and Spaeth grading systems are the only two such systems that have been widely embraced and used in daily clinical practice. The simpler Shaffer grading system was introduced in 1960[14] and the more complex but more informative grading approach by Spaeth in 1971 (Figures 4-11a-d).[15,16] These grading systems have proven invaluable in pinpointing narrow angles that are potentially occludable as well as in describing other clinical entities such as angle recession and pigmentary dispersion syndrome (PDS).

The Shaffer system was developed using the Goldmann contact lens.[15] Only one variable was singled out: the most posterior structure of the angle that could be directly visualized. Grade 4 is designated when the ciliary band is seen easily. For Grade 3, only the scleral spur can be identified. With a Grade 2 angle, the trabecular meshwork is visible. Schwalbe's line and perhaps the anterior portion of the meshwork is identified in a Grade 1 angle. Only peripheral cornea and Schwalbe's line are discerned with a Grade 0 angle. Grades 3 and 4 are deemed open and not occludable angles. Grade 2 has a low possibility, and Grade 1 is a very high possibility for angle closure. Grade 0 indicates that angle closure is present (Table 4-3).

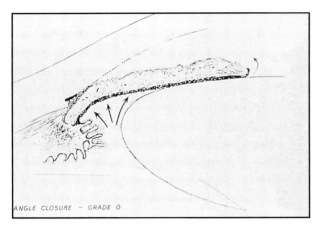

Figure 4-11a. Shaffer grading system. Grade 0 = angle closed.

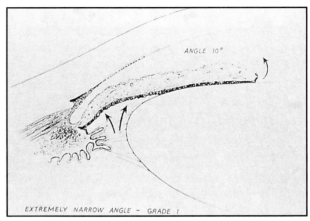

Figure 4-11b. Shaffer grading system. Grade 1 = narrow occludable angle.

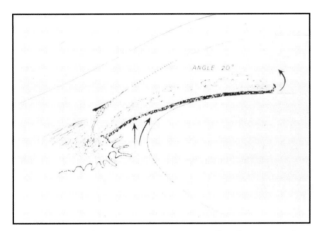

Figure 4-11c. Shaffer grading system. Grade 2 = moderately open.

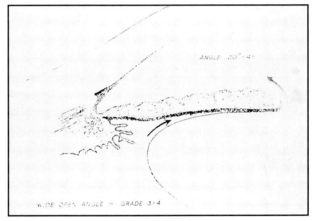

Figure 4-11d. Shaffer grading system. Grades 3 and 4 = wide open angles.

The Spaeth angle classification is based on the assessment of three variables. It requires that the observations be made with indentation gonioscopy. As with the Shaffer system, the first variable documents the most posterior angle structure visualized; however, that observation is two phased: pre- and post-indentation gonioscopy. The site at which the iris inserts is labeled A through E (Figures 4-12a-f). E is for extremely deep at the level of the ciliary body exposing a large ciliary body band. D is for deep, with the iris insertion exposing a moderate to a small amount of the ciliary body band. When the iris stops at the scleral spur, this is designated as C. B symbolizes iris insertion behind Schwalbe's line. Finally, A depicts an anterior insertion at Schwalbe's line or higher. However, in some patients the iris may be seen to rest against a higher level along the angle, although the true anatomical insertion is more posterior. This level of appositional closure is

Table 4-3

Shaffer Angle Grading System

Grade	Most Posterior Part of Angle Seen	Angle in Degrees
0	Cornea	Closed
1	Schwalbe's	10
2	Trabecular meshwork	20
3	Scleral spur	25
4	Ciliary body	Greater than 30

noted in parentheses before the level of true insertion revealed by compression gonioscopy. For example, if on first viewing the peripheral iris is against the middle of the trabecular meshwork, but during compres-

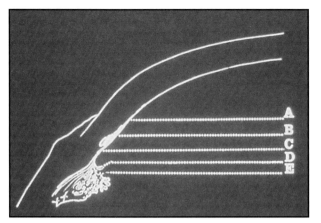

Figure 4-12a. Spaeth angle classification. First variable = insertion of iris.

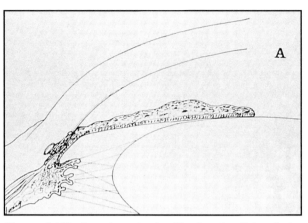

Figure 4-12b. Spaeth angle classification. A = Schwalbe's.

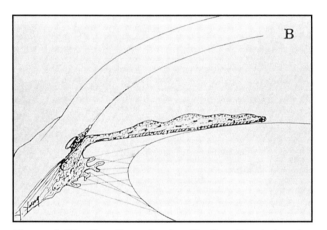

Figure 4-12c. Spaeth angle classification. B = trabecular meshwork.

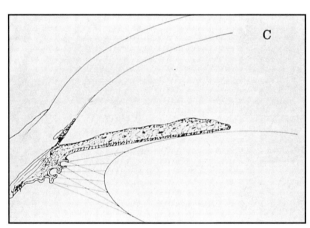

Figure 4-12d. Spaeth angle classification. C = scleral spur.

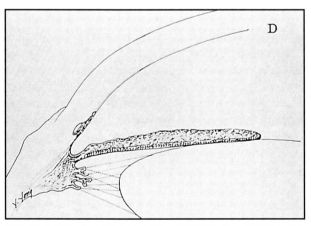

Figure 4-12e. Spaeth angle classification. D = ciliary body.

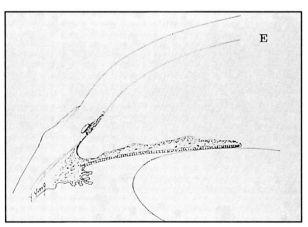

Figure 4-12f. Spaeth angle classification. E = low ciliary body.

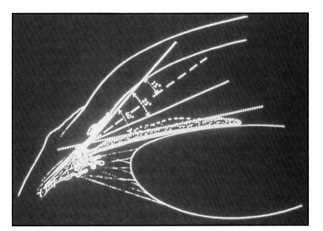

Figure 4-13. Spaeth angle classification. Second variable = angle width (degrees).

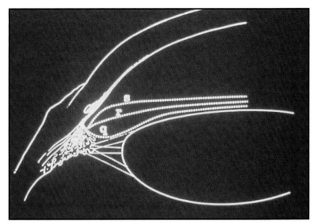

Figure 4-14. Spaeth angle classification. Third variable = peripheral iris configuration, (q) Concave posterior bow, (r), slight convex anterior bow, (s) markedly steep (plateau iris).

sion the angle opens to reveal an iris insertion into the ciliary body, the classification would be (B) D.

The second variable is estimation of the angle width in degrees (Figure 4-13). The width is established by creating imaginary lines from the peripheral corneal undersurface and the peripheral anterior iris surface. A 15 degree or less angulation implies a narrow angle. When 30 degrees or more, it is wide (it may be open or closed depending on the level of iris insertion).

The third variable estimate is the peripheral iris configuration (Figure 4-14). An r (regular) is applied to the most common shape, which is flat or a gradual anterior bowing. An s (steep) designates an extremely bowed initial anterior iris rise which levels off sharply. Lastly, a q (queer) configuration is a posteriorly bowed concavity of the iris. This last finding is typical for PDS or lens subluxation.

A quick and accurate record of the angle with the Spaeth classification can be readily noted in a patient's chart. This allows for meaningful future comparisons, even when other physicians examine the angle. Sample notations would be (A) D 10r, a narrow, potentially occludable angle; and E 45 q, a wide open angle seen with a posterior bowing.

PATHOLOGICAL ANGLES
Primary Angle Closure—Narrow Angles

Narrow angles may be open or closed with peripheral anterior synechias. After completion of indentation gonioscopy, a clinical judgment is rendered as to whether an angle may be occludable, potentially lead-

ing to an acute or chronic angle-closure glaucoma. Presentation with an acute angle-closure attack demands examination of the contralateral eye. This examination is vitally important in making the correct diagnosis. If the contralateral eye does not have a narrow angle, then a secondary angle-closure glaucoma should be suspected in the involved eye, such as inflammatory or neovascular glaucoma. In asymptomatic patients, despite "normal" IOPs, the presence of peripheral anterior synechias is a hallmark of progressive chronic angle-closure glaucoma (Figures 4-15a-c). Until a prophylactic laser iridotomy is performed, creeping synechial angle closure tends to be progressive. These adhesions in the angle initially appear superiorly because that is, typically, the most narrow region of the angle.

Assessment of the response to laser iridotomy or instillation of pilocarpine requires gonioscopic confirmation of angle deepening. Patency of laser iridotomies can occasionally be verified by seeing the lens capsule through the iridotomy. However, a transillumination defect alone can be misleading. The laser iridotomy may not fully penetrate the iris while dusting off much of the posterior pigment epithelial layer. This situation creates a window defect on retroillumination, but the iridotomy remains imperfect. Assurance of definitive angle deepening and success of the iridotomy is only obtained through confirmatory gonioscopy. If the angle is still occludable then either the iridotomy is not patent or a plateau iris configuration exists (Figures 4-16a and b). The latter condition is not due to a pupillary block mechanism, but instead results from a very steep iris

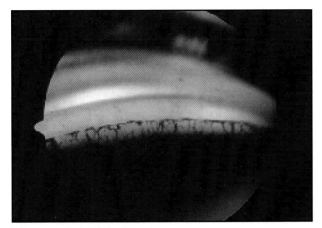

Figure 4-15a. Differentiation between iris processes and PAS. Iris processes (thin).

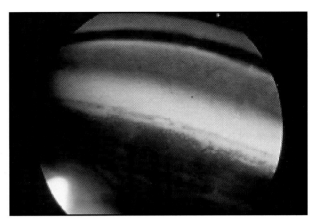

Figure 4-15b. Differentiation between iris processes and PAS. Iris processes (confluent).

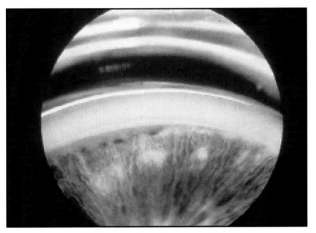

Figure 4-15c. Differentiation between iris processes and PAS.

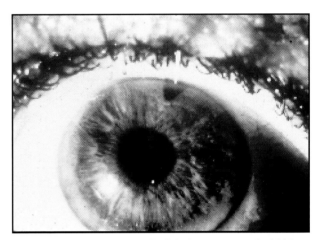

Figure 4-16a. Plateau iris. Definitely patent surgical iridectomy.

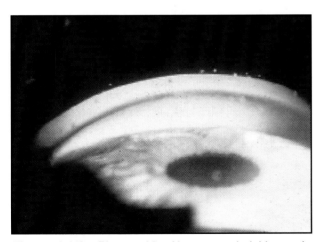

Figure 4-16b. Plateau iris. Narrow occludable angle despite iridectomy.

configuration due to a high iris insertion and partially rotated ciliary body. These eyes do not benefit from an iridotomy and should be treated with miotics and/or laser iridoplasty to flatten and pull away the peripheral iris from the angle structures.

When patients are placed on pilocarpine drops rather than being treated with an iridotomy for a narrow angle, there is a variable and unpredictable response. Most patients benefit with angle deepening in response to miotic use, but some develop an even more narrow angle, increasing the risk of angle closure. This further narrowing may be due to relaxation of the lens iris diaphragm, shallowing of the anterior chamber, and enhanced lens iris pupillary block. Other forms of angle closure glaucoma include nanophthalmos, retinopathy of prematurity, and microspherophakia—all of which occur in relatively

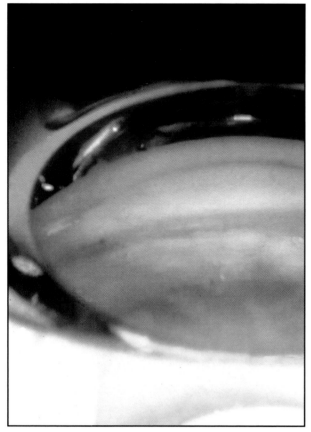

Figure 4-17a. Angle neovascularization. Fine branching angle vessels crossing onto trabecular meshwork.

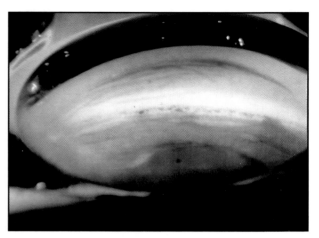

Figure 4-17b. Angle neovascularization. Associated PAS with angle neovascularization.

young patients. In nanophthalmos, the eyes are quite hyperopic although in the other two, the eyes are very myopic. With nanophthalmos, there is a normal size lens within a short globe, whereas in retinopathy of prematurity the axial length is average but the lens is extraordinarily large.

Secondary Angle Closure

When angle-closure glaucoma is unilateral, a secondary etiology should be considered. In most of these cases there is no pupillary block component and, therefore, an iridectomy would be of no benefit. Neovascular glaucoma presents with angle neovascularization preceding synechial angular closure (Figures 4-17a and b). If panretinal photocoagulation is promptly performed to minimize the ischemia-induced release of an angiogenesis factor, then further synechial development often can be arrested. When detected at a relatively early stage, the IOP may not become significantly elevated and may be controlled

with medical therapy. In some cases, angle neovascularization may be visible prior to any pupillary iris neovascularization. Therefore, gonioscopy is necessary to diagnose and monitor the response to therapy in neovascular glaucoma.

Iridocorneal endothelial syndrome (ICE) has characteristic very high, broad areas of peripheral anterior synechias. The adhesions often are higher than Schwalbe's line. The other eye displays a relatively normal appearing angle. There are three variants of ICE syndrome. In essential iris atrophy, there may be polycoria and corectopia. In Cogan's iris nevus syndrome there are multiple iris "nevi"; however, Chandler's syndrome may have quite subtle slit lamp findings in contrast to the dramatic gonioscopic findings of broad synechial angle closure.

Inflammatory glaucomas lead to the development of broad synechias characteristically starting inferiorly. Sometimes a sterile hypopyon, angle keratic precipitates, or angle granulomas my be observed. With complete 360 degree posterior synechias of the pupillary border to the lens capsule, no aqueous is allowed through the pupil and iris bombe may ensue. The peripheral iris billows up closing off the angle. The pupillary block can be alleviated by a peripheral laser iridotomy.

Ciliary body rotation occurs with inflammatory diseases such as scleritis, uveal effusion syndrome, and AIDS-associated choroidal detachments. The iatrogenic causes of ciliary body rotation include tight scleral buckles for retinal detachments and extensive panretinal laser photocoagulation. Cycloplegia and anti-inflammatory therapy help reverse the secondary

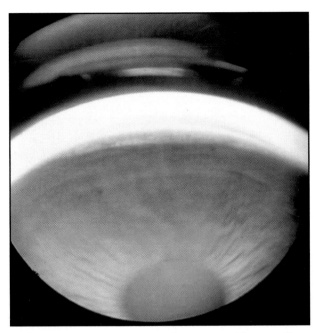

Figure 4-18. Focal angle recession—extra wide gray ciliary body band.

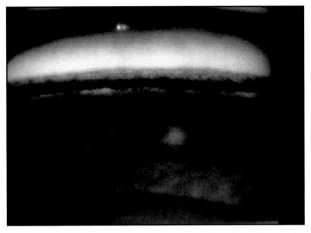

Figure 4-19. Heavy black pigmentation of trabecular meshwork in pigmentary dispersion syndrome.

angle closure. In these cases, an iridotomy would be of no help because there is no pupillary block element.

Aniridia typically does not have complete absence of the iris; there is a rudimentary iris stump. The iris characteristically rotates anteriorly leading to an angle-closure glaucoma. The angle may be difficult to visualize because of corneal pannus and epitheliopathy. These corneal changes are most common in patients that develop aniridia at a relatively young age.

Secondary Open-Angle Glaucomas

Trauma to the globe can result in a tear in the ciliary body band (resulting in angle recession) or a separation of the ciliary body from the scleral spur (cyclodialysis cleft). Traumatic angle recession is identified by a deepening of the angle and low iris insertion with exposure of a wide segment of the ciliary body band. It may be focal over only part of the angle, making it readily apparent when performing gonioscopy on that eye alone (Figure 4-18). If there is a 360 degree angle recession, comparison with the contralateral eye often proves helpful. An additional clue is the paucity of iris processes in the area of concern, because the iris processes often get sheared off at the time of trauma. The recessed angle is the result of blunt trauma which leads to a tear within the body

of the ciliary band. There is an associated trabecular sclerosis identified histologically, implying a higher resistance to aqueous outflow. Clinically the response to pilocarpine and argon laser trabeculoplasty is poor compared to primary open-angle glaucoma.

Many distinguishing features of PDS are observed on gonioscopy. The trabecular meshwork often is so pigmented that the area is obliterated by the dense pigmentation, which is uniform over the entire angle (Figure 4-19). Some pigment even may be deposited on the posterior lens capsule at the zonular insertion site. The peripheral angle configuration may have a q convexity with a posterior bow. A reverse pupillary block mechanism has been invoked to explain this finding. A laser peripheral iridotomy has been advocated by some as a treatment for pigmentary dispersion so as to "normalize" the q to an r iris configuration. Theoretically, there would be less iris zonular chafing and pigmentary release. The pigment granules are thought to be damaging or obstructive to the aqueous inflow system. With less pigment in the trabecular meshwork, theoretically, there would be a decreased chance of progressive IOP elevation. Nevertheless, there are no definitive studies demonstrating that iridotomies are beneficial to patients with pigmentary glaucoma.

Persistent or intermittent uveitis and secondary glaucoma following trauma may be caused by a retained intraocular foreign body. Gonioscopy may be the only method permitting the visualization of the foreign body in the angle (Figures 4-20a-c). Removal of the foreign body often leads to resolution of these problems. Accurate localization of the foreign body permits successful removal in the operating room.

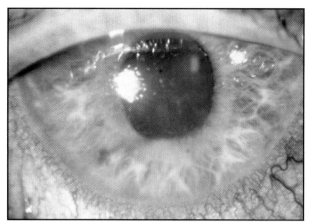

Figure 4-20a. Secondary glaucoma with intraocular foreign body. Small full thickness corneal scar.

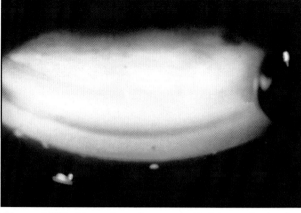

Figure 4-20b. Secondary glaucoma with intraocular foreign body. Angle foreign body.

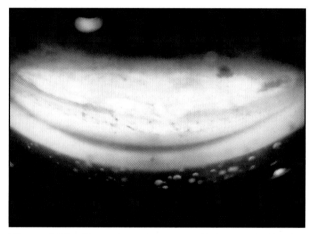

Figure 4-20c. Secondary glaucoma with intraocular foreign body. After surgical removal of foreign body.

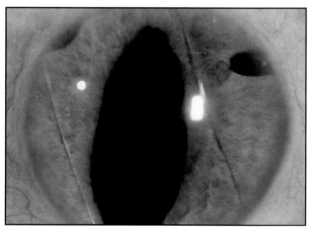

Figure 4-21a. UGH syndrome. Vision 20/20 with anterior chamber implant.

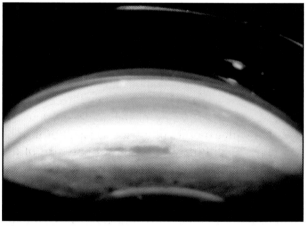

Figure 4-21b. UGH syndrome. Small inferior hyphema.

After intraocular lens implantation, some patients suffer from "uveitis-glaucoma-hyphema" (UGH) syndrome. Typical cases are easy to diagnose, however, frequently the presentation is subtle. Patients may complain of intermittent blurring, which may be due to intermittent hyphema and transient IOP elevation. Examination of the angle may reveal a tiny residual hyphema not seen by slit lamp microscopy (Figures 4-21a and b).

A thickening of Schwalbe's line with anterior displacement has been termed a *posterior embryotoxin* (Figures 4-22a and b). This finding can be seen as a white line in the peripheral cornea best visualized nasally and temporally. If there are iris processes extending to Schwalbe's line, Axenfeld's anomaly is diagnosed. These findings, when accompanied by corectopia and polycoria, comprise Rieger's anomaly.

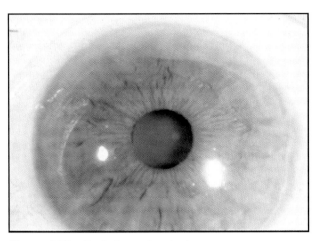

Figure 4-22a. Posterior embryotoxin.

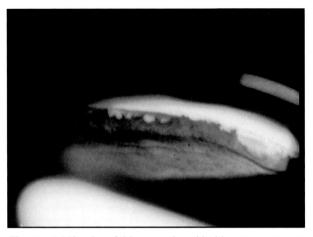

Figure 4-22b. Axenfeld anomaly with iris processes to Schwalbe's line.

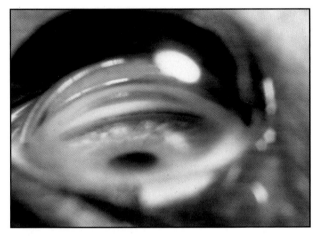

Figure 4-23a. Blood in Schlemm's canal associated with elevated episcleral venous pressure.

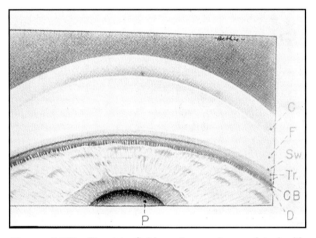

Figure 4-23b. Blood in Schlemm's canal associated with elevated episcleral venous pressure.

There may be systemic manifestations such as oligodontia, microdontia, maxillary hypoplasia, and a prominent umbilicus. About 50% of these eyes develop glaucoma by young adulthood.

Episcleral venous pressure may be raised above the normal 7 to 9 mmHg to levels of 30 to 35 mmHg in the presence of cavernous sinus-carotid fistula, dural shunts, Sturge-Weber syndrome, and thyroid ophthalmopathy. This "back" pressure elevates the IOP resulting in reflux of blood into Schlemm's canal, which often can be seen when observing the trabecular meshwork gonioscopically (Figures 4-23a and b).

In contradistinction to PDS, in exfoliation syndrome there is a non-homogenous dense, coarse pigmentation of the trabecular meshwork being most heavily pigmented inferiorly (Figures 4-24a-c). Frequently, there is a narrow, potentially occludable angle. A dense, fine wavy pigmentary line may be deposited anterior to Schwalbe's line; this is referred to as *Sampaolesi's line*.

With Fuchs heterochromic iridocyclitis there occasionally may be spontaneous hyphemas seen on gonioscopy.[17] These occur because of the angle neovascularization that accompanies this clinical entity. Surprisingly, there are almost never any peripheral anterior synechiae in association with angle neovascularization in Fuchs heterochromia.

Seeding from ciliary body or iris tumors may give rise to asymmetric pigmentation of the trabecular meshwork in the affected eye compared to the contralateral eye. Some ciliary body tumors may be best seen on gonioscopy. Accurate localization is important in planning treatments such as iridocyclectomy or radiation.

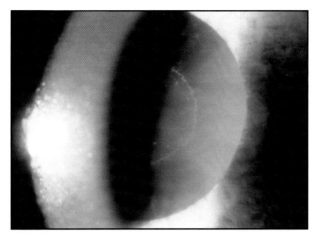

Figure 4-24a. PEX syndrome. Deposits on lens capsule.

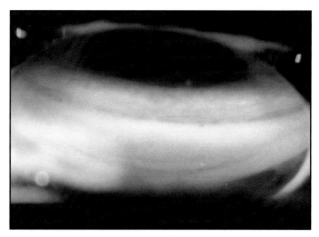

Figure 4-24b. PEX syndrome. Superior angle.

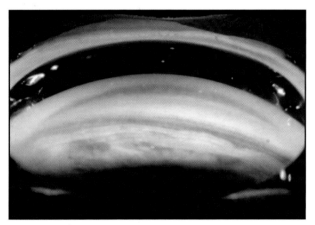

Figure 4-24c. PEX syndrome. Inferior angle with Sampaolesi line.

Hypotony

When confronted with persistent hypotony and decreased vision following trauma or surgery, a search should be made for a cyclodialysis cleft (Figure 4-25). With blunt trauma, there may be a separation of the ciliary body from its attachment to the scleral spur. This injury allows aqueous to pass directly into the suprachoroidal space, and leads to profound IOP reduction. With a soft globe, meaningful gonioscopy may be difficult. The angle can be better examined and the cleft precisely located if the eye is repressurized by injecting viscoelastic into the anterior chamber. Argon laser application to the cleft, or the gap between the ciliary body and scleral spur, occasionally helps seal the cleft, and permanently re-elevate the IOP.

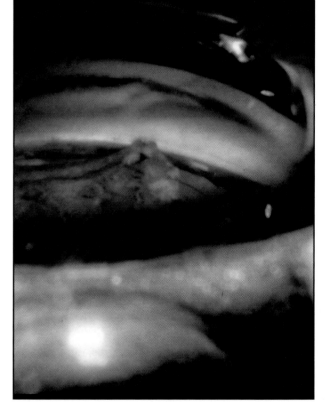

Figure 4-25. Traumatic cyclodialysis cleft.

TREATMENT

There are a variety of treatments in ophthalmology that require facility with gonioscopy. Direct visualization allows the safe and effective use of lasers, and proper technique with surgical instruments.

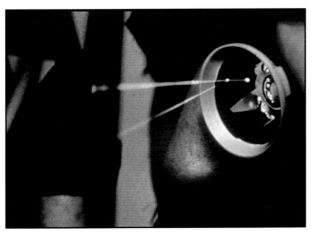

Figure 4-26. Application of argon laser trabeculoplasty with Goldmann goniolens.

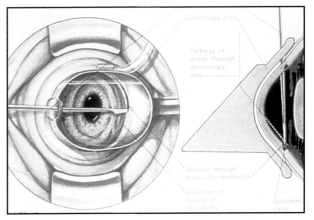

Figure 4-27. Goniotomy with Barkan direct goniolens.

Argon Laser Trabeculoplasty

Argon laser trabeculoplasty requires precise placement of the laser burns under direct visualization of the trabecular meshwork (Figure 4-26). In addition, the end point is the visible tissue reaction to the laser energy. The ideal laser placement is at the junction of the pigmented and non-pigmented trabecular meshwork. Anterior shots may be ineffective. Posterior placement, besides being painful for the patient, can lead to iritis and peripheral anterior synechias. The visible end point is minimal blanching of the trabecular meshwork with little if any bubble formation. Excessive laser absorption is a concern because experimental glaucoma can be induced in animal models from planned excessive laser application to the angle. Clinically, the power should be adjusted to a level that provides the ideal response. The amount of trabecular meshwork pigmentation and corneal clarity are critical determinants of the amount of energy required.

Goniotomy

Clear visualization of the angle is crucial for safe, effective guidance of a goniotomy blade in surgery for congenital glaucoma (Figure 4-27). The blade is swept across the point of iris insertion, which is unusually anteriorly displaced. Using a Barkan or similar direct goniolens while performing the goniotomy allows precise observation of the procedure. A posterior shift of the iris insertion should be seen following the sweep with the blade. The gonioto-

my is not performed by touch; it is a purely visually directed operation.

Sclerostomy Blockage

Occasionally, a filtering operation fails because of internal occlusion of the sclerostomy site, either by iris, fibrotic membrane, pigment, or an endothelial sheet (Figures 4-28a-d). These obstructions may occur early or late after filtering surgery. Laser application to the exact site of blockage sometimes can re-establish filtration without resorting to another operative intervention.

Hypotony

A cyclodialysis cleft may be responsible for persistent hypotony following surgery or trauma. If the vision is diminished then closure of the cleft should be undertaken. Argon laser application at the site may induce fibrin formation and promote closure. If that treatment is unsuccessful, surgical repair by direct suturing of the ciliary body to the scleral wall under a scleral flap may be necessary. This procedure may be supplemented by cryo application in the region to provide a firm adhesion. Cessation of aqueous flow to the suprachoroidal space results in IOP elevation usually with an accompanying improvement in vision. The initial IOP rise following successful closure often is rapid resulting in transiently high postoperative pressures.

Gonioscopy has become firmly established as a vital diagnostic tool in glaucoma diagnosis and thera-

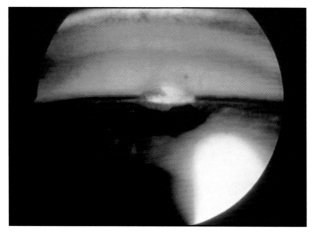

Figure 4-28a. Internal sclerostomy following trabeculectomy. Patent internal opening.

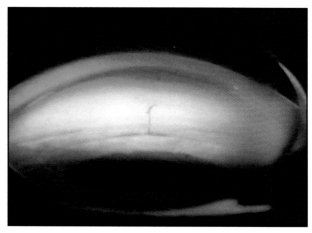

Figure 4-28b. Internal sclerostomy following trabeculectomy. Wisp of iris to sclerostomy.

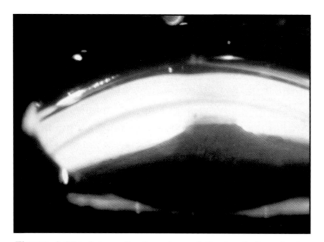

Figure 4-28c. Internal sclerostomy following trabeculectomy. Large iris incarceration in sclerostomy (inadequate peripheral iridectomy at time of surgery).

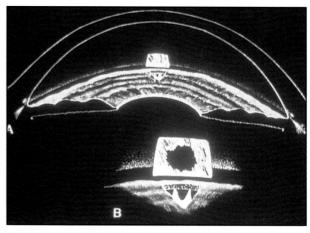

Figure 4-28d. Internal sclerostomy following trabeculectomy. Internal revision of sclerostomy with YAG laser through indirect goniolens.

py. In addition, mastery of gonioscopy is essential in many laser and operative techniques currently used.

REFERENCES

1. Trantas A. Ophthalmoscopie de la region ciliaire et retrociliaire. *Arch Ophthalmol.* 1907;27:581.
2. Trantas A. L'Ophthalmoscopie de l'angle iridioreen (gonioscopie). *Arch Ophthalmol.* 1918;36:257.
3. Becker SC. *Clinical Gonioscopy.* St Louis, Mo: CV Mosby Co; 1972.
4. Alward WLM. *Color Atlas of Gonioscopy.* Barcelona, Spain: Mosby; 1994.
5. Troncoso MU. Gonioscopy and its clinical applications. *Am J Ophthalmol.* 1925;8:433-449.
6. Goldmann H. Ur Technick der Spaltlampenmicroskopie. *Ophthalmologica.* 1938;96:90-97.
7. Becker SC. *Clinical Gonioscopy: A Text and Steroscopic Atlas* (pp. 37-80). St Louis, Mo: CV Mosby Co; 1972.
8. Smith CA, Pepose JS. Disinfection of tonometers and contact lenses in the office setting: are current techniques adequate? *Am J Ophthalmol.* 1999;127:77.
9. Kolker AE, Hetherington J. Gonioscopic and microscopic anatomy of the anterior chamer of the eye. In: *Becker-Shaffer's Diagnosis and Therapy of the Glaucomas.* 5th ed. St Louis, Mo: CV Mosby; 1983.
10. Fellman RL, Spaeth GL, Starita RJ. Gonioscopy: key to successful management of glaucoma. American Academy of Ophthalmology. Focal points 1984: clinical modules for ophthalmologists. No. 7. San Francisco, Calif: American Academy of Ophthalmology; 1984:1-8.
11. Lichter PR. Iris processes in 340 eyes. *Am J Ophthalmol.* 1969;68:872-878.

12. Henkind P. Angle vessels in normal eyes. A gonioscopic evaluation in anatomic correlation. *Br J Ophthalmol.* 1964;48:551-557.

13. Van Herick W, Shaffer RN, Schwartz A. Estimation of the width of angle of anterior chamber. *Am J Ophthalmol.* 1969;68:626.

14. Shaffer RN. Gonioscopy, ophthalmoscopy, and perimetry. *Trans Am Acad Ophthalmol Otolaryngol.* 1960;64:112-127.

15. Spaeth GL. The normal development of the human anterior chamber angle: a new system of descriptive grading. *Trans Ophthalmol Soc UK.* 1971;91:709-739.

16. Spaeth GI. Gonioscopy: uses old and new. The inheritance of occludable angles. *Trans Am Acad Ophthalmol Otolaryngol.* 1978;85:222-232.

17. Amsler M, Verrey F. Heterochromic de Fuchs et Fragilite Vasculaire. *Ophthalmologica.* 1946;3:177.

Chapter Five

ULTRASOUND BIOMICROSCOPIC FEATURES OF THE GLAUCOMAS

Jeffrey M. Liebmann, MD
Hiroshi Ishikawa, MD
Robert Ritch, MD

INTRODUCTION

The development of new imaging systems is rapidly altering our understanding of ocular anatomy and pathophysiology. High frequency ultrasound biomicroscopy (UBM, Paradigm Medical Industries, Inc, Salt Lake City, Utah) produces high resolution in vivo images of the anterior segment. The structures surrounding the posterior chamber, previously hidden from clinical observation, can be imaged and their anatomic relationships assessed. Ocular anatomy in health and disease can then be assessed. The purpose of this chapter is to explore the role of UBM in the diagnosis and management of anterior segment disease.

EQUIPMENT AND TECHNIQUE

The resolution, depth of penetration, and tissue resolution of ultrasonography are affected by transducer frequency. Higher frequency transducers permit increased resolution, but only at the expense of decreasing tissue penetration depth. The original ultrasound biomicroscope, developed by Pavlin and colleagues, is based on 50 to 100 MHz transducers incorporated into a B-mode clinical scanner.[1] The commercially available UBM unit is most often configured with a 50 MHz transducer and provides a tissue resolution of approximately 50 µm and a penetration depth of 5 mm. Virtually all anterior segment structures can be visualized at this frequency. At 60 MHz, the zonular apparatus is slightly better imaged. Increasing the transducer frequency to 100 MHz increases the tissue resolution to approximately 20 µm, but the decreased penetration depth limits scanning to the cornea, which is useful in the evaluation of refractive surgery. The decreased penetration depth afforded with a 42 MHz transducer permits visualization of the entire ciliary body and may prove useful in studies of accommodation. The images shown in this chapter were obtained with the standard 50 MHz transducer.

The technique of UBM has been reported in detail elsewhere and is similar to traditional immersion B-scan ultrasonography.[2-4] A 20-mm eye cup is inserted between the lids and holds the methylcellulose[2,4] or normal saline[5] coupling medium. After insertion of the probe into the coupling medium, the real-time image is displayed on a video monitor and can be stored on videotape for later analysis. Good qualitative information can be obtained by inexperienced examiners with minimal practice. However, ultrasonography is an art, and acquisition of highly reproducible distance measurements are strongly dependent on examiner technique and experience. The plane of section, distance from the center of the anterior chamber, and the orientation of the probe with respect to the perpendicular may affect the apparent structural configuration of the anterior segment.

As mentioned above, quantitative interpretation of anterior segment relationships using UBM scan information is more difficult than qualitative assessment. Pavlin et al described and quantified a series of anterior segment parameters for investigations with the UBM,[2] although interobserver error partially limits their application.[6,7] Factors that contribute to the variability of UBM image acquisition include room illumination, fixation, and accommodative effort, each of which affects anterior segment anatomy by altering pupillary size, ciliary body architecture, or probe orientation.[6-9] These should be held constant, particularly when quantitative information is being gathered.[6,7] In our laboratory, patients are asked to fixate with the fellow eye at a ceiling-mounted target to minimize changes in accommodation and eye position. Room illumination is held constant. Because the probe itself is in constant motion during scanning, soft contact lenses may be used to prevent potential corneal injury or for patients with significant corneal surface disease or recent surgery.[10]

THE NORMAL EYE

An understanding of the normal anatomy of the intact human eye in vivo is necessary to appreciate pathologic states. In the normal eye, the cornea, anterior chamber, posterior chamber, iris, ciliary body, and anterior lens surface can be recognized easily (Figure 5-1). Localizing the position of scleral spur, trabecular meshwork, Schwalbe's line, and the zonular apparatus requires more precision and attention to technique on the part of the examiner. Little attention has yet been paid to biometric differences among normal

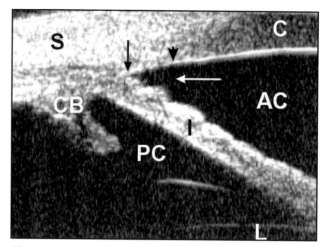

Figure 5-1. The UBM of a normal eye. The cornea (C), anterior chamber (AC), iris (I), lens (L), posterior chamber (PC), angle (white arrow), scleral spur (thin arrow), Schwalbe's line (arrowhead) sclera (S), and ciliary body (CB) are visible.

eyes, which might be investigated by UBM.[7]

The anatomic relationships of the structures of the anterior segment are often more important than their specific anatomy. In many normal individuals, the iris has a slightly convex configuration, consistent with the relative pupillary block present in most eyes. The response of the eye to a variety of stimuli, such as light or accommodative targets, alters these relationships, and will be described more fully below.

ANGLE-CLOSURE GLAUCOMA

Accurate diagnosis of the angle-closure glaucomas is critical to both their detection and treatment.[11] Failure to accurately diagnose angle closure often is an important factor in eyes with labile or poorly controllable intraocular pressure (IOP). Although gonioscopic evaluation of the anterior chamber angle with a Goldmann or Koeppe lens provides information about angle anatomy, clinical examination of the angle with the Zeiss indentation gonioprism permits dynamic evaluation of angle configuration and allows the clinician to differentiate between synechial and appositional closure.[12] Although the trabecular meshwork itself cannot be visualized with UBM, identification of the scleral spur during imaging localizes its posterior margin. Scleral spur can be seen as the innermost point of the line separating the ciliary body and the sclera at its point of contact with the anterior chamber. The trabecular meshwork is located directly anterior

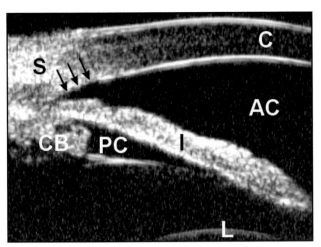

Figure 5-2a. Changing illumination alters angle configuration. Under normal conditions, the miotic response to light causes the angle to open. Aqueous has access to the trabecular meshwork (arrows).

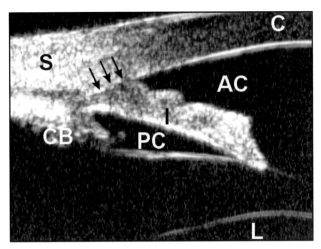

Figure 5-2b. If the room illumination is dimmed during scanning of the patient in 5-2a, pupillary dilation may cause the peripheral iris to crowd the angle and become apposed to the trabecular meshwork, causing angle closure.

to this structure and posterior to Schwalbe's line, which is the most peripheral portion of Descemet's membrane. It is advantageous to obtain at least one good image containing Schwalbe's line and scleral spur in each quadrant, so that regional differences in anatomy can be detected.

An important, though often overlooked, feature of angle anatomy is that it may be affected by the physiological state of the individual, ambient illumination, and accommodative status. For example, increasing room illumination or use of a bright slit-lamp beam results in miosis, which tends to widen the angle. Conversely, movement of the peripheral iris during pupillary dilation tends to crowd the angle. Although provocative testing for assessment of angle closure is now rarely used, gonioscopy should always be performed in a darkened room to maximize the likelihood that angle closure in an eye with an anatomically narrow angle will be detected. We perform gonioscopy in a room with the lights extinguished and the door closed using the smallest amount of slit-lamp illumination that permits a view of the angle.[13] The slit-lamp beam should not be directed through the pupil as this will cause miosis. The degree of angle narrowing under these conditions is often much greater than expected and can be demonstrated by UBM, which provides information on the state of the angle under normal light conditions and its tendency to occlude spontaneously under dark conditions (Figures 5-2a and b).

Evaluation of UBM images in the practice setting is useful for both the physician and the patient. The images are extremely useful for explaining the nature of disease processes and the rationale of treatment to patients who may be confused about the difference between open-angle and angle-closure glaucomas and different types of laser surgery.

Pupillary Block

Pupillary block is the most common form of angle-closure glaucoma and is responsible for more than 90% of cases. In pupillary block, resistance to aqueous flow through the pupil creates a relative pressure gradient between the anterior and posterior chambers, and forces the iris anteriorly, causing anterior iris bowing, narrowing of the angle, and acute or chronic angle-closure glaucoma (Figure 5-3a). The anterior segment structures and their anatomic relationships appear otherwise normal.

Laser iridotomy eliminates the pressure differential between the anterior and posterior chambers and relieves the iris convexity. This treatment results in several changes in anterior segment anatomy. The iris assumes a flat or planar configuration and the iridocorneal angle widens (Figure 5-3b). The region of iridolenticular contact actually increases, as aqueous flows through the iridotomy rather than the pupillary space.[12,14]

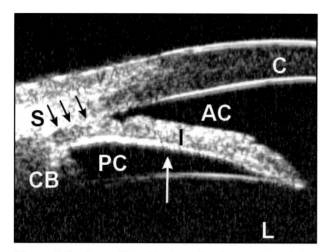

Figure 5-3a. In pupillary block angle closure, the relative pressure differential between the posterior and anterior chambers causes an iris convexity (white arrow). The angle is closed (black arrows).

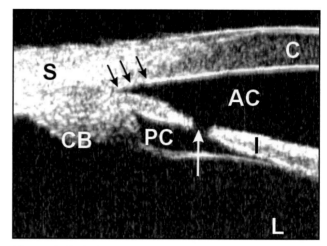

Figure 5-3b. Following laser iridotomy (white arrow), aqueous has free access to the anterior chamber and the pressure gradient is eliminated. The iris assumes a flat (planar) configuration and the angle opens (black arrows).

Plateau Iris

In plateau iris, abnormal ciliary body position or development leads to angle closure because of anteriorly positioned ciliary processes, which force the peripheral iris into the angle (Figure 5-4a).[3,11,15,16] On gonioscopy, the iris root angulates forward and then centrally. The iris root may be short and inserts anteriorly on the ciliary face, producing a shallow, narrow angle with a sharp drop-off of the peripheral iris. Before iridotomy, the anterior chamber is usually of medium depth and the iris surface mildly convex. Laser iridotomy either fails to open the angle or opens it only partially. Argon laser peripheral iridoplasty, however, provides the definitive treatment (Figure 5-4b).[12,14,17,18]

Plateau iris syndrome refers to the development of angle closure, either spontaneously or after pupillary dilation, in an eye with plateau iris configuration despite the presence of a patent opening in the iris. Some patients may develop acute angle-closure glaucoma. The extent, or the "height" to which the plateau rises, determines whether the angle will close completely or only partially. The angle can narrow further with age due to enlargement of the lens, so that an angle with plateau configuration, which does not close after iridotomy, may do so some years later. Periodic gonioscopy is required.

Lens-Induced Glaucoma

Anterior lens subluxation or intumescence may precipitate acute angle-closure glaucoma (phacomorphic glaucoma) due to the lens pressing against the iris and ciliary body and forcing them anteriorly.

Malignant Glaucoma

Also known as ciliary block, angle closure is caused by forces posterior to the lens which push the lens-iris diaphragm forward. It presents the greatest diagnostic and treatment challenge of the angle-closure glaucomas. Analogous to pupillary block, in which the angle is occluded by iris because of a pressure differential between the posterior and anterior chambers, in ciliary block, a pressure differential is created between the vitreous and aqueous compartments by aqueous misdirection into the vitreous.[19-21]

Alternatively, swelling or anterior rotation of the ciliary body with forward rotation of the lens-iris diaphragm and relaxation of the zonular apparatus may cause anterior lens displacement, which in turn causes direct angle closure by physically pushing the iris against the trabecular meshwork. UBM often reveals a shallow supraciliary detachment not evident on routine B-scan examination (Figure 5-5).[11] This effusion appears to be the cause of the anterior rotation of the ciliary body and the forward movement of the lens-iris diaphragm.

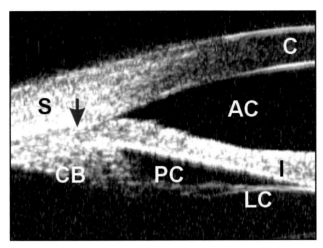

Figure 5-4a. The physical presence of the ciliary body forces the peripheral iris into the angle and closes the angle in plateau iris syndrome. The scleral spur is visible (arrow).

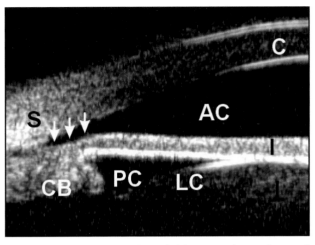

Figure 5-4b. Laser iridoplasty (white arrows) may be used in plateau iris syndrome to relieve appositional angle closure.

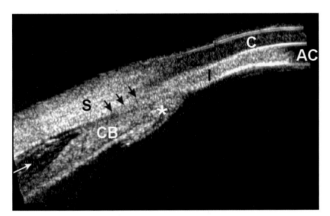

Figure 5-5. Malignant glaucoma can result from aqueous misdirection or from annular ciliary body detachment. In the latter case, fluid is visible in the supraciliary space (white arrow). In either case, anterior rotation of the ciliary body about its insertion into the scleral spur may cause a secondary angle-closure glaucoma (black arrows).

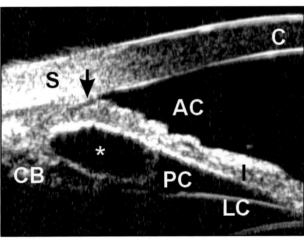

Figure 5-6. Iridociliary cysts (asterisk) may cause focal angle-closure and are characterized by an echolucent interior. The angle is closed (arrow).

Other Causes of Angle Closure

Iris cysts, ciliary body cysts, or both can produce either acute or chronic angle-closure glaucoma. These conditions usually are easily diagnosed, as the angle is closed either focally or, if cysts are multiple, intermittently. When angle closure mimicking pupillary block occurs, however, a high index of suspicion and careful gonioscopic evaluation are required. UBM is extremely helpful in making the diagnosis in these patients. The angle may be closed by other disease processes, including anterior subluxation of the lens, iris or ciliary body cysts (Figure 5-6), enlargement of the ciliary body due to inflammation or tumor infiltration,

and air or gas bubbles after intraocular surgical procedures.[22-25]

PIGMENT DISPERSION SYNDROME (PDS) AND PIGMENTARY GLAUCOMA

The abnormal iris configuration in PDS has been extensively studied using UBM.[8,9,26,27] PDS is an autosomal-dominant disorder in which mechanical friction between the posterior iris surface and anterior zonular bundles results in disruption of iris pigment epithelial cells. Liberated pigment particles accumulate throughout the anterior segment, which results in

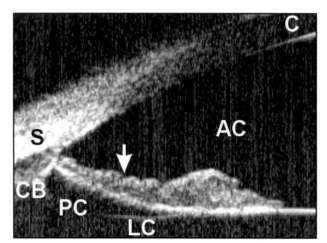

Figure 5-7a. PDS. Concave iris configuration (arrow).

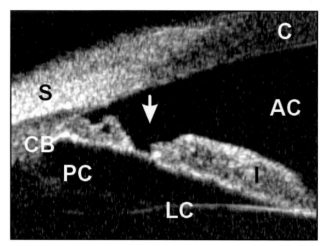

Figure 5-7b. Planar configuration after laser iridotomy (arrow).

trabecular dysfunction and elevated IOP. The classic diagnostic triad consists of a Krukenberg spindle, slit-like, mid-peripheral, radial iris transillumination defects, and pigment deposition on the trabecular meshwork. The iris tends to have a concave configuration on gonioscopy and its insertion on the ciliary face typically is posterior. Myopia is present in about 80% of affected individuals and predisposes to the phenotypic expression of the disorder.

UBM illustrates a widely open angle. The iris configuration typically is concave, with a variable amount of iridozonular contact. The iris is in apposition to a larger region of anterior lens capsule than refraction-matched controls. This diffuse apposition acts as a flap-valve, which does not permit flow of aqueous from the anterior chamber to the posterior chamber (Figures 5-7a and b). Due to a relatively higher pressure within the anterior chamber compared to the posterior chamber, the iris is forced posteriorly into proximity with the zonular bundles, a condition termed *reverse pupillary block*, in order to distinguish it from the pupillary block typically seen in angle closure.

Miotic agents relieve the reverse pupillary block, which permits accumulation of aqueous within the posterior chamber and forces the iris into a more anterior position. Laser iridotomy eliminates reverse pupillary block by allowing free movement of aqueous between the anterior and posterior chambers and causes the iris to flatten. Both miotic therapy and laser iridectomy eliminate reverse pupillary block. In this way, iridozonular contact is diminished with either therapy, which should theoretically halt pigment liberation.

The iris configuration in PDS and normal individuals may be affected by accommodation,[28] resulting in a concavity similar to that seen in PDS (Figures 5-8a and b). The displaced aqueous is forced into the angle recess and can exacerbate a preexisting iris concavity in individuals with PDS.

JUVENILE PRIMARY OPEN-ANGLE GLAUCOMA

Juvenile primary open-angle glaucoma, defined as primary open-angle glaucoma appearing between the ages of 10 and 35 years, often is familial and accompanied by markedly elevated IOP. Several large pedigrees have been described and genetic analysis in unrelated families suggests a defect in the q21-q31 region of chromosome 1. UBM investigation of these patients revealed the trabecular meshwork to be shorter in antero-posterior dimension than in eyes with similar degrees of myopia.[29] This suggests that a structural as well as functional component to the elevated IOP is present in these eyes and that it may be possible, based upon the UBM image analysis, to identify those individuals more likely to develop elevated IOP prior to its rise.

OCULAR TRAUMA

Hyphema resulting from anterior segment trauma often is accompanied by angle recession. The ciliary body face is torn at the iris insertion, resulting in the gonioscopic appearance of an abnormally wide ciliary

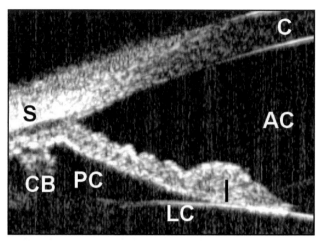

Figure 5-8a. Prior to accommodation, the iris is planar.

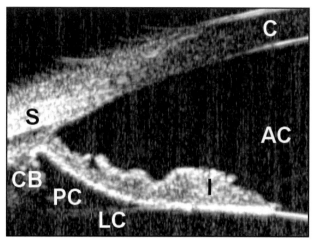

Figure 5-8b. Increased iris concavity during accommodation.

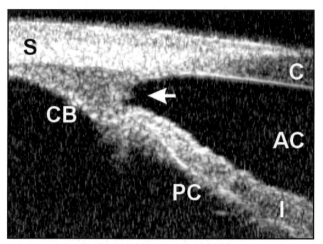

Figure 5-9. In trauma, injury causes a tear into the face ciliary body in angle recession (white arrow), but the iris remains attached to scleral spur and there is no direct communication from the anterior chamber to the supraciliary space.

body band (Figure 5-9). On the other hand, in cyclodialysis the ciliary body is avulsed from its normal attachment at the scleral spur, creating a direct communication from the anterior chamber to the supraciliary space (Figures 5-10a and b). When visible gonioscopically, a cyclodialysis appears as a cleft beginning at the scleral spur and continuing to the ciliochoroidal space. Although cyclodialysis clefts may be diagnosed by direct visualization during gonioscopy, the attempt may be unrewarding in recently operated and traumatized eyes when hazy media, distorted anatomy, or hypotony are present. The displacement of aqueous into the angle recess during indentation gonioscopy can aid in exposing clefts when the peripheral anterior chamber is flat.

When hazy media or abnormal anterior segment architecture prevent or limit adequate visualization during gonioscopy, UBM can be used to differentiate the angle recession and cyclodialysis.[30-32] In addition, the presence of supraciliary fluid and visualization of a connection from the anterior chamber to the supraciliary space confirms the latter diagnosis. Early diagnosis and appropriate management of cyclodialysis clefts are important because visual recovery may occur with resolution of hypotony and is dependent on its extent and duration. Iridodialysis also can be detected.

IRIS AND CILIARY BODY ABNORMALITIES

UBM can be used to differentiate solid from cystic lesions of the iris and ciliary body (Figure 5-11).[33] The dimensions of iris tumors can be measured and the extent to which they do or do not invade the iris root and ciliary face can be determined.

In eyes with hypotony, UBM may reveal or confirm the presence of low-lying ciliochoroidal effusion. The ciliary body may become edematous during cyclitis or enlarged in Sturge-Weber syndrome.

INTRAOCULAR LENS (IOL) POSITION

IOL position can be evaluated with UBM. IOL haptics are readily distinguishable from surrounding structures. Because the capsular bag cannot always be visualized, the most peripheral portion of the haptic defines its position. Haptic position location can be identified as being in the capsular bag (Figure 5-12), ciliary sulcus, or dislocated (Figure 5-13).

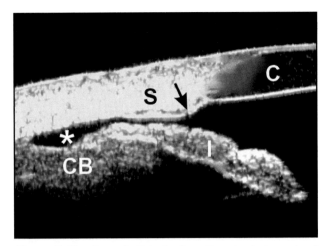

Figure 5-10a. In cyclodialysis, the ciliary body is avulsed from its attachment to the scleral spur (black arrows), allowing aqueous to flow from the anterior chamber across the cleft into the ciliochoroidal space (asterisk).

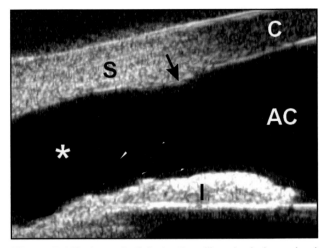

Figure 5-10b. In cyclodialysis, the ciliary body is avulsed from its attachment to the scleral spur (black arrow), allowing aqueous to flow from the anterior chamber across the cleft into the ciliochoroidal space (asterisk).

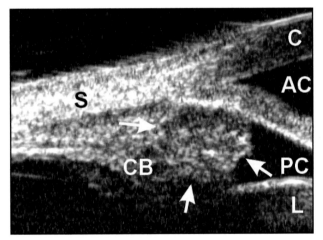

Figure 5-11. Tumors or infiltration of the iris (white arrow) or ciliary body may also cause angle closure and are characterized by uneven internal echoes when compared to cystic structures.

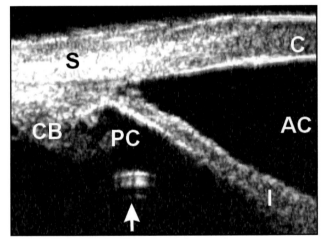

Figure 5-12. The most peripheral portion of the haptic is positioned within the capsular bag and is located central to the ciliary body (white arrow).

EYES WITH OPAQUE MEDIA

UBM permits visualization, localization, measurement, and documentation of anterior segment anatomy and pathology in eyes with opaque corneas.[34] Corneal thickness can be measured, although this is more accurately done with pachymetry. The status of the crystalline lens, the position of an IOL in the anterior or posterior chambers, decentration or tilt of the IOL lens optic, and haptic location can be assessed. The position of the iris and presence or absence of peripheral anterior synechiae can be determined. Hyphemas or other space-occupying material in the anterior chamber can be identified.

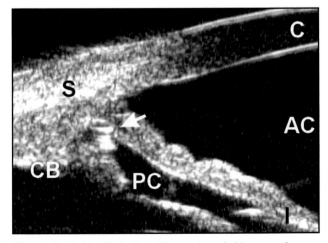

Figure 5-13. Haptic in the ciliary sulcus (white arrow).

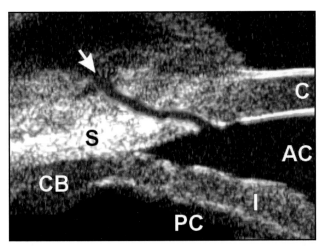

Figure 5-14. In this functioning filtering bleb, the outflow pathway from the anterior chamber, through the internal ostium, beneath the scleral flap (arrow), and into the subconjunctival space is visible.

UBM is an important tool in surgical planning prior to penetrating keratoplasty, anterior segment reconstruction, and IOL removal, repositioning, or implantation. It allows the surgeon to assess the need and/or extent of anterior segment reconstruction at the time of keratoplasty and to explain with greater confidence the potential risks and benefits of the planned procedure to patients and their families. Intraoperative inspection of the anterior and posterior chambers and iridocorneal angle with UBM may permit the results of surgical manipulation to be immediately evaluated, assessed, and corrected. Postoperative imaging allows more accurate diagnosis and timely treatment of surgical complications.

FILTERING BLEBS

One goal of the glaucoma surgeon is to recognize early filtration failure and treat it appropriately. Failing or failed filtering procedures can sometimes be rescued and a second procedure avoided. A functioning filtration bleb is characterized by a diffuse sonographically reflectant granular density and a fluid track. Tenon's cysts appear as sonographically lucent cavities within a compact outer layer, although a fluid connection between the anterior chamber and the bleb cavity often can still be recognized (Figure 5-14). Failed blebs often are flat and have no visible connection between the anterior chamber and the bleb cavity.

Accurate localization of the site of obstruction to fluid flow can be facilitated by UBM. Sites of poten-

tial blockage include the internal ostium (within the eye), beneath the scleral flap (within the surgical drainage tunnel), at the episclera (due to scarring immediately above the scleral flap) and bleb encapsulation (in the surrounding tissues).

SUMMARY

UBM has revolutionized current understanding of a wide variety of disorders of the anterior segment. Future applications of this technology will yield important information regarding accommodation, normal ocular physiology, and disease pathophysiology.

Note: Supported by a grant from the New York Glaucoma Research Institute, New York, NY.

REFERENCES

1. Pavlin CJ, Sherar MD, Foster FS. Subsurface ultrasound microscopic imaging of the intact eye. *Ophthalmology.* 1990;97:244-250.
2. Pavlin CJ, Harasiewicz K, Eng P, Foster FS. Ultrasound biomicroscopy of anterior segment structures in normal and glaucomatous eyes. *Am J Ophthalmol.* 1992;113:381-389.
3. Pavlin CJ, Foster FS. Ultrasound biomicroscopy in glaucoma. *Acta Ophthalmol.* 1992;70(suppl 204):7-9.
4. Pavlin CJ, Foster FS. *Ultrasound Biomicroscopy of the Eye.* New York, NY: Springer-Verlag; 1995.
5. Tello C, Liebmann J, Ritch R. An improved coupling medium for ultrasound biomicroscopy. *Ophthalmic Surg.* 1994;25:410-411.
6. Tello C, Liebmann J, Potash SD, et al. Measurement of ultrasound biomicroscopy images: intraobserver and interobserver reliability. *Invest Ophthalmol Vis Sci.* 1994;35:3549-3553.
7. Ishikawa H, Liebmann JM, Ritch R. Quantitative ultrasound biomicroscopy. *Ophthalmic Practice.* 1998;16:133-138.
8. Potash SD, Tello C, Liebmann J, Ritch R. Ultrasound biomicroscopy in pigment dispersion syndrome. *Ophthalmology.* 1994;101:332-339.
9. Liebmann JM, Tello C, Chew S-J, et al. Prevention of blinking alters iris configuration in pigment dispersion syndrome and in normal eyes. *Ophthalmology.* 1995;102:446-455.
10. Tello C, Potash S, Liebmann J, Ritch R. Soft contact lens modification of the ocular cup for high resolution ultrasound biomicroscopy. *Ophthalmic Surg.* 1994;24:563-564.
11. Ritch R, Liebmann J, Tello C. A construct for understanding angle-closure glaucoma: the role of ultrasound biomicroscopy. *Ophthalmol Clin N Amer.* 1995;8:281-293.
12. Caronia RM, Liebmann JM, Stegman Z, et al. Iris-lens contact increases following laser iridotomy for pupillary block angle-closure. *Am J Ophthalmol.* 1996;122:53-57.
13. Stegman Z, Ishikawa H, Liebmann JM, et al. The dark room provocative test revisited: The role of ultrasound biomicroscopy. *Invest Ophthalmol Vis Sci.* 1996;37(suppl):S818.

14. Liebmann JM, Ritch R. Laser iridotomy. *Ophthalmic Surg Lasers.* 1996;27:209-227.

15. Liebmann JM, Ritch R. Ultrasound biomicroscopy of the anterior segment. *J Am Optom Assoc.* 1996;67:469-479.

16. Pavlin CJ, Ritch R, Foster FS. Ultrasound biomicroscopy in plateau iris syndrome. *Am J Ophthalmol.* 1992;113:390-395.

17. Ritch R, Liebmann JM. Laser iridotomy and iridoplasty. In: Ritch R, Shields MB, Krupin T, eds. *The Glaucomas.* 2nd ed (pp. 1549-1573). St Louis, Mo: CV Mosby Co; 1996.

18. Ritch R. Argon laser peripheral iridoplasty. *Asia-Pacific J Ophthalmol.* 1990;2:95-99.

19. Katz NR, Finger PT, McCormick SA, et al. Ultrasound biomicroscopy in the management of malignant melanoma of the iris. *Arch Ophthalmol.* 1995;113:1462-1463.

20. Tello C, Chi T, Shepps G, et al. Ultrasound biomicroscopy in pseudophakic malignant glaucoma. *Ophthalmology.* 1993;100:1330-1334.

21. Trope G, et al. Malignant glaucoma: clinical and ultrasound biomicroscopic characteristics. *Ophthalmology.* 1994;101:1030-1035.

22. Garcia-Feijoo J, Martin-Cabajo M, Benitez del Castillo JM, Garcia-Canchez J. Ultrasound biomicroscopy in pars planitis. *Am J Ophthalmol.* 1996;121:214-215.

23. Cohen RG, Wu HK, Schuman JS. Glaucoma with inflammatory precipitates on the trabecular meshwork: a report of Grant's syndrome with ultrasound biomicroscopy of precipitates. *J Glaucoma.* 1996;5:266-270.

24. Gohdo T, Tsukahara S. Ultrasound biomicroscopy of shallow anterior chamber in Vogt-Koyanagi-Harada syndrome. *Am J Ophthalmol.* 1996;122:112-115.

25. Gentile RC, Tello C, Liebmann JM, et al. Ciliary body enlargement and cyst formation in uveitis. *Br J Ophthalmol.* In press.

26. Sokol J, Stegman Z, Liebmann JM, Ritch R. Location of the iris insertion in pigment dispersion syndrome. *Ophthalmology.* 1996;103:289-293.

27. Pavlin CJ, Macken P, Trope G, et al. Ultrasound biomicroscopic features of pigmentary glaucoma. *Can J Ophthalmol.* 1994;29:187-192.

28. McWhae JA, Crichton ACS, Reimer J. A dynamic study of accommodation using ultrasound biomicroscopy. In press.

29. Stegman Z, Sokol J, Liebmann JM, et al. Reduced trabecular meshwork height in juvenile primary open-angle glaucoma. *Arch Ophthalmol.* 1996;114:660-663.

30. Gentile RC, Pavlin CJ, Liebmann JM, et al. Accurate diagnosis of traumatic cyclodialysis clefts by ultrasound biomicroscopy. *Ophthalmic Surg Lasers.* 1996;27:97-105.

31. Berinstein DM, Gentile RC, Sidoti PA, et al. Ultrasound biomicroscopy in anterior ocular trauma. *Ophthalmic Surg Lasers.* 1997;28:201-207.

32. Karwatowski WSS, Weinreb RN. Imaging of cyclodialysis cleft by ultrasound biomicroscopy. *Am J Ophthalmol.* 1994;117:541-543.

33. Augsburger JJ, Affel LL, Benarosh DA. Ultrasound biomicroscopy of cystic lesions of the iris and ciliary body. *Trans Am Ophthalmol Soc.* 1996;94:259-274.

34. Milner MS, Liebmann JM, Tello C, et al. High-resolution ultrasound biomicroscopy of the anterior segment in patients with dense corneal scars. *Ophthalmic Surg.* 1994;25:284-287.

Chapter Six

The Pathophysiology of Glaucomatous Optic Neuropathy and Normal Tension Glaucoma

Madhu S. R. Gorla, MD

Nasreen A. Syed, MD

Evan Benjamin Dreyer, MD, PhD

The hallmark of glaucoma is damage to the optic nerve and to the ganglion cells whose axons comprise it. A solid understanding of the pathophysiologic changes that take place in the nerve, both those changes observable clinically and on a microscopic level, is vitally important in managing the patient with glaucoma. The accurate diagnosis of the patient with glaucoma depends, in large measure, on an ability to evaluate the optic nerve. Determining whether glaucomatous damage has occurred occasionally is simple, however, usually it requires careful observation and attention.

Other authors in this text have described some of the newer and more sophisticated technologies for evaluating the optic nerve and nerve fiber layer. In this chapter, we intend to illustrate some of the clinical changes that take place in the glaucomatous nerve, and to review several of the theories that have been put forth to account for the damage glaucoma causes to the optic nerve. We also will review the salient features of normal pressure glaucoma.

As a general rule, the optic nerve should be examined on every visit; for an accurate evaluation, one should use either the 78 or 90 D lens at the slit lamp through the dilated pupil. This technique provides a stereoscopic view and allows for a careful assessment of nerve contour, color, the location of vessels, and for the preparation of an accurate drawing. In our opinion, however, one cannot follow glaucoma patients properly without optic nerve photographs, to allow for valid comparison over a period of years. Because changes in the optic nerve may well precede any visual field loss, if one can accurately determine that the optic nerve is changing with time, one can intervene to further lower the intraocular pressure (IOP), and hopefully retard the glaucomatous process. By the same token, if the nerve is stable, then both patient and physician can be reassured that the glaucomatous process is slowed or stopped.

Optic nerve changes indicative of glaucoma include the presence of optic nerve cup asymmetry, evidence of progressive enlargement of the optic cup, notching or undermining of the nerve rim, vertical elongation of the cup, splinter hemorrhage, or nasal displacement of the vessels. The experienced observer knows that these findings may be subtle and require careful examination for their detection.

The features characteristic of the glaucomatous optic nerve, which will be discussed in this chapter, are depicted in Figures 6-1 through 6-5.

Figure 6-1 illustrates end stage glaucoma; almost no healthy tissue can be visualized in this nerve. This nerve is effectively "cupped out." Curiously, this patient retains 20/25 acuity in this eye, albeit with split fixation. The goal of glaucoma therapy is to prevent the development of such advanced damage.

Figures 6-2a and b illustrate a subtle form of asymmetry. The cup in the right eye is slightly larger than that in the left. Although the finding is not diagnostic of glaucoma, it is strongly indicative.

Figure 6-3 depicts an optic nerve hemorrhage. These splinter hemorrhages may be more common in normal pressure glaucoma, but can be seen in all forms of the disease. Such hemorrhages are characteristic of the presence of glaucoma, although, of course, exceptions exist.

Figure 6-4 illustrates both vertical elongation of the cup and nasalization of the vessels. This displacement of blood vessels toward the nasal aspect of the disc is thought to result from a loss of supporting tissue.

Figure 6-5 depicts baring of the lamina cribrosa and undermining of the rim. At the slit lamp, with three-dimensional viewing techniques, one can detect that the tissue immediately behind the edge of the cup has been lost.

There are many variants of these findings. It is only by careful and repeated observation that one can distinguish glaucomatous pathology. Frequently, it is not possible on a first visit to establish whether or not a patient has glaucomatous optic neuropathy. Sometimes it is only with serial photographs over a period of years can one determine if the nerve is changing.

The histopathologic features of glaucomatous neuronal insult at the light microscopic level include loss of ganglion cells in the retinal ganglion cell layer with associated thinning of the retinal nerve fiber layer. Those ganglion cells located in the superotemporal and inferotemporal regions of the retina in the midperipheral sector are the earliest to be damaged. Also, larger ganglion cells are at higher risk of damage compared with small ganglion cells (discussed

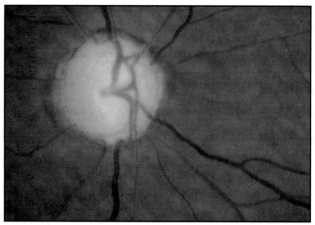

Figure 6-1. End stage glaucoma. This nerve is effectively "cupped out."

further below). In the optic nerve, as illustrated in Figures 6-6a and b, the most obvious change is that of progressive enlargement of the optic cup and thinning of the retrolaminar axonal bundles. Eventually, posterior bowing of the lamina cribrosa occurs with loss of organization of the axonal bundles and glial proliferation both in the optic nerve and in the retinal ganglion cell layer. Markedly elevated IOP prior to removal of an eye with end stage glaucoma demonstrates focal ischemia in the prelaminar and laminar portions of the disc. This results in a cystoid change in the nerve parynchema known as Schnabel's cavernous optic atrophy. These features may be found in cases of advanced glaucoma and may be present regardless of the mechanism of glaucoma (ie, open or closed angle).

Almost 600 papers have been written in the past 20 years on the pathophysiology of glaucomatous optic neuropathy. Nevertheless, there remains much that is unknown about why the optic nerve is damaged by glaucoma. Far more heat than light has been generated by debates on this topic. In fairness, the pathophysiology of most chronic diseases is not well understood. Our understanding of the glaucomatous process has been greatly limited by two factors:

1. The only well-established animal model is the monkey
2. Pathologic analysis of human tissue has been hampered by the scarcity of tissue for analysis, and the fact that those eyes available for analysis have either had very advanced glaucomatous damage or other confounding ophthalmic conditions.

Nevertheless, theories abound as to the etiology of optic nerve and ganglion cell loss in glaucoma.

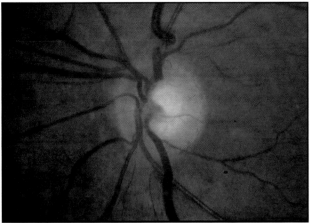

Figure 6-2a. Subtle glaucomatous asymmetry.

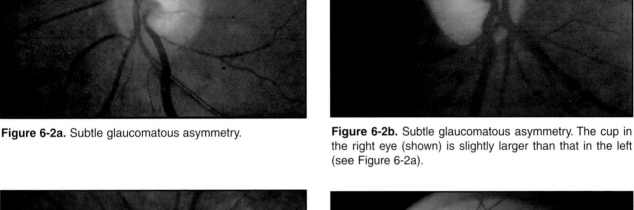

Figure 6-2b. Subtle glaucomatous asymmetry. The cup in the right eye (shown) is slightly larger than that in the left (see Figure 6-2a).

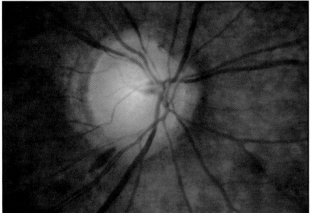

Figure 6-3. An optic nerve hemorrhage.

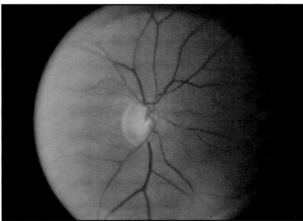

Figure 6-4. Vertical elongation of the cup, and nasalization of the vessels.

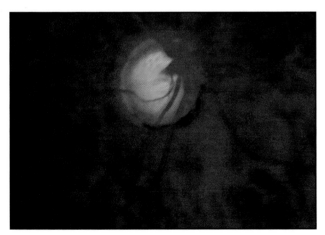

Figure 6-5. Baring of the lamina cribrosa and undermining.

Although probably first described by Hippocrates, the association of "hardening" of the eye with visual loss dates to the British oculist, Roger Banister. The theories explaining the etiology of the optic nerve loss date properly to 1858, when two separate and distinct explanations were offered. H. Müller suggested that the increased pressure seen in this disease directly compromised the nerve, and that the cell loss was due to mechanical trauma.[1] Von Jaeger, in the same year, proposed instead that vascular compromise was at fault, and that neurons died in response to a paucity of blood flow.[2] Some 150 years later, both the traumatic and vascular theories have their strong proponents. This debate remains unresolved.

Glaucomatous optic nerve damage has long been observed clinically and anatomically as changes in the prelaminar region of the optic nerve, including pro-

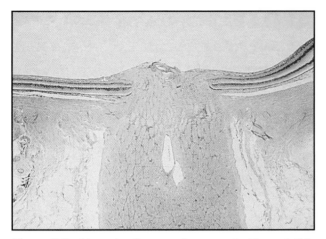

Figure 6-6a. Normal optic nerve (compare to Figure 6-6b).

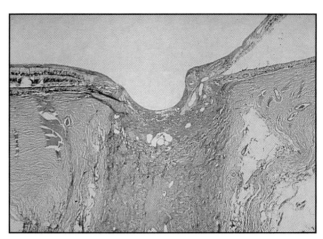

Figure 6-6b. Pathophysiologic changes in the glaucomatous optic nerve.

gressive cupping and compression. The sequence of events that occur before the clinical evidence of glaucomatous change, however, is less certain. Several theories exist at the molecular, cellular, and anatomical levels, which may describe potential factors involved in glaucomatous damage.

Changes in neurons, the lamina cribrosa, glial cells, and blood vessels all have been observed with glaucomatous change of the optic nerve. The fact that less surrounding connective tissue is available to support axons at the superior and inferior poles of the may lead to earlier damage there.[3] Eventually, damage also occurs at other regions of the nerve. Eventually, no axon is spared from eventual damage in the untreated eye. Nerve damage occurs in the nasal and temporal quadrants in late stages of the disease. Changes in the lamina cribrosa include compression of its sheets early on, with a bowing outward at its attachment to the sclera. The bowing appears to be earlier superiorly and inferiorly.[4] The supporting cells of the nerve are not lost in glaucoma; instead the glial cells remain (although they do undergo non-specific changes) even in advanced cases. There appears to be no loss of the capillaries of the optic nerve head in glaucomatous eyes.[5] Nevertheless, glaucomatous patients may have areas within the optic nerve that are predisposed to hypoperfusion in certain circumstances. Hayreh has noted that 60% of glaucomatous eyes have watershed areas in the temporal optic nerve region, which may predispose this region to earlier damage.[6]

All currently recognized therapies for the treatment of glaucoma are based on the observations that lowering IOP may slow or stop the progression of glaucomatous damage. The direct mechanical theory of optic nerve damage is based on the early observation by Müller that high IOP leads to compression and death of optic nerve neurons.[1] The theory states that increased IOP leads to backward bowing of the lamina cribrosa sheets. This tissue distortion may lead to compression of the nerves, which then may decrease retrograde axoplasmic transport.[1]

Experiments have shown that axonal damage is diffuse rather than focal, however, which one may expect in a nerve with a localized kinking defect due to mechanical factors.[7]

As noted above, a competing theory to explain the cause of glaucomatous damage indicates that vascular factors may be most responsible for glaucomatous changes. Data from fluorescein angiograms have shown that in glaucomatous eyes there are regions of transient hypoperfusion corresponding to areas of visual field loss.[8]

In 1968, investigators began to consider that glaucoma might in some way interfere with axoplasmic flow, probably at the level of the lamina cribrosa.[9] Impaired axoplasmic flow might prevent the appropriate trophic factors from reaching the ganglion cell body, and ultimately result in cell death. Ganglion cell death appears to be caused at least in part by loss of trophic factor influence following blockage of retrograde axonal transport. The blockage of retrograde transport may cause the cells to initiate a suicide response consistent with apoptosis. This response is found at normal IOP levels but is increased with raised IOP.[10] More recently, Quigley and co-workers have shown that the ganglion cell death seen in glaucoma is apoptotic in nature, consistent with the kind of cell loss one sees with trophic factor deprivation.[11] The cells show chromatin condensation and other features characteristic of apoptosis. Delivery of trophic factors and manipulation of ganglion cell genetic expression of controlling influences over programmed cell death may be two methods of preventing glaucomatous injury.[11]

Nitric oxide also may be an important mediator in retinal ganglion cell death. Increased levels of nitric oxide isoforms in the optic nerve head of patients with primary open-angle glaucoma (POAG) suggests that nitric oxide may have a neurodestructive effect on the optic nerve head. One isoform, NOS-3, appears to be increased in glaucomatous eyes, and may serve to be neuroprotective by causing increased blood flow. Inhibitors to NOS-1 and NOS-2 potentially may be useful in the treatment of glaucomatous nerve disorders.[12]

In our laboratory, we have established that the excitatory amino acid, glutamate, is elevated in the vitreous of glaucoma patients.[13]

Studies in the central nervous system over the past three decades have found that both traumatic and ischemic neuronal injury, two etiologies that may explain the optic nerve damage in glaucoma, can be mediated by excessive levels of glutamate and other excitatory amino acids.[14] Glutamate mediated excitotoxicity has been demonstrated in a broad assortment of central nervous system disorders, including stroke, trauma, epilepsy, Huntington's disease, amyotrophic lateral sclerosis, and AIDS dementia.[14] Because the neuron damaged in glaucoma, the retinal ganglion cell, is a bona fide neuron of the central nervous system, perhaps excitatory amino acids also might play a role in the retinal ganglion cell loss seen in glaucoma.

The rise in IOP associated with glaucoma may lead directly to a secondary increase in vitreal glutamate, or there might be other pathologic steps involved. However, if the glutamate level in the rat eye is chronically doubled (by serial injections), 50% of the retinal ganglion cells are killed after 3 months. Therefore, even if glutamate elevation is only an epiphenomenon associated with glaucoma, it may contribute to ganglion cell loss in humans. If one can identify interventions that retard the toxic effects of glutamate, one should be able to slow or prevent glaucomatous visual loss.

The toxic potential of glutamate to cells in the mammalian retinal ganglion cell layer is well-known.

Two British investigators, Lucas and Newhouse reported the effects of glutamate on the mammalian eye in 1957.[15] Although they were trying to block retinal degenerations, they found that subcutaneous injection of glutamate in mice led to massive destruction of the inner retinal layers, most notably the retinal ganglion cell layer. John Olney, Washington University, demonstrated similar glutamate-induced retinal toxicity in neonatal mice, and called this lesion *excitotoxic* due to excess stimulation by an excitatory amino acid.[16] Sisk and co-workers injected glutamate into the vitreous of adult rats and reported degeneration of the ganglion cell layer.[17,18] Azuma and co-workers demonstrated that intraocular glutamate can cause cupping of the optic nerve.[19] The retinal changes throughout these studies are markedly similar to the histopathology seen in glaucoma.

Although there are several classes of glutamate receptors, excitotoxic retinal ganglion cell loss is mainly due to glutamate binding to the N-methyl-D-aspartate (NMDA) subtype.[20-22] NMDA toxicity to retinal ganglion cells is true in vivo as well. A single intravitreal injection of only 20 nanomoles of NMDA can kill 70% of the retinal ganglion cells in the adult rat retina, sparing the other retinal layers.[23]

In our work, we have shown that glutamate is elevated to toxic levels in the vitreous of glaucoma patients.[13] We found a glutamate concentration of 28.3 ± 5.2 µM compared to 10.3 ± 2.4 µM in control eyes. No other amino acids differed between the two eyes.

Vitreous glutamate increases with glaucoma (r = .78, P < 0.001). Cataract type, age, sex, race, axial length of the eye, preoperative acuity, type or duration of glaucoma therapy, IOP (either at presentation or during the course of treatment), and preoperative acuity were not significant variables in the analysis of vitreous glutamate levels. Ambati et al have confirmed that glutamate is elevated in the vitreous of glaucoma patients.[24]

Similar results are found in a form of rabbit glaucoma.[25] First described a century ago, buphthalmia in the rabbit is associated with markedly enlarged corneas (up to 17 mm in diameter at 1 year of age, compared to 14 mm in controls[26]). These rabbit eyes also have iridocorneal angle structure abnormalities, ciliary process atrophy, and deep excavation of the optic nerve.[26-33] We explored whether an elevation in vitreal glutamate was present in the buphthalmic, glaucomatous rabbit eye.

The glutamate levels in the buphthalmic rabbit eye was 135 ± 13 µM/L, compared to 23 ± 13 µM/L in control eyes (P < 0.001). These results indicate that the buphthalmic rabbit eye has an elevated vitreous glutamate concentration of approximately six times normal.

In collaboration with Dr. Dennis Brooks (University of Florida), we have further found that glutamate levels are elevated in the vitreous of dogs with glaucoma.[34]

As alluded to above, in recent groundbreaking work, Quigley and co-workers have shown that ganglion cell death in glaucoma proceeds through an apoptotic mechanism rather than necrosis.[11]

Excitotoxicity to retinal ganglion cells is mediated by overstimulation of the NMDA subtype of glutamate receptor, which in turn leads to excessive levels of intracellular calcium.[21,22,35] The excessive levels of calcium thus engendered have been shown to correlate with eventual cell death.[36,37] This association of excessive calcium levels with cellular toxicity suggests that a causal relationship exists, perhaps mediated through calcium-dependent enzymes. These enzymes include those translational and transcriptional enzymes that have been implicated with apoptotic death.[38] We, therefore, considered whether agents that can interfere with translation or transcription also are effective at preventing NMDA excitotoxicity.[39]

In the presence of NMDA, cycloheximide or actinomycin D each could prevent the NMDA-mediated cell loss; however, blockade of either translation or transcription effectively prevented retinal ganglion cell death resulting from exposure to low concentrations of NMDA. These agents could be added 2 hours after the initial NMDA insult and still could protect against excitotoxicity. The addition of 25 μM NMDA to retinal ganglion cells initiates a cascade of cellular events, including both translational and transcription events, leading to cell death. As noted above, interruption of this schema with either actinomycin D or cycloheximide is sufficient to prevent cellular toxicity.

The low dose of glutamate that we have postulated may play a role in glaucomatous loss appears to trigger an apoptotic death, which is the mechanism of cell death in glaucoma.

As we reviewed above, although a bolus of glutamate is acutely toxic to mammalian retinal ganglion cells and other central neurons,[15,16,40,41] less is known about chronic perturbations of glutamate levels (as might be seen in glaucoma). We therefore explored the toxicity of a 2- to 3-fold increase in intravitreal glutamate, as well as the ability of the NMDA antag-

onist, memantine, to protect against any such toxicity.[42] The glutamate level in the rat eye was elevated to ~30 mM by serial injections, and ganglion cell survival assessed.[42] There was a significant loss of ganglion cells after 3 months of glutamate injections, from a control value of 96,500 ± 8500 retinal ganglion cells per eye to 56,000 ± 9600 cells in the glutamate treated eyes (P < 0.001). When animals were treated with both chronic glutamate and an NMDA antagonist, memantine, 83,000 ± 4900 ganglion cells remained after 3 months. Therefore, memantine is protective in this paradigm. It appears that a relatively minor but chronic elevation of glutamate (similar to what we have observed in the human eye with glaucoma) over endogenous levels can be toxic to retinal ganglion cells.[42]

One unusual aspect of glaucomatous optic neuropathy is that larger retinal ganglion cells are preferentially damaged in this disease.[3] The distribution of retinal ganglion cell size (and implications for cell function) has been extensively explored in the mammalian retina,[43] but less is known about whether cell size affects sensitivity to glutamate. Previous investigators have demonstrated that larger retinal ganglion cells show greater susceptibility to glutamate-induced cell stress.[44] We therefore chose to explore whether larger retinal ganglion cells were more sensitive to glutamate-mediated neuronal cell death in vitro and in vivo.[45]

Most surprisingly, smaller retinal ganglion cells were not sensitive to the addition of exogenous glutamate. Exogenous glutamate had little effect on cell viability for cells smaller than 7.7 mm. In vitro, only larger retinal ganglion cells were killed with exogenous glutamate.

These findings held true in the whole animal eye as well. Rodent eyes were injected with NMDA, and the animal sacrificed. When viable cells were scored by size, the mean cell size in the control eyes was 9.6 ± 0.3 mm, larger than the mean of 8.2 ± 0.4 mm seen in eyes treated with NMDA (P < 0.01). As in vitro, NMDA had little effect on retinal ganglion cells smaller than 7.7 mm in diameter. Cells larger than this diameter were killed by intraocular NMDA.

Larger retinal ganglion cells are more sensitive to NMDA receptor-mediated neurotoxicity both in vivo and in vitro. If glutamate does indeed play a role in retinal ganglion cell loss secondary to glaucoma, this may partially explain why in this disease larger retinal ganglion cells are lost first. One of the surprising aspects of glutamate toxicity in the retina is its marked selectively for ganglion cells. Retinal ganglion cells are unique in the retina in having extremely long processes (extending to the lateral geniculate). This fact raises the possibility that long neurites predispose retinal ganglion cells to excitotoxic damage. The precise role played by various subclasses and locales of glutamate receptors, however, remains obscure. We, therefore, explored whether NMDA receptors located on neurites were likely to contribute to excitotoxicity.[46]

Retinal ganglion cells with processes were far more sensitive to NMDA-mediated excitotoxicity than retinal ganglion cells without such neurites. Furthermore, susceptibility to NMDA toxicity increased with process length.

The data reviewed above suggest that glutamate is elevated in the vitreous of glaucoma eyes (human, dogs, and rabbits) to a level that might be toxic to retinal ganglion cells. Glutamate is more toxic to neurons with longer processes and to larger retinal ganglion cells. The low doses of glutamate that we propose are implicated in glaucoma can cause apoptotic-like death, as has been described in glaucoma. This is by no means convincing evidence that blocking glutamate toxicity can prevent glaucomatous blindness. Future lines of investigation may help to establish whether agents that block excitotoxicity may play a role in the management of this disease, and to identify the source of the elevated glutamate in patients with glaucoma.

In any event, the pathophysiology underlying glaucomatous optic neuropathy remains something of an enigma; one can only hope that the next 600 papers will shed light on the true etiology of the ganglion cell loss and blindness that unfortunately accompanies this disease.

NORMAL TENSION GLAUCOMA

Normal tension glaucoma (NTG) is, perhaps, best described as "a condition in which cupping of the optic nerve head, loss of the retinal nerve fiber layer, and visual field defects similar to those seen in other forms of chronic glaucoma are seen, and in which an IOP level outside the statistically normal range without treatment has not been documented, nor is any other cause for these changes apparent."[47] The incidence probably is more than what was previously thought, and may be about equal to the incidence of POAG. This disease has been described variously as a

variant of POAG with no documented elevated increased IOPs, or as a glaucoma with other major factors involved (including vascular). Patients with normal tension glaucoma tend to have a wider diurnal IOP fluctuation than normal controls. Visual field loss tends to be worse in the eye with the higher IOP, suggesting a mechanism related to IOP levels.[48] Retinal and choroidal hemodynamics may differ between patients with POAG and NTG; retinal circulation is delayed in patients with POAG, whereas choroidal circulation is slower in patients with NTG.[49]

Clinically, there is an apparent mismatch between the amount of optic nerve head cupping and visual field loss in NTG.[50] NTG eyes may have increased cupping compared to POAG patients in eyes with similar visual field loss. In addition, these eyes have a higher incidence of optic disc hemorrhages,[51] shallower cups, greater frequency and amount of peripapillary atrophy, and larger optic nerves in comparison to POAG eyes. Similar to POAG, risk factors include increasing age and family history. There is equivocal data regarding gender as a risk factor. There is a higher rate of NTG within the Asian and African American populations. There may be an increased prevalence of immune-related disorders in these patients, including arthritis, hypothyroidism, and Raynaud's disease.[52]

Possible associated factors include an increased incidence of vasospastic symptoms such as migraine and cold fingers. Similar events may be occurring within the optic nerve circulation leading to decreased perfusion and ultimately damage. One study has found a greater extent of cerebral infarcts and corpus callosum atrophy in these patients, indicating possible ischemic neuronal degeneration.[53]

The current methods of treatment are similar to that of POAG and involve lowering IOP. Medical and surgical techniques have been shown to lower the rate of visual field progression[54]; however, therapy may be accompanied by its own complications. Treatment is generally indicated when there is progression of the disease as shown by worsening in visual fields, optic disc appearance, optic disc hemorrhage, and/or increased IOP. Calcium channel blockers have been shown to reverse cold-induced visual field loss as well as improve contrast sensitivity in eyes with NTG.[55] An understanding of the possible contributing vascular processes may provide effective treatment modalities for this disease in the future.

REFERENCES

1. Müller H. Anatomische Beitrage zur Ophthalmologie: Ueber Nervean-Veranderungen an der Eintrittsstelle des Schnerven. *Arch Ophthalmol.* 1858;4:1.
2. vonJaeger E. Ueber Glaucom und seine Heilung durch Iridectomie. *Z Ges der Aertze zu Wien.* 1858;14:484.
3. Quigley H, Sanchez R, Dunkelberg G, Hernault N, Baginski T. Chronic glaucoma selectively damages large optic nerve fibers. *Invest Ophthalmol Vis Sci.* 1987;28:913.
4. Quigley HA, Hohman RM, Addicks EM. Morphologic changes in the lamina cribrosa correlated with neural loss in open-angle glaucoma. *Am J Ophthalmol.* 1983;95:673.
5. Quigley HA, Hohman RM, Addicks EM, Green WR. Blood vessels of the glaucomatous optic disc in experimental primate and human eyes. *Invest Ophthalmol Vis Sci.* 1984;25:918-931.
6. Hayreh SS. Pathogenesis of cupping of the optic disc. *Br J Ophthalmol.* 1974;58:863-876.
7. Radius RL, Anderson DR. Rapid axonal transport in primate optic nerve. Distribution of pressure-induced interruption. *Arch Ophthalmol.* 1981;99:650-654.
8. Schwartz B, Rieser JC, Fishbein SL. Fluorescein angiographic defects of the optic disc in glaucoma. *Arch Ophthalmol.* 1977;95:161.
9. Lampert PW, Vogel MH, Zimmerman LE. Pathology of the optic nerve in experimental acute glaucoma. Electron microscopic studies. *Invest Ophthalmol.* 1968;7:199-213.
10. GarciaValenzuela E, Gorczyca W, Darzynkiewicz Z, Sharma SC. Apoptosis in adult retinal ganglion cells after axotomy. *J Neurobiol.* 1994;25:431-438.
11. Quigley HA, Nickells RW, Pease ME, et al. Retinal ganglion cell death in experimental monkey glaucoma and axotomy occurs by apoptosis. *Invest Ophthalmol Vis Sci.* 1995;36:774-786.
12. Neufeld AH, Hernandez MR, Gonzalez M. Nitric oxide synthase in the human glaucomatous optic nerve head. *Arch Ophthalmol.* 1997;115:497-503.
13. Dreyer EB, Zurakowski D, Schumer RA, Podos SM, Lipton SA. Elevated glutamate in the vitreous body of humans and monkeys with glaucoma. *Arch Ophthalmol.* 1996;114:299-305.
14. Choi DW. Glutamate neurotoxicity and diseases of the nervous system. *Neuron.* 1988;1:623-634.
15. Lucas DR, Newhouse JP. The toxic effect of sodium L-glutamate on the inner layers of the retina. *Am Med Assoc Arch Ophthalmol.* 1957;58:193-201.
16. Olney JW. Glutamate-induced retinal degeneration in neonatal mice: electron microscopy of the acutely evolving lesion. *J Neuropath Exp Neurol.* 1969;28:455-474.
17. Sisk DR, Kuwabara T, Kirsch AD. Behavioral recovery in albino rats with glutamate-damaged retinas. *Invest Ophthalmol Vis Sci.* 1984;25:1124-1128.
18. Sisk DR, Kuwabara T. Histologic changes in the inner retina of albino rats following intravitreal injection of monosodium L-glutamate. *Graefes Arch Clin Exp Ophthalmol.* 1985;223:250-258.
19. Azuma N, Kawamura M, Kohsaka S. Morphological and immunohistochemical studies on degenerative changes of the retina and the optic nerve in neonatal rats injected with monosodium-L-glutamate. *Nippon Ganka Gakkai Zasshi.* 1989;93:72-79.
20. Sucher NJ, Wong LA, Lipton SA. Redox modulation of NMDA receptor-mediated Ca2+ flux in mammalian central neurons. *Neuroreport.* 1990;1:29-32.
21. Sucher NJ, Lei SZ, Lipton SA. Calcium channel antagonists attenuate NMDA receptor-mediated neurotoxicity of retinal ganglion cells in culture. *Brain Res.* 1991;551:297-302.
22. Sucher NJ, Aizenmann E, Lipton SA. N-Methyl-D-Aspartate antagonists prevent kainate neurotoxicity in rat retinal ganglion cells in vitro. *J Neurosci.* 1991;11:966-971.
23. Siliprandi R, Canella R, Carmignoto G, et al. N-methyl-D-aspartate induced neurotoxicity in the adult rat retina. *Vis Neurosci.* 1992;8:567-573.
24. Ambati J, Chalam KV, Chawla DK, et al. Elevated gamma-aminobutyric acid, glutamate, and vascular endothelial growth factor levels in the vitreous of patients with proliferative diabetic retinopathy. *Arch Ophthalmol.* 1997;115:1161-1166.
25. Dreyer EB. Amino acid abnormalities in the vitreous of the buphthalmic rabbit. *Veterinary and Comparative Ophthalmology.* 1997;7:192-195.
26. Kolker AE, Moses RA, Constant MA, Becker B. The development of glaucoma in rabbits. *Invest Ophthalmol.* 1963;2:316-321.
27. McMaster PRB. Decreased aqueous outflow in rabbits with hereditary buphthalmia. *Am Med Assoc Arch Ophth.* 1960;64:388-391.
28. Pilcher A. Spontanes Glaukom beim Kaninchen. *Arkh vergl Ophth.* 1909;1:175.
29. Schloesser C. Acutes Secundar-Glaucom beim Kaninchen. *Ztschr vergl Augenh.* 1886;4:79.
30. Smith JH. The blood-aqueous barrier in hydrophthalmic rabbits. *Ophthalmologica.* 1944;108:293.
31. Vogt A. Hydrophthalmus hereditaire chez le lapin. *Clin Ophthalmol.* 1919;23:667.
32. Rochon-Duvigneaud A. Un cas de buphthalmie chez le lapin. *Ann Ocul.* 1921;158:401.
33. Hanna BL, Sawin PB, Sheppard B. Recessive buphthalmos in the rabbit. *Genetics.* 1962;47:519.
34. Brooks DE, Garcia GA, Dreyer EB, Zurakowski D, Franco-Bourland RE. Vitreous body glutamate concentrations in dogs with glaucoma. *American Journal of Veterinary Research.* 1997;58:864-867.
35. Hahn JS, Aizenman E, Lipton SA. Central mammalian neurons normally resistant to glutamate toxicity are made sensitive by elevated extracellular Ca2+ toxicity is blocked by the N-methyl-D-aspartate antagonist MK-801. *Proc Natl Acad Sci USA.* 1988;85:6556-6560.
36. Eimerl S, Schramm M. The quantity of calcium that appears to induce neuronal death. *J Neurochem.* 1994;62:1223-1226.
37. Hartley DM, Kurth MC, Bjerkness L, Weiss JH, Choi DW. Glutamate receptor-induced calcium accumulation in cortical cell culture correlates with subsequent neuronal degeneration. *J Neurosci.* 1993;13:1993-2000.

38. Goldstein P, Ojcius DM, Young JDE. Cell death mechanisms and the immune system. *Immunol Rev.* 1991;121:29-65.

39. Dreyer EB, Zhang D, Lipton SA. Transcriptional or translational inhibition blocks low dose NMDA-mediated cell death. *Neuroreport.* 1995;6:942-944.

40. Rothman SM, Olney JW. Excitotoxicity and the NMDA receptor. *Tr Neurosci.* 1987;10:299-302.

41. Mosinger JL, Price MT, Bai HY, et al. Blockade of both NMDA and non-NMDA receptors is required for optimal protection against ischemic neuronal degeneration in the in vivo adult mammalian retina. *Exp Neurol.* 1991;113:10-17.

42. Vorwerk CK, Lipton SA, Zurakowski D, et al. Chronic low dose glutamate is toxic to retinal ganglion cells; toxicity blocked by memantine. *Invest Ophthalmol Vis Sci.* 1996;37:1618-1624.

43. Dräger UR, Olsen JF. Ganglion cell distribution in the retina of the mouse. *Invest Ophthalmol Vis Sci.* 1981;20:285-293.

44. Caprioli J, Kitano S. Large retinal ganglion cells are more susceptible to excitotoxic and hyopoxic injury than small cells. *Invest Ophthalmol Vis Sci.* 1993;34:1429.

45. Dreyer EB, Pan ZH, Storm S, Lipton SA. Greater sensitivity of larger retinal ganglion cells to NMDA-mediated cell death. *Neuroreport.* 1994;5:629-631.

46. Heng JE, Moscaritolo K, Dreyer EB. NMDA sensitivity is neurite enhanced. *Neuroreport.* 1995;6:1890-1892.

47. Werner EB. Normal tension glaucoma. In: Ritch R, Shields MB, Krupin T, eds. *The Glaucomas.* 2nd ed. 1996;769.

48. Cartwright MJ, Anderson DR. Correlation of asymmetric damage with asymmetric intraocular pressure in normal-tension glaucoma (low-tension glaucoma). *Arch Ophthalmol.* 1988;106:898-900.

49. Duijm HF, vandenBerg TJ, Greve EL. A comparison of retinal and choroidal hemodynamics in patients with primary open-angle glaucoma and normal-pressure glaucoma. *Am J Ophthalmol.* 1997;123:644.

50. Gramer E, Althaus G, Leydhecker W. Localization and depth of glaucomatous visual field defects in relation to the size of the neuroretinal rim area of the disc in low-tension glaucoma, glaucoma simplex, and pigmentary glaucoma: clinical study with the Octopus 201 perimeter and the Optic Nerve Head Analyzer. *Klin Monatsbl Augenheilkd.* 1986;189:190.

51. Kitazawa Y, Shirato S, Yamamoto T. Optic disc hemorrhage in low-tension glaucoma. *Ophthalmology.* 1986;93:853-857.

52. Cartwright MJ, Grajewski AL, Friedberg ML, Anderson DR, Richards DW. Immune-related disease and normal-tension glaucoma. A case-control study. *Arch Ophthalmol.* 1992;110:500-502.

53. Ong K, Farinelli A, Billson F, Houang M, Stern M. Comparative study of brain magnetic resonance imaging findings in patients with low-tension glaucoma and control subjects. *Ophthalmology.* 1995;102:1632-1638.

54. Bhandari A, Crabb DP, Poinoosawmy D, et al. Effect of surgery on visual field progression in normal-tension glaucoma. *Ophthalmology.* 1997;104:1131-1137.

55. Bose S, Piltz JR, Breton ME. Nimodipine, a centrally active calcium antagonist, exerts a beneficial effect on contrast sensitivity in patients with normal-tension glaucoma and in control subjects. *Ophthalmology.* 1995;102:1236-1241.

Chapter Seven

Optic Nerve Imaging Techniques in Glaucoma

Iftikhar M. Chaudhry, MD
Joel S. Schuman, MD

INTRODUCTION

Essential in the diagnosis of glaucoma is the evaluation of the optic nerve head and nerve fiber layer. Since 1851, when Helmholtz first invented the ophthalmoscope, ophthalmologists have been evaluating the optic nerve for characteristic changes in glaucoma.[1] Though critical, this assessment is subjective and intraobserver as well as interobserver variability is high.[2,3] In addition, other parameters of glaucoma diagnosis including automated perimetry and intraocular pressure (IOP) measurement can also be limited and miss the diagnosis and progression of glaucoma, especially at the early stages.[4] In fact, up to 40% of nerve fibers may be lost without detection of glaucoma by the above parameters.[5]

Because optic nerve damage is irreversible, early detection is crucial. The objective of imaging of the optic nerve and nerve fiber layer is to precisely quantify, with a maximum of reproducibility, the status of these tissues and thereby detect early glaucoma.

OPTIC NERVE HEAD IMAGING

Stereoscopic Optic Nerve Head Photography

An important advance from subjective individual drawings of the optic nerve was the advent of fundus photography. The first stereoscopic fundus camera, the Nordenson, was introduced in the early 20th century. Stereoscopic photography allowed the physician to document the longitudinal change in the optic nerve head[6]; however, the interpretation of these pictures is quite subjective. Even experts looking at photographs disagree about degree and progression of disease.[3]

Automated Optic Nerve Head Analyzers

Optic nerve head analyzers were the first automated instruments invented to overcome some of the subjectivity of fundus examination and photography. Using standard camera optics, these instruments attempt to quantitate cupping, neural rim area, and other parameters of the optic nerve head. The first of these, the PAR IS 2000 (later the Topcon IMAGEnet, Topcon Instruments, Paramus, NJ), used stereoscopic fundus photos or 35 mm slides and created a three-dimensional map of the optic nerve head.[7] The operator determined the disc margin by four individual points and the computer determined the cup margin, which was set as 120 microns from the disc margin.

A similar optic nerve head analyzer, the Humphrey Retinal Analyzer (Humphrey Instruments, Inc, San Leandro, Calif), used a red-free stereoscopic video camera. It required the operator to determine eight or more points to define the disc.[8]

Similar to the PAR and Humphrey, the Rodenstock Optic Nerve Analyzer (Rodenstock Instruments, Danbury, Conn) projected two sets of seven evenly spaced lines on the optic nerve head. Along these 14 vertical stripes, depth was calculated at 140 different points. This analyzer calculated the cup to be 150 microns posterior to the disc.[9]

All of the above instruments required a constant plane of reference of which there was none in the posterior fundus. They used this plane to calculate the cup depth. This method of arbitrarily describing the cup as a certain distance posterior to the rim appeared to overestimate small cups and underestimate larger cups. Variability tended to be high and magnification errors also were present.[10]

A newer instrument that tended to improve on the older optic nerve head analyzers was the GlaucomaScope (Ophthalmic Imaging Systems, Sacramento, Calif). Using a technique of computed raster stereography, it projected a series of equidistant, parallel, straight lines onto the optic disc at oblique angles.[11] Cupping was measured based on the amount of deflection of the lines, which was proportional to the amount of excavation. The lines had a reference point that was 350 µm nasal and temporal to the disc. The operator again outlined the disc margin and selected a reference point, which was used for future image registration. The cup was defined as 140 µm or more below the reference plane. Ninety-one hundred real data points as well as thousands of interpolated points were used to plot out a numeric and gray scale printout. Each number in the printout represented the average depth in a cell 75 microns by 100 microns in size (Figures 7-1 and 7-2). Variability occurred secondary to differences in patient alignment, topographic fluctuations around steep slopes and blood vessels on the optic nerve head, and the inherent variability associated with the instrument and computer calculations.[11-13]

The optic nerve head analyzers attempted to be objective but were limited by variability, lack of reproducibility, and the subjectivity of the operator.[14-23] The most reliable measured parameter by these instruments was the neural rim area, however, overall variation of optic nerve head topography was 165 microns.[8,24]

Confocal Scanning Laser Ophthalmoscopy (CSLO)

Using a double scanning confocal optical system, coronal optical sections of the retina and optic nerve head are produced (Figure 7-3).[25] The laser is scanned on the retina along with the detector system. At a time, just one spot on the retina is illuminated through a pinhole. The reflected light is then received by another pinhole aperture. Most other reflections from out of focus plane areas are blocked.[26,27] This technique reduces scatter and improves contrast as compared to non-confocal systems. Laser scanning uses a lower level of illumination compared to ophthalmoscopy and fundus photography. The pupil can remain undilated and thus patient comfort is enhanced. The non-confocal systems were the early scanning laser ophthalmoscopes in which the display and detection apertures were separate and inverted.

Several confocal laser scanning systems were produced, some of which are still available. The Rodenstock confocal scanning laser ophthalmoscope (no longer available) used a He-Ne or argon laser to scan a retinal plane. Image analysis was performed using reflectometry to measure the differences in wavelength reflection. It produced high quality tissue sections and could be used through an undilated pupil to measure three-dimensional structures with good reproducibility.[25]

The Heidelberg Laser Tomographic Scanner (Heidelberg Instruments, Heidelberg, Germany, no longer available) obtained 32 evenly spaced coronal sections of the optic nerve head using a He-Ne laser to image. The Zeiss Laser Tomographic Scanner (LTS, Zeiss Instruments, Thornwood, NJ, no longer available) also used the He-Ne laser.[28]

The available CSLOs include the Topographic Scanning Systems (TopSS, Laser Diagnostic Technologies, Inc, San Diego, Calif) and the Heidelberg Retinal Tomograph (HRT, Heidelberg Engineering GmbH, Heidelberg, Germany).[29,30]

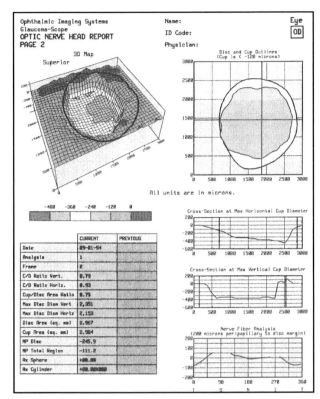

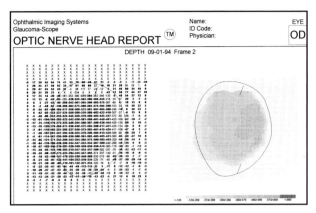

Figure 7-2. Glaucoma-Scope gray scale and numerical displays of an eye with advanced cupping. Reprinted with permission from Schuman JS, Noecker RJ. Imaging of the optic nerve head and nerve fiber layer in glaucoma. *Ophthalmol Clin North Am.* 1995;8(2):259-279.

Figure 7-1. Glaucoma-Scope report on an eye with advanced cupping. Reprinted with permission from Schuman JS, Noecker RJ. Imaging of the optic nerve head and nerve fiber layer in glaucoma. *Ophthalmol Clin North Am.* 1995;8(2):259-279.

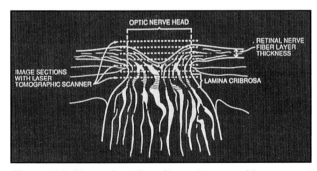

Figure 7-3. Plane of section of laser tomographic scanners (coronal). Courtesy of Robert N. Weinreb, MD. Reprinted with permission from Schuman JS, Noecker RJ. Imaging of the optic nerve head and nerve fiber layer in glaucoma. *Ophthalmol Clin North Am.* 1995;8(2):259-279.

In the HRT, the laser scans the optic disc and retina in two dimensions and in 32 different coronal focal planes. The images are acquired within 32 ms with a repetition rate of 20 Hz. The images are digitized into a frame of 256 x 256 pixels with 8-bit resolution each and are displayed on the computer monitor. The com-

puter then generates a three-dimensional image; the whole process takes about 1.5 seconds and can be performed on undilated eyes. To obtain topographic parameters, the operator outlines the optic disc margin. A reference point as defined by the HRT software is defined as a plane 50 µm posterior to the peripapillary retinal surface. Some of the topographic parameters measured include cup/disc area, cup area, cup/disc area ratio, cup volume, rim volume, mean cup depth, cup shape measure (the third moment of the mean), peripapillary retinal height, and indirect nerve fiber layer thickness. Some studies show significant correlation between HRT parameters like rim area and cup shape measure among others with visual field indices.[31] Key questions regarding the specific stereometric parameters that are important for glaucoma detection are still being addressed.

The nerve fiber layer thickness also can be indirectly calculated using the HRT, albeit indirectly. This measurement is not the absolute thickness but is a measure of the distance between a defined retinal reference plane and the vitreal surface of the retina.

Figures 7-4a and b illustrate a normal optic nerve head. Notice the depth-of-focus image of the optic nerve head and the outline of the rim performed by the operator. Next to it is the horizontal cross-section of the optic nerve head. The optic nerve head and rim appear normal. In the color-coded topography image, light colors indicate depressed structures and dark colors indicate elevated structures. The pink color indicates the size of the cup and the green indicates the

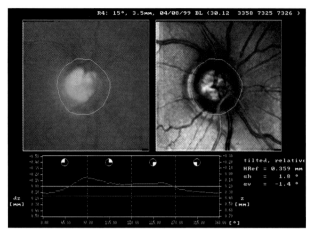

Figure 7-4a. Display of healthy optic nerve head with HRT.

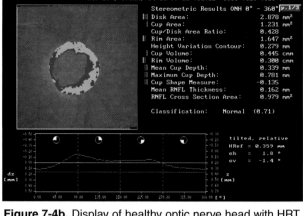

Figure 7-4b. Display of healthy optic nerve head with HRT.

neural rim. A relative nerve fiber layer thickness for each quadrant also is shown. A list of topographic parameters is displayed.

Figures 7-5a and b illustrate a glaucomatous optic nerve head as imaged by HRT. The color-coded topography image shows marked cupping, as illustrated by the pink colored area. This rendering of the optic nerve appearance can be a good teaching tool for patients, as well as an objective, quantitative measure for the physician.

The CSLOs provide enhanced imaging and analysis of the optic nerve head and indirect measurements of the nerve fiber layer. These data are more precise than those available with the optic nerve head analyzers. The CSLOs have a variability as high as 102 microns[24]; however, the HRT has a variability of 25 to 40 microns with a single scan, which can be improved, with a series of three scans.[30,32-34] Misalignment between the patient and laser scanner may account for significant variability with the HRT.[35] The axial resolution is 300 microns; for this reason CSLOs are not well-suited for precise cross-sectional imaging of the retina.[28]

NERVE FIBER LAYER IMAGING

Thinning of the nerve fiber layer is a sensitive indicator of glaucomatous damage, preceding both visual field loss and detectable changes in optic nerve head appearance.[36,37] Since Hoyt and Newman first reported nerve fiber layer atrophy in patients with glaucoma, a much-improved understanding of the importance of the nerve fiber layer has evolved.[38] The

nerve fiber layer normally tends to thin with age.[39-41] The optic nerve and nerve fiber layer are composed of axons of ganglion cells. These cells are damaged in glaucoma and thus produce vision loss. The axons of ganglion cells are less compact in the retinal nerve fiber layer and thus easier to evaluate. Even a reduction of 10 to 20 :m in nerve fiber layer thickness may be a significant sign of glaucoma damage and may be an early indication of impending visual loss.[5] Therefore, accurate and reproducible measurements of the nerve fiber layer are important in glaucoma diagnosis and management.

Similar to optic nerve head examination and photography, nerve fiber layer examination and photography are important but subjective methods. The optic nerve head analyzer as discussed above can be used to measure peripapillary nerve fiber layer defects but needs a steady reference plane over time in the retina, of which there is none.[16]

The Nerve Fiber Analyzer

The Nerve Fiber Analyzer (NFA, GDx, Laser Diagnostic Technologies, San Diego, Calif) is a confocal scanning laser ophthalmoscope with a polarization modulator, a cornea polarization compensator, and a polarization detection unit. Using scanning laser polarimetry, a method that provides quantitative assessment of the nerve fiber layer, the laser measures the rotation of the polarized light reflected from the retina.[28,42] The birefringence of the nerve fiber layer causes a change in the polarization of the light beam called *retardance* (Figure 7-6).[32-34] The polarized light

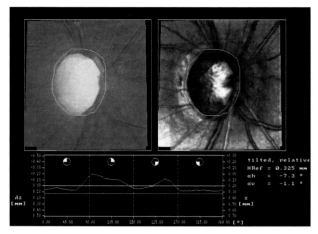

Figure 7-5a. Display of glaucomatous optic nerve head with HRT.

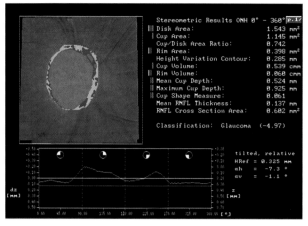

Figure 7-5b. Display of glaucomatous optic nerve head with HRT.

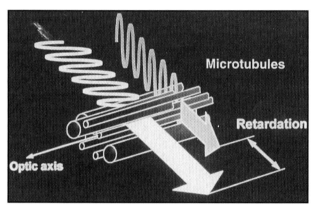

Figure 7-6. Graphic depiction of retardance, the delay of polarized light by refringent fibers. Courtesy of Laser Diagnostic Technologies, Inc. Reprinted with permission from Schuman JS, Noecker RJ. Imaging of the optic nerve head and nerve fiber layer in glaucoma. *Ophthalmol Clin North Am.* 1995;8(2):259-279.

rotation is assumed to be in proportion to the nerve fiber layer thickness. Other assumptions that are made are that the nerve fiber layer is the main birefringent tissue in the retina and that the birefringence of the nerve fiber layer is homogeneous. The NFA employs a compensation scheme for any polarization effects of other tissues anterior to the limiting membrane, such as the cornea and the lens. The NFA has shown significantly lower nerve fiber layer thickness in ocular hypertensives and glaucoma patients, however, there is overlap. In a glaucoma population, NFA showed statistically significant nerve fiber layer thinning in the lower quadrant.[43] In vitro, its resolution is 13 :m.[32] Studies show that the NFA provides reproducible measurements but further research is needed to define

its use in the management of glaucoma patients, however, early results are promising.[34,43,44] The relationship of nerve fiber layer measurements to visual field indices and the sensitivity of scanning laser polarimetry to detect change over time are still being studied.[45]

Optical Coherence Tomography

Optical coherence tomography (OCT, Humphrey Instruments, San Leandro, Calif) is a new technique for high-resolution imaging of the human retina and nerve fiber layer.[46-59] Cross-sectional images can be obtained with a resolution of 10 microns, which is superior to that of other currently available instruments. Reproducibility is in the range of 15 microns. OCT provides resolution significantly higher than that of other techniques (eg, the resolution of clinical ultrasound is limited by the wavelength of sound in ocular tissue to approximately 150 µm). Ultrasound biomicroscopy has a spatial resolution of 20 µm but is limited to imaging of the anterior segment by its penetration depth of only 4 mm. Ocular aberrations and the maximum entrance pupil diameter of the eye limit the resolution of the scanning laser ophthalmoscope to approximately 300 µm. Traditional imaging systems such as computed tomography and magnetic resonance imaging have limited utility in ophthalmic imaging as the spatial resolution of these systems are on the order of several hundred microns. The high-resolution cross-sectional imaging provided by OCT is particularly useful in the evaluation of macular disease, glaucoma, and other optic nerve diseases.[48,52,53,56]

The limitations of OCT include the inability to obtain high-quality images through media opacities such as dense cataract or vitreous hemorrhage. The use of OCT also is limited to cooperative patients who are able to maintain fixation for the full acquisition time of 1 to 2.5 seconds. Computer image processing techniques eliminate eye movement due to fluctuations in the IOP produced by variations in pulse pressure, mild tremor, and microsaccades, but can not eliminate image degradation from patients with excessive movement.

The operation of OCT is based on the principle of low coherence interferometry. In this technique, the distances and sizes of different structures in the eye are determined by measuring the "echo" time it takes for light to be backscattered from different structures at various axial distances, or the time of flight of reflected or backscattered light. This technique is analogous to A-mode ultrasound, in which the axial length of the eye is measured using sound rather than light.[46,47]

The OCT hardware utilizes a fiber optic equipped standard slit-lamp and allows for structures to be imaged without direct contact with the ocular surface (Figure 7-7). The OCT unit is made by Humphrey Instruments and is commercially available. A light source consisting of a superluminescent diode projects a partially coherent, continuous, near-infrared light at a wavelength of 810 nm. The power of the light source is approximately 200 mW, which is well within acceptable levels set by the American National Standards Institute for retinal radiation. The light is focused onto the retina by a standard mounted +78 D condensing lens. The optical beam from the light source is directed onto a partially reflective mirror (optical beam splitter). This mirror splits the light into two beams. One beam is directed into the eye and is reflected from intraocular structures at various distances. This reflected beam consists of multiple echoes and provides information about the distance and thickness of various fundus structures. The second beam is reflected from a reference mirror at a known spatial location. This beam travels back to the beam splitter where it combines with the optical beam reflected from the eye. When the two light beams coincide they produce a phenomenon known as *interference*, which is measured by a photodetector.[46,47]

The beam of light reflected from the reference mirror coincides with the beam of light reflected from a given structure in the eye only if both pulses arrive at the same time. It occurs when the distance that light

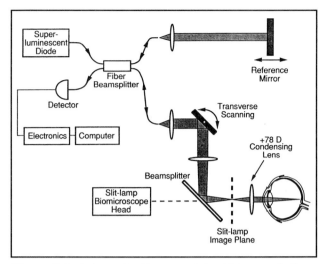

Figure 7-7. Schematic diagram of the high-speed, fiber-optic OCT scanner. Reprinted with permission from Schuman JS, Noecker RJ. Imaging of the optic nerve head and nerve fiber layer in glaucoma. *Ophthalmol Clin North Am.* 1995;8(2):259-279.

travels to and from the reference mirror equals the distance that light travels when it is reflected from a given fundus structure. The position of the reference mirror can be adjusted so that the time delay of the reference light beam matches the time delay of light echoes from the fundus structures. Thus, the interferometer can precisely measure the echo delay of fundus structures.

By measuring the echo delay of various fundus structures, a translated axial image similar to A-mode ultrasonography is produced. When successive axial measurements at different transverse points are combined, a tomographic or cross-sectional image of tissue is obtained. OCT images are displayed in false color to enhance differentiation of structures. Bright colors (red to white) correspond to tissues with high relative optical reflectivity, whereas darker colors (blue to black) correspond to areas of minimal or no optical reflectivity.

A single OCT scan consists of 100 to 200 axial scans. Nerve fiber layer thickness measurements are automated and displayed by quadrant, clock hour, and as an overall mean.[56] Nerve fiber layer measurements of 125 to 130 microns in the superior and inferior quadrants are deemed to be normal, though a large normative database stratified by age is not yet available (Figure 7-8).[55] OCT confirms that the nerve fiber layer does thin with age. Glaucoma patients demonstrate nerve fiber layer thinning that is significant, especially in the lower quadrant.[56] Small focal defects detect-

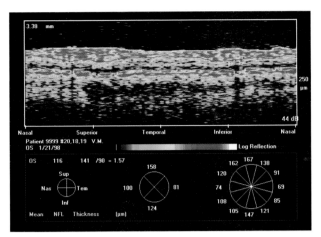

Figure 7-8. Circular OCT scan of healthy eye. Note the nerve fiber layer is thickest superiorly and inferiorly as seen by the anteriormost red reflection in the false color image. This is also evident with the quadrant and clock hour measurements of the nerve fiber layer.

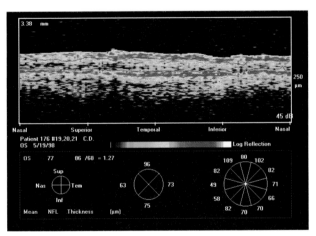

Figure 7-9b. OCT of same eye shows diffuse loss of nerve fiber layer.

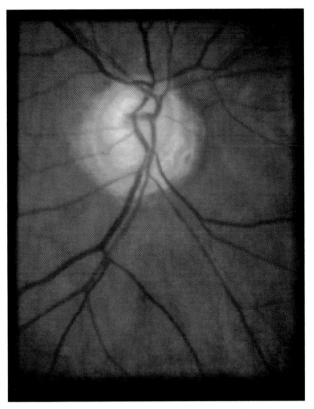

Figure 7-9a. Stereo optic disc photograph with advanced cupping.

CONCLUSION

Optic nerve imaging techniques have come a long way since the initial descriptions of the optic nerve head in the 19th century. At the dawn of the new millennium, newer imaging techniques of the optic nerve head and nerve fiber layer will help in the early detection of glaucoma and its management. Hopefully, significant functional visual loss will be prevented thereby paving the way to a bright future when blindness from glaucoma can be minimized or even eliminated.

ed by OCT, which correspond to visual field defects, can be seen. Progression of glaucoma can be seen in humans and the glaucomatous monkey model. Diffuse nerve fiber layer thinning is evident in severely glaucomatous eyes (Figures 7-9a and b). The precision and reproducibility of the OCT can aid in the detection of glaucoma at an earlier stage, potentially prior to visual field loss. The progression of optic nerve head damage with minimal loss of functional vision also may be diagnosed.

Table 7-1 lists the imaging devices discussed and their features.

Table 7-1

Comparison of Features of Selected Optic Nerve Head and Nerve Fiber Layer Imaging Devices

Instrument	Target	Imaging Principle	Price ($)	Minimum Pupil Size (mm)	Measurement Time	Resolution Lateral/Axial	Reference Plane?	Advantages	Disadvantages
IMAGEnet	ONH	Stereoscopic videographic imaging	79,000	7	2 seconds	100/300μ	yes	Works with existing fundus camera	Pupil dilation, long processing times
GlaucomaScope	ONH/NFL	Raster stereography	24,900	4.5	2 minutes	50/300μ	yes	Relatively inexpensive	Long imaging times
Retinal Tomograph	ONH/NFL	Confocal laser scanning	45,900	1	1.5 seconds	20/300μ	yes	No dilation	Complicated software, uses reference plane
TopSS	ONH/NFL	Confocal laser scanning	From 34,500	1	0.9 seconds	20/300μ	yes	No dilation, easy software	Measures only optic nerve head topography and NFL height currently
Nerve Fiber Analysis	NFL	Laser scanning polarimetry	54,000	1	0.7 seconds	20/13μ	no	High resolution of NFL measurement	Calculates NFL thickness using birefringence
Optical Cohererence Tomography	NFL	Optical coherence	75,000	4	2.5 seconds	20/10μ	no	Direct cross sectional imaging with highest resolution of NFL	Not yet commercially available

Reprinted with permission from Schuman JS, Noecker RJ. Imaging of the optic nerve head and nerve fiber layer in glaucoma. *Ophthalmol Clin North Am.* 1995;8(2):259-279.

REFERENCES

1. Helmholtz H. *Beschreiburg eines augenspiegels zur untersuchung der netzhaut in lebenden augi.* Berlin, Germany: A Forstner; 1851.
2. Lichter PR. Variability of expert observers in evaluating the optic disc. *Trans Am Ophthalmol Soc.* 1976;74:532-535.
3. Tielsch JM, Katz J, Quigley HA. Intraobserver and interobserver agreement in measurement of optic disc characteristics. *Ophthalmology.* 1988;95:350-356.
4. Anderson DR. Glaucoma: the damage caused by pressure. *Am J Ophthalmol.* 1989;108:121.
5. Quigley HA, Addicks EM, Green WR. Optic nerve damage in human glaucoma. *Arch Ophthalmol.* 1982;100:135-146.
6. Drance SM, Fairclugh M, Butler DM, et al. The importance of disc hemorrhage in the prognosis of chronic open angle glaucoma. *Arch Ophthalmol.* 1977;95:226-228.
7. Varma R, SpaethGL. The PAR IS 2000: a new system for retinal digital analysis. *Ophthalmic Surg.* 1988;19:1183.
8. Dandona L, Quigley HA, Jampel HD. Reliability of optic nerve head topographic measurements with computerized image analysis. *Am J Ophthalmol.* 1989;108:414-421.
9. Bishop KI, Werner EB, Krupin T, et al. Variability and reproducibility of optic disc topographic measurements with the Rodenstock Optic Nerve Head Analyzer. *Am J Ophthalmol.* 1988;106:696-702.
10. Echelman DA, Shields MB. Optic nerve head imaging. In: Albert DA, Jakobiec FJ, eds. *Principles and Practice of Ophthalmology.* Philadelphia, Pa: WB Saunders; 1993.
11. Belyea DA, Dan JA, Lieberman MF, et al. The Glaucomascope: reproducibility and accuracy of results. *Invest Ophthalmol Vis Sci.* 1994;35:429.
12. Hamzavis S, Stewart WC, Thompson TL. Inter and intraobserver variation of the optic nerve head in cadaver eyes using the Glaucoma-scope. *Invest Ophthalmol Vis Sci.* 1994;35(suppl):427.
13. Hoskins HD, Hetherington J, Glenday M, et al. Repeatability of the Glaucoma-scope measurements of optic nerve head topography. *Glaucoma.* 1994;3:177-185.
14. Airaksinen PF, Drance SM, Schulzer M. Neuroretinal rim area in early glaucoma. *Am J Ophthalmol.* 1985;99:1.
15. Balazsi GA, Drance SM, Schulzer M, et al. Neuroretinal rim area in suspected glaucoma and early chronic open-angle glaucoma. *Arch Ophthalmol.* 1984;102:1011-1014.
16. Caprioli J. The contour of the juxtapapillary nerve fiber layer in glaucoma. *Ophthalmology.* 1990;97:358-66.
17. Caprioli J, Klingbeil U, Sears M, et al. Reproducibility of optic disc measurements with computerized analysis of stereoscopic video images. *Arch Ophthalmol..* 1986;104:1035.
18. Caprioli J, Miller JM. Videographic measurements of optic nerve topography in glaucoma. *Invest Ophthalmol Vis Sci.* 1988;29:1294.
19. Caprioli J, Ortiz-Colberg R, Miller JM, Tressler C. Measurements of peripapillary nerve fiber layer contour in glaucoma. *Am J Ophthalmol.* 1989;108:404-413.
20. Mikelberg FS, Airaksinen PJ, Douglas GR, et al. The correlation between optic disc topography measured by the video-ophthalmograph (Rodenstock analyzer) and clinical measurement. *Am J Ophthalmol.* 1985;100:417.
21. Shields MB, Martone JF, Shelton AR, et al. Reproducibility of topographic measurements with the optic nerve head analyzer. *Am J Ophthalmol.* 1987;104:581.
22. Shields MB. The future of computerized image analysis in the management of glaucoma. *Am J Ophthalmol.* 1989;108:319-323.
23. Shields MB, Tiedeman JS, Miller KN, et al. Accuracy of topographic measurements with the optic nerve head analyzer. *Am J Ophthalmol.* 1989;107:273-279.
24. Cioffi GA, Robin AL, Eastman RD, et al. Confocal laser scanning ophthalmoscope: reproducibility of optic nerve head topographic measurements with the confocal laser scanning ophthalmoscope. *Ophthalmology.* 1993;100:57-62.
25. Webb RH, Hughes GW, Delori FC. Confocal scanning laser ophthalmoscope. *Applied Optics.* 1987;26:1492.
26. Kino GS, Corle TR. Confocal scanning optical microscopy. *Physics Today.* 1989;42:55.
27. Shuman H, Murray JM, DiLullo C. Confocal microscopy: an overview. *Biotechniques.* 1989;7:154.
28. Dreher AW, Tso PC, Weinreb RN. Reproducibility of topographic measurements of the normal and glaucomatous optic nerve head with the laser tomographic scanner. *Am J Ophthalmol.* 1991;111:221.
29. Kruse FE, Burk RO, Volcker HE, et al. Reproducibility of topographic measurements of the optic nerve head with laser tomographic scanning. *Ophthalmology.* 1989;96:1320-24.
30. Weinreb RN, Dreher AW, Bille J. Quantitative assessment of the optic nerve head with the laser tomographic scanner. *Int J Ophthalmol.* 1989;13:125-129.
31. Iester M, Mikelberg FS, Courtright P, Drance SM. Correlation between visual field indices and Heidelberg retina tomograph parameters. *J Glaucoma.* 1997;6(2):78-82.
32. Weinreb RN, Dreher AW, Coleman A, et al. Histopathologic validation of Fourier-ellipsometry measurements of retinal nerve fiber layer thickness. *Arch Ophthalmol.* 1990;108:557.
33. Weinreb RN, Lusky M, Bartsch DU, et al. Effect of repetitive imaging on topographic measurements of the optic nerve head. *Arch Ophthalmol.* 1993;111:636.
34. Zangwill L, Berry CA, Garden VS et al. Reproducibility of retardation measurements with the nerve fiber analyzer II. *J Glaucoma.* 1997;6(6):384-389.
35. Orgul S, Cioffi GA, Bacon DR, Van Buskirk EM. Sources of variability of topometric data with a scanning laser ophthalmoscope. *Arch Ophthalmol.* 1996;114(2):161-164.
36. Sommer A, Katz J, Quigley HA, et al. Clinically detectable nerve fiber atrophy preceded by the onset of glaucomatous field loss. *Arch Ophthalmol.* 1991;109:77-83.
37. Sommer A, Miller NR, Pollack I, et al. The nerve fiber layer in the diagnosis of glaucoma. *Arch Ophthalmol.* 1977;95:2149-2156.
38. Hoyt WF, Newman NM. The earliest observable defect in glaucoma? *Lancet.* 1972;1:692-693.

39. Balazsi AG, Rootman J, Drance SM, et al. The effect of age on the nerve fiber population of the human optic nerve. *Am J Ophthalmol*. 1984;97:760-766.

40. Chi Q, Tomita G, Inazumi K, et al. Evaluation of the effect of aging on the retinal nerve fiber layer thickness using scanning laser polarimetry. *J Glaucoma*. 1995;4:406-413.

41. Johnson BM, Miao M, Sadun AA. Age-related decline of human optic nerve axon populations. *Age*. 1987;10:5-9.

42. Dreher AW, Reiter K, Weinreb RM. Spatially resolved birefringence of the retinal nerve fiber layer assessed with a retinal laser ellipsometer. *Applied Optics*. 1992;31:3730-3735.

43. Marraffa M, Mansoldo C, Morbio R et al. Does nerve fiber layer thickness correlate with visual field defects in glaucoma? A study with the nerve fiber layer analyzer. *Ophthalmologica*. 1997; 211(6):338-40.

44. Anton A, Yamagishi N, Zangwill L et al. Mapping structural to functional damage in glaucoma with standard automated perimetry and confocal scanning laser ophthalmoscopy. *Am J Ophthalmol*. 1998 125 (4):436-446.

45. Tjon-Fo-Sang MJ, Lemij HG. The sensitivity and specificity of nerve fiber layer measurements in glaucoma as determined with scanning laser polarimetry. *Am J Ophthalmol*. 1997; 123(1):62-69.

46. Hee MR, Izatt JA, Swanson EA, et al. Optical coherence tomography for micron- resolution ophthalmic imaging. *IEEE Engineering in Medicine and Biology*. 1995;14(1): 67-75.

47. Hee MR, Izatt JA, Swanson EA, et al. Optical coherence tomography of the human retina. *Arch Ophthalmol*. 1995;113:325-332.

48. Hee MR, Puliafito CA, Wong C, et al. Optical coherence tomography of macular holes. *Ophthalmology*. 1995;102: 748-756.

49. Huang D, Stinson WG, Schuman JS, et al. High-resolution measurement of retinal thickness using optical coherence domain reflectometry. *Invest Ophthalmol Vis Sci*. 1991;32 (suppl):S1019.

50. Huang D, Swanson EA, Lin CP, et al. Optical coherence tomography. *Science*. 1991;254:1178.

51. Puliafito CA, Hee MR, Lin CP, et al. Imaging of macular diseases with optical coherence tomography. *Ophthalmology*. 1995;102:217-229.

52. Roh S, Noecker RJ, Schuman JS, et al. Effect of optic nerve head drusen on nerve fiber layer thickness. *Ophthalmology*. 1998;105(5):875-878.

53. Roh S, Noecker RJ, Schuman JS. Evaluation of coexisting optic nerve head drusen and glaucoma with optical coherence tomography. *Ophthalmology*. 1997;104(7):1138-44.

54. Schuman JS. Imaging of the optic nerve head and nerve fiber layer in glaucoma. In: Epstein DL, Allingham RR, Schuman JS, eds. *Chandler and Grant's Glaucoma*. Baltimore, Md: Williams and Wilkins; 1997.

55. Schuman JS. Optical Coherence Tomography for imaging and quantitation of nerve fiber layer thickness. In: Schuman JS, ed. *Imaging in Glaucoma*. Thorofare, NJ: SLACK Incorporated; 1997.

56. Schuman JS, Hee MR, Puliafito CA, et al. Quantification of nerve fiber layer thickness in normal and glaucomatous eyes using optical coherence tomography: a pilot study. *Arch Ophthalmol*. 1995;113:586-596.

57. Schuman JS, Noecker RJ. Imaging of the optic nerve and nerve fiber layer in glaucoma. *Ophthalmol Clin North Am*. 1995;8:259-279.

58. Swanson EA, Huang D, Hee MR, et al. High-speed optical coherence domain reflectometry. *Opt Lett*. 1992;17:151-153.

59. Swanson EA, Izatt JA, Hee MR, et al. In vivo retinal imaging using optical coherence tomography. *Opt Lett*. 1993;18: 1864-1866.

Chapter Eight

GLAUCOMA VISUAL FIELDS

Elliot B. Werner, MD

Glaucoma is treated in order to preserve vision. Tests of visual function, thus, are of critical importance in evaluating the glaucoma patient and in guiding treatment. Despite recent advances in optic nerve and retinal nerve fiber layer evaluation, and despite many recent studies of a variety of visual functions in glaucoma, white light perimetry remains the most reliable widely used tool to detect functional impairment as a result of glaucoma.

As a pure diagnostic tool, perimetry has a number of shortcomings. Other modalities maybe more useful for population screening. Automated perimetry, however, compares favorably with other clinical techniques for detecting glaucomatous damage. Perimetry is indispensable as an indication of the extent of glaucomatous damage and as an aid in determining if an individual with glaucoma is deteriorating.

There are two steps in diagnosing glaucomatous visual field loss using automated perimetry. The first is to determine whether the visual field is normal or not. The second step is to decide if any visual field abnormality is due to glaucoma or something else. The second step actually is the easier of the two. Differentiating the normal from the abnormal field is not straightforward. It requires a knowledge of the range of visual field responses in the normal population, an understanding of probability, and the ability to interpret detailed statistical analysis of the visual field data. The essential purpose of visual field testing in glaucoma is to determine the extent of functional visual loss and whether or not it is progressive.

When applied to perimetry, the term *normal* actually describes the range of test results found in the non-diseased population. The range of normal has been determined experimentally, and the results are stored in the computer memory of most automated perimeters. This database allows the comparison of an individual patient's visual field with the expected normal values. Because of the wide range of normal, one cannot say with certainty that a particular visual field is normal or abnormal. One can, however, determine the likelihood of finding a particular visual field result in a normal individual. If that likelihood is very small, one assumes that visual field probably is abnormal. Specific examples of visual fields in this chapter are taken from the Humphrey Visual Field Analyzer. Similar results and analytic software are available with the Octopus and other automated perimeters.

The determination that a visual field is within the normal range cannot be made by simple inspection. Statistical analysis is necessary. Statistical software packages available with some perimeters provide probability statements about the visual field data that allow the clinician to determine whether a particular visual field falls within the normal range. If all statistical parameters are within the normal range, chances are that the visual field is normal. The sensitivity of automated threshold perimetry for detecting visual field defects is very high. It is extremely unlikely that a patient with a clinically significant visual field defect would have a normal result. The opposite, however, is not always true.

Many otherwise normal patients will have a visual field that appears abnormal because of the large number of artifacts that can occur during automated visual field testing. In other words, the specificity of automated perimetry is not as high as clinicians would like. When performing perimetry on patients suspected of having glaucoma, it is important to distinguish the visual field that appears abnormal because of artifact from the visual field that truly is abnormal as a result of glaucoma or some other disease such as cataract, retinal disease, neurologic lesions, etc. Statistical analysis must be combined with other clinical findings, experience, and the ability to recognize specific patterns of visual field loss related to specific diseases or artifacts.

RELIABILITY INDICES

The Reliability Indices are found in the upper left hand corner of the STATPAC 2 printout of the Humphrey Visual Field Analyzer (Figure 8-1). Reliability is tested by presenting "catch trial" targets designed to measure fixation losses and false positive and false negative responses. The fixation loss rate relates to the number of times a patient responds to a target placed in the blind spot. If the fixation loss rate exceeds 33%, it is flagged (Figure 8-2). The false positive error rate refers to the number of times a patient responds when no target is presented. The false nega-

tive error rate refers to the number of times a patient fails to respond to a suprathreshold (very bright) target placed in a seeing area of the visual field. The false positive and false negative errors are flagged if either exceeds 33% (Figures 8-3 and 8-4).

The Reliability Indices are an indicator of the extent to which a particular patient's results may be reliably compared to the normal range of values stored in the computer memory. The Reliability Indices often are misinterpreted as an indicator of how accurate and believable a patient's test results are. In fact, many patients who are flagged by the perimeter as having low reliability appear to have very accurate and reproducible visual field results (see Figure 8-2). On the other hand, some patients who appear to be very reliable have highly variable results.

Some types of visual field defects are themselves associated with changes in the Reliability Indices. For example, glaucoma causes an increase in the false negative response rate, and very large defects may be associated with very low fixation loss rates. Much useful information can, however, still be obtained from many patients despite a high fixation loss or false negative rate.

A high false positive rate often is associated with the patient who responds frequently even when targets are not presented, the so-called "trigger happy" patient. This tendency may result in a visual field with abnormally high decibel thresholds that obviously is not interpretable (see Figure 8-3).

GLOBAL INDICES

The four Global Indices are found in the lower right hand corner of the Humphrey STATPAC 2 printout (see Figure 8-1). The mean deviation (MD) is a measure of the average departure of each test location from the age-corrected normal value. The pattern standard deviation (PSD) is the standard deviation of the differences between the threshold value at each test location and the expected value. It is a measure of the extent to which the threshold determinations at different locations in the visual field differ from each other. The short-term fluctuation (SF) represents the variability of the patient's responses during the test. The corrected pattern standard deviation (CPSD) is similar to the PSD but is adjusted downward by subtracting that portion of the PSD that actually is due to the SF. The corrected loss variance (CLV) of the

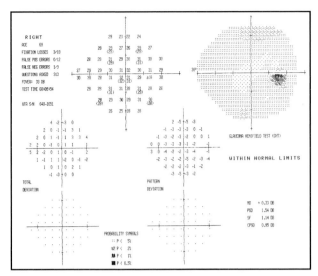

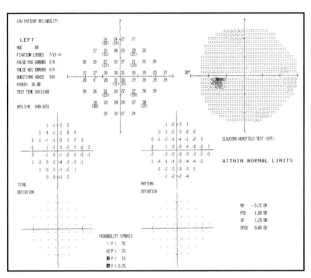

Figure 8-1. Printout of a normal visual field from the Humphrey Visual Field Analyzer. The reliability indices, fixation losses, false-positive errors, and false-negative errors are found in the upper left-hand corner just below the patient's age. The global indices are found in the lower right-hand corner just below the gray scale interpolation of the threshold values. None of the global indices (MD, PSD, SF, CPSD) is flagged with a "P" value, indicating that all are within the expected range of normal. The numeric and graphic representations of the total and pattern deviations are found where indicated in the left and center lower portion of the printout. There are no probability symbols in either the total or pattern deviation, indicating that the threshold value of each test location is within the normal range for the patient's age. The Glaucoma Hemifield Test result is found just below the gray scale interpolation and is *Within Normal Limits.*

Figure 8-2. Visual field showing an elevated fixation loss rate of 7/19. This rate exceeds 33% and is flagged with "xx" as well as a statement *Low Patient Reliability.* The visual field otherwise appears entirely normal. The presence of a reliability index outside of the "normal range" does not necessarily mean that the results of the test are invalid. Repeatability and correlation with other clinical findings are more important criteria.

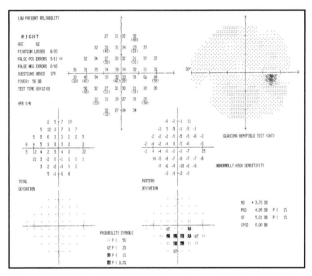

Figure 8-3. Visual field of a "trigger happy" patient who frequently responds at times when no test target is presented. The result of such actions is a high false-positive error rate, an unphysiologically elevated mean deviation (MD), and an abnormally high sensitivity that is seen as white areas in the gray scale interpolation, the so-called white field artifact. Note the foveal sensitivity of 56 DB. The Glaucoma Hemifield Test shows *Abnormally High Sensitivity.*

Octopus system, although calculated differently, provides similar information. The calculation of the global indices is weighted to give greater importance to the test locations near fixation and less importance to more peripheral locations.

If a global index is outside the expected normal range, a "P" value appears next to it (see Figure 8-4). The "P" value represents the proportion of normal subjects in whom an index of that value is found. For example, if P < 1% appears next to the MD, fewer than 1% of normal subjects of that age will have an MD at that level. Any global index with a P value less than 5% has a high probability of being abnormal

The MD is mainly an index of the size of a visual field defect. It is not, as is widely believed, an indicator of generalized depression of the visual field. The MD is very sensitive to generalized loss of sensitivity, but purely localized defects that are large enough also affect the MD.

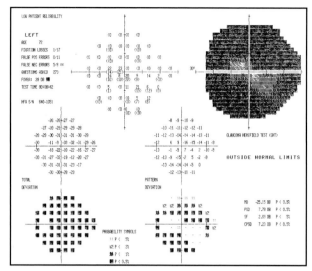

Figure 8-4. Visual field of a patient with very advanced field loss. The false-negative error rate is flagged and the message *Low Patient Reliability* appears. High false-negative response rates are common in patients with glaucomatous field loss and do not necessarily indicate poor reliability. The global indices are flagged with "P" values indicating a high probability that they are abnormal.

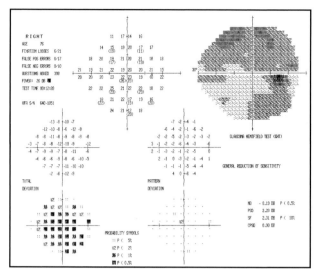

Figure 8-5. Visual field of a patient with a nearly pure generalized loss due to cataract. The MD is significantly below the expected range of normal at the P <0.5% level while the PSD and CPSD are within the normal range. The total deviation shows many probability symbols most of which are not found in the pattern deviation. The Glaucoma Hemifield Test shows *Generalized Reduction of Sensitivity*.

The PSD and CPSD are indices of localized nonuniformity of the surface of the hill of vision. They are extremely sensitive to localized visual field defects and are not affected by purely generalized loss of sensitivity.

By looking at the MD and PSD (or CPSD if the SF is excessive), it is possible to anticipate the nature of any visual field defect before inspecting the rest of the visual field data. If both the MD and PSD are within the normal range, the visual field is probably normal or very minimally disturbed (see Figure 8-1). If the MD is abnormal but the PSD is normal, there is probably a pure generalized depression (Figure 8-5). If the MD is normal but the PSD is abnormal there is a small, purely localized defect or artifact (Figure 8-6). If both are abnormal, there is a large defect present with a significant localized component (Figures 8-7 and 8-8). When both are abnormal, however, it is impossible to determine whether there is any significant generalized depression without inspecting the remainder of the visual field data. The interpretation of the global indices is summarized in Table 8-1.

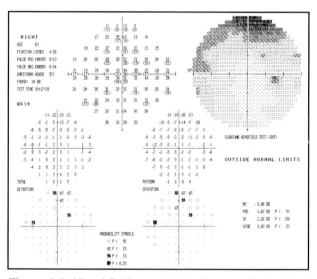

Figure 8-6. Visual field consistent with a small, localized defect. The MD is within the normal range, while the PSD and CPSD are outside the expected range of normal. The total and pattern deviation plots show almost identical arrays of probability symbols. The Glaucoma Hemifield Test, which is very sensitive to small differences in threshold between the superior and inferior hemifields, shows *Outside Normal Limits*.

TOTAL AND PATTERN DEVIATION

The total and pattern deviations are found as arrays of numbers and graphic plots in the center and

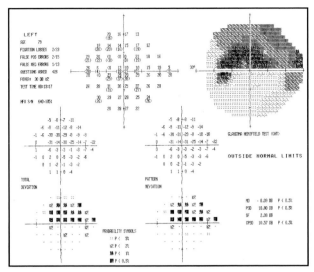

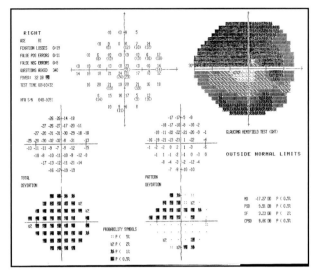

Figure 8-7. Visual field consistent with a large defect with a significant localized component. Both the MD and PSD are outside the expected range of normal at the P <0.5% level. Inspection of the global indices alone does not allow a determination of the relative amounts of generalized and localized loss. The number and distribution of probability symbols in the total and pattern deviation are very similar indicating that this is almost a pure localized defect. The Glaucoma Hemifield Test is *Outside Normal Limits* reflecting the marked difference in sensitivity between the superior and inferior hemifields.

Figure 8-8. Visual field consistent with a large defect with a significant localized component. The MD and PSD are both outside the expected range of normal. The graphic representation of the total and pattern deviation shows many probability symbols in the total deviation. The symbols in the inferior half of the field are not seen in the pattern deviation, but the symbols in the superior half of the field are found in both plots. These findings are typical of a mixed generalized and localized defect (contrast Figure 8-7). The Glaucoma Hemifield Test is *Outside Normal Limits*. This type of field defect is often seen in glaucoma patients who also have a cataract or a small pupil.

Table 8-1

Interpretation of the Global Indices on the Humphrey Visual Field Analyzer*

MD	PSD (or CPSD)	Interpretation
Normal	Normal	Visual field probably normal
Abnormal	Normal	Generalized loss of sensitivity
Normal	Abnormal	Small localized defect
Abnormal	Abnormal	Large defect with a significant localized component

*Artifacts may cause the global indices to be abnormal in the absence of any pathologic cause for visual field loss.

lower portions of the STATPAC 2 printout (see Figure 8-1). The total deviation represents the difference between the measured threshold of each individual test location and the age-corrected normal value for that location. Visual field thresholds decline with age at the rate of between 0.5 and 1.0 decibels per decade. Statements about whether or not the threshold of a particular test location is normal must take into account the patient's age. An abnormal result for a patient age 20 may be well within the normal range for a patient age 80. The actual measured thresholds are shown in the array of numbers in the upper central portion of the printout to the left of the gray scale.

The pattern deviation represents the difference between an adjusted threshold of each individual test location and the age-corrected normal value for that location. The pattern deviation is derived from the total deviation by adjusting the measured thresholds upward or downward by an amount that reflects any generalized change in the threshold of the least damaged portion of the visual field. The information in the total deviation, thus, may be thought of as a combination of generalized plus localized change. The information in the pattern deviation represents purely localized change. Although the interpretation of the pattern deviation and pattern standard deviation is similar, and the similarity of the names may be confusing, they are not identical and should not be confused.

The graphic probability plots indicate how frequently a total or pattern deviation value at a particular test location would be found in the normal population. There are four symbols ranging from P < 5% to P < 0.5%. A black square, for example, indicates the total or pattern deviation value for that test location will be found in fewer than 0.5% of normal subjects. Groupings of symbols in a portion of the visual field, therefore, indicate a high probability of an abnormality there.

If there are no symbols in either the total or pattern deviation plot, the visual field is probably normal (see Figure 8-1). If the array of symbols in the total and pattern deviation is very similar, the defect is probably a purely localized one (see Figures 8-6 and 8-7). If there are many symbols in the total deviation and none or very few in the pattern deviation, the defect is a purely generalized one (see Figure 8-5). If there are many symbols in the total deviation and a smaller but still significant number in the pattern deviation, there is a mixed generalized and localized defect (see Figure 8-8). Symbols in the pattern deviation, which are not found in the total deviation, are usually seen in the trigger happy patient (see Figure 8-3) with a high false-positive error rate and abnormally high sensitivity (see discussion of the Glaucoma Hemifield Test).

The location and distribution of the symbols in the total and pattern deviation plots also can help define the location of the lesion responsible for the visual field defect and distinguish glaucomatous from non-glaucomatous visual field loss.

THE GLAUCOMA HEMIFIELD TEST

The Glaucoma Hemifield Test is a recent innovation and attempts to provide information about the difference between the superior and inferior halves of the visual field. The Glaucoma Hemifield Test evaluates the differences in threshold of mirror image groups of points on either side of the horizontal midline. There are six interpretive messages that may appear depending on the relationship of the thresholds in the superior and inferior halves of the field.

1. *Within Normal Limits* (see Figure 8-1) means that there is no significant difference between the superior and inferior halves of the visual field and the overall sensitivity of the field is normal.
2. *Outside Normal Limits* (see Figure 8-7) appears when there are significant differences in the threshold of the superior and inferior halves of the visual field.
3. *Borderline* (Figure 8-9) appears when there are threshold differences between the superior and inferior halves of the visual fields, but they do not reach statistical significance.
4. *General Reduction of Sensitivity* (see Figure 8-5) appears when the overall sensitivity of the least damaged portion of the visual field is depressed below normal, but there is no significant difference between the superior and inferior halves of the field.
5. *Abnormally High Sensitivity* (see Figure 8-3) appears when the overall sensitivity is higher than expected. This message most often is found in the presence of a high false positive rate and usually represents an artifact of testing.
6. *Borderline* combined with *General Reduction of Sensitivity* (Figure 8-10) appears in patients with a significant generalized loss of sensitivity and a residual moderate difference in the sensitivity of the superior and inferior hemifields.

The specificity and sensitivity of the Glaucoma Hemifield Test for detecting nerve fiber bundle visual field defects are quite high, especially if consistently abnormal results are obtained after repeat testing. In the absence of the messages *outside normal limits* or *borderline,* it is very unlikely that a visual field defect of the type seen in glaucoma is present. On the other hand, although an abnormal Glaucoma Hemifield Test may be due to an artifact, the presence of a glaucomatous visual field defect is possible and should be carefully evaluated.

The management of glaucoma includes perimetry at regular intervals. All glaucoma patients capable of cooperating for the test should be tested at the time of initial diagnosis. Perimetry should then be repeated within a few weeks in order to have at least two baseline tests for comparison with subsequent tests. In patients with inconsistent results or with a significant

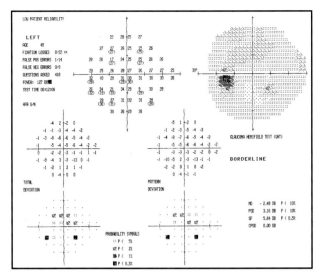

Figure 8-9. *Borderline* Glaucoma Hemifield Test consistent with a small difference in sensitivity between the superior and inferior hemifields. This is an unusual field. The global indices suggest a generalized loss with a large short-term fluctuation (SF), while the total and pattern deviations suggest a localized defect. The presence of a high SF, a high fixation loss rate, and a low foveal sensitivity despite 20/20 vision indicate that patient reliability may be a problem. Clinically, the approach to this patient would be to evaluate the fundus carefully and repeat the field.

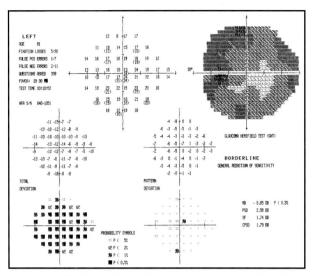

Figure 8-10. *Borderline—General Reduction of Sensitivity* Glaucoma Hemifield Test results in a patient with what appears to be a mostly generalized loss. The markedly depressed paracentral test location just superior and nasal to fixation is enough to trigger the *Borderline* result.

learning effect, more than two baseline tests may be required. For ocular hypertensive patients or other patients with normal fields, an annual visual field may be adequate. In patients with visual field loss, the frequency of testing depends on the severity of the patient's glaucoma and the risk for future progression. For such patients, two or more visual fields per year may be indicated.

Some patients are incapable of performing automated perimetry. Sometimes the patient's vision is so poor that perimetry yields little useful information. In other patients, an adequate examination cannot be conducted because of age or physical or psychological problems. There is no point in forcing such patients to undergo perimetry repeatedly if useful clinical information is not being generated. Many patients, however, who have problems with automated perimetry at first can learn to perform adequately with proper coaching and experience.

The standard test program used in glaucoma patients is the 30-2. The 24-2 eliminates the peripheral test locations of the 30-2 program except for the most nasal portion of the field. Many clinicians now routinely use the 24-2 in glaucoma patients because it

seems to provide as much clinically useful information as the 30-2 and saves about 5 minutes testing time per eye. The shorter testing time may reduce patient fatigue and encourage cooperation and compliance with the examination. The 10-2 program is useful in patients with very advanced field loss who only have a small island of vision persisting near fixation. The foveal sensitivity is also a very useful piece of information and should be turned "ON" when performing threshold perimetry in glaucoma patients.

FASTPAC

FASTPAC (Figure 8-11), a technique for measuring perimetric thresholds, is available with the Humphrey Visual Field Analyzer. The major advantage of FASTPAC is the reduced testing time. FASTPAC, however, seems to be associated with an increased variability of patient responses and a difference in Mean Deviation measurement that may affect the detection of visual field defects.

The Glaucoma Hemifield Test is not available when FASTPAC is used, nor is the Glaucoma Change Probability Program. FASTPAC appears to be most useful in patients unable to tolerate full threshold testing without undue fatigue. Humphrey has recently introduced a new testing algorithm called SITA (Swedish Interactive Testing Algorithm), which may provide full threshold accuracy with significantly shorter testing time.

GLAUCOMATOUS VISUAL FIELD DEFECTS

Most visual field defects seen in glaucoma are of the nerve fiber bundle type. As a result of glaucomatous damage to ganglion cell axons at the optic nerve head, there is a loss of retinal nerve fiber bundles. This loss may be either diffuse, localized, or both. The characteristic shape and location of the visual field defects seen in glaucoma result from the anatomy of the retinal nerve fiber layer. The defects seen in an individual patient depend on the location of the damaged nerve fibers, and whether the damage is predominantly localized or diffuse.

The most characteristic feature of the nerve fiber bundle visual field defect is the tendency to respect the horizontal meridian, especially in the nasal portion of the field. Isolated nerve fiber bundle defects rarely cross the nasal horizontal midline. Even in patients with more advanced visual field loss due to glaucoma there often is a detectable difference in the measured threshold on either side of the nasal horizontal midline.

Another feature of nerve fiber bundle visual field defects is the tendency to occur in the Bjerrum area, which is found between 10 and 20 degrees from fixation temporally and fans out to between 2 and 25 degrees nasally. Scotomas in this area often assume an arcuate shape with the circumferential diameter greater than the radial diameter. Fixation itself is usually spared unless the defect is far advanced. Nerve fiber bundle defects may, however, come to within 1 degree of fixation.

Clinically, nerve fiber bundle defects may appear as paracentral or arcuate scotomas, nasal steps, temporal sector defects, or various combinations (Figures 8-12 through 8-16). Any visual field defect, which has nerve fiber bundle characteristics in a patient with optic disc cupping, may safely be assumed to be glaucomatous in nature.

Generalized loss of retinal sensitivity, enlargement of the blind spot, and selective loss of sensitivity in the nasal periphery without specific nerve fiber bundle characteristics have been described in glaucoma. There are many other causes for these types of visual field defects. Although any of them may occur as an isolated finding in glaucoma, more commonly they are associated with a nerve fiber bundle defect.

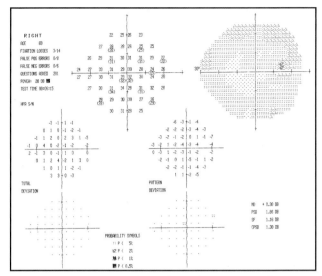

Figure 8-11. Example of a FASTPAC visual field. The test time is only 6 minutes, 15 seconds. This is considerably shorter than the time required for a comparable full threshold field. The Glaucoma Hemifield Test is not available with FASTPAC.

ARTIFACTS

There are a number of artifacts of visual field testing that can produce results resembling true visual field defects. An artifact does not reflect abnormal visual function. Rather, it results from the way the patient responds to the testing situation. Generalized depressions such as these are seen in patients with cataracts or small pupils are not artifacts. They are true visual field defects that reflect diminished visual function. Artifacts and nonglaucomatous visual field defects must be distinguished from each other as well as from defects due to glaucoma.

The learning effect is a common artifact seen in patients undergoing their first visual field examination. Typically, it appears as a loss of sensitivity that is most pronounced in the more peripheral portions of the field. The defect either disappears or markedly improves after the second or third examination.

An apparent depression in the superior peripheral portion of the field may resemble an arcuate scotoma in the gray scale. The superior portion of the visual field normally has lower sensitivity and higher variability. Careful inspection of the total and pattern deviation as well as the Glaucoma Hemifield Test will help identify this artifact. Blepharoptosis, however, even when very mild may produce significant depressions in the superior visual field resembling the defects seen in glaucoma. Some of these defects may be quite close to fixation.

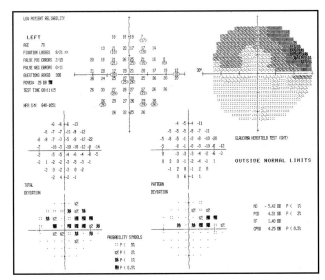

Figure 8-12. A superior nerve fiber bundle defect that is most pronounced near the nasal horizontal meridian.

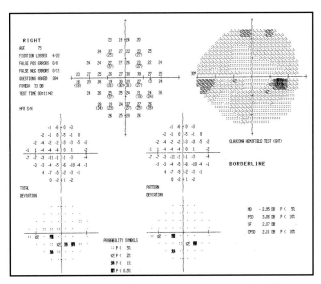

Figure 8-13. An early inferior nerve fiber bundle defect.

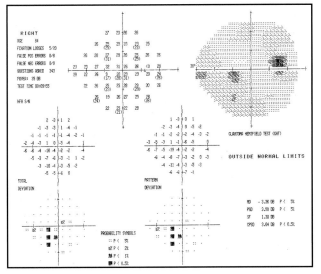

Figure 8-14. An inferior paracentral scotoma.

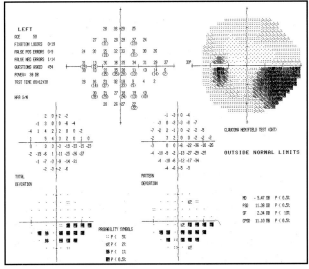

Figure 8-15. A large inferior nerve fiber bundle defect that is densest in the nasal quadrant but displays an arcuate shape.

In order to obtain accurate central visual fields, the patient's refractive correction must be placed in the perimeter. If this is not done, the visual field may appear abnormal. In general, about one decibel of loss will appear for each diopter of over- or undercorrection placed in the perimeter. The loss due to incorrect refractive correction tends to be most pronounced in the central visual field.

If the pupil is smaller than 2.5 mm, an otherwise normal visual field may appear to be depressed, and an abnormal visual field may appear worse than it really is. Strictly speaking, this is not an artifact because the changes in the visual field result from an alteration of the visual pathway. A small pupil will, however, make interpretation of the visual field difficult. The pupil size should be recorded each time the visual field is tested. If an effect of miosis on the visual field is suspected, the pupil should be dilated prior to the examination. Many clinicians routinely dilate pupils less than 3 mm for perimetry.

The rim of the lens holder may produce a scotoma by obscuring a portion of the patient's view of the perimeter bowl (Figure 8-17). The lens holder should be placed as close to the patient's eye as possible and

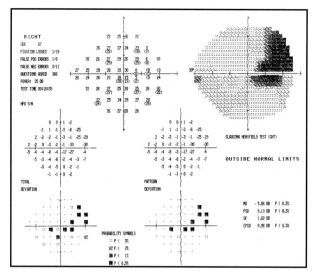

Figure 8-16. A dense superior temporal sector defect combined with a relative inferior arcuate scotoma.

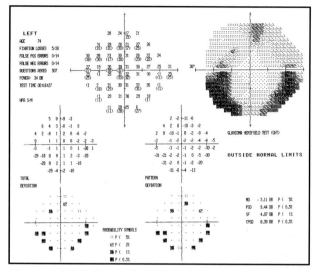

Figure 8-17. A dense visual field defect due to a lens rim artifact. This field defect completely disappeared when the patient and the lens holder were properly positioned.

the patient's eye should be well-centered behind the lens. Fatigue and an unduly long examination time also may be associated with depressed sensitivity and apparent visual field defects.

DETECTION OF PROGRESSIVE VISUAL FIELD LOSS

The detection of progressive glaucomatous visual field loss with automated perimetry is an extremely complex problem, which has not been satisfactorily solved. The visual fields of both normal individuals and glaucoma patients are subject to a large degree of long-term fluctuation, which is defined as variation in measured visual thresholds of examinations performed on different days. Long-term fluctuation has been extensively studied and shown to be larger in glaucoma patients than in normals, larger in more extensively damaged areas of the visual field, larger in the periphery of the field than near fixation, and larger in the superior half of the field.

Because of the large amount of long-term fluctuation found in the visual fields of glaucoma patients, it is often difficult to decide if the difference between two fields is due to true progressive field loss or random variation. Investigators have been grappling with this problem since the inception of automated perimetry. Even experienced clinicians often have difficulty in determining whether or not visual field defects are progressing and frequently do not agree with statisti-

cal tests applied to the visual field data. Recent techniques have improved agreement among clinicians and statistical tests in detecting progressive field loss, but we still lack a generally accepted "gold standard" definition of progression that has been validated.

Despite these problems, it has become apparent that multiple visual field examinations are required to separate fluctuation from progression, and that progression is more easily detected when a series of visual fields are graphically displayed in a single printout. Clinicians should probably not even attempt to diagnose progression with fewer than six examinations. One should also not rely on simple inspection of individual visual field printouts.

The STATPAC 2 software provides three ways to display serial visual field data to assist in determining the presence of progression:
1. Overview printout
2. Change analysis printout
3. Glaucoma change probability analysis.

The overview printout (Figures 8-18a and b) simply displays the gray scale, measured thresholds, and total and pattern deviations, usually on a single sheet of paper. Trends over time may be more easily demonstrated with this printout, but no statistical analysis is performed.

The change analysis printout (Figure 8-19) displays serial visual field data as a set of frequency distributions of the actual measured threshold data in the form of box plots. The normal distribution is shown as

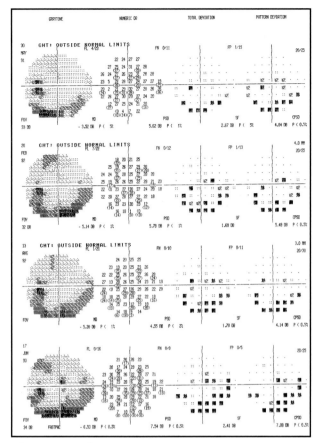

Figure 8-18a. Overview printout showing progressive glaucomatous visual field loss. The enlargement and deepening of the defect is well seen in the gray scale, total and pattern deviation displays.

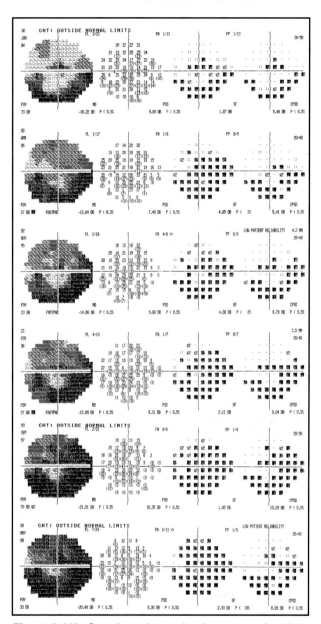

Figure 8-18b. Overview printout showing progressive glaucomatous visual field loss. The enlargement and deepening of the defect is well seen in the gray scale, total and pattern deviation displays.

a sample box plot to the left of the display. The actual values are presented in chronological order in the graph. The numbers along the "Y" axis of the graph represent the difference between the actual measured threshold and the age-corrected normal, in other words, the departure from normal. Positive values represent test locations with thresholds above normal and negative values, test locations with thresholds below normal. The highest value in the box plot, the top of the "T," is the best point in the visual field. It is the test location with the highest value compared to the normal. The top of the box is the 85th percentile. Fifteen percent of the test locations have values higher, and 85% have values lower than that represented by the top of the box. The thick bar in the middle of the box is the median value. Fifty percent of the thresholds are above and 50% below this value. The bottom of the box is the 15th percentile, while the bottom of the "T" is the worst point in the field. The box plot does not

take into consideration the location of the test points, only their threshold values compared to normal. When a large number of fields are available, downward trends in any part of the box plot can often be easily distinguished from random fluctuation to allow a diagnosis of progression. Progression may not necessarily be the result of glaucoma because cataracts, other media opacities, and retinal disease also cause progressive deterioration of the visual field.

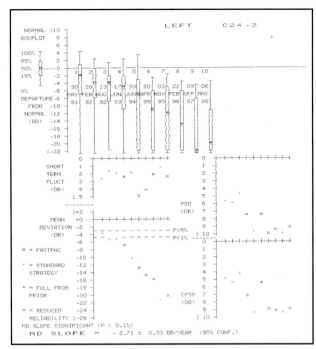

Figure 8-19. Change analysis printout of the same patient in Figures 8-18a and b showing a progressing visual field. The boxplot frequency distributions demonstrate a downward trend between May 1991 and May 1998. The negative slope of the MD regression line is significant. Visual inspection of the PSD and CPSD plots also shows a steady decline. Compare the gray scale and total deviation displays in Figures 8-18a and b.

Below the box plots, the global indices are displayed over time. If more than four visual fields are available, a linear regression on the MD over time is presented with the slope of the regression line and a statement regarding statistical significance. Visual inspection of the PSD or CPSD plot over time may show progressive deepening or enlargement of a localized defect, particularly in patients with early field loss. The usefulness of this type of analysis in detecting progression is questionable.

The glaucoma change probability analysis printout (Figure 8-20) displays the gray scale, total deviation, and change in threshold from baseline for each test location of a series of fields on a single sheet of paper. To the right of this data is a graph representing the probability that changes in each individual test location are outside the expected range of random fluctuation. Clear triangles represent test locations showing improvement while solid black triangles represent test locations showing deterioration.

Progression is usually represented by a cluster of black triangles in the same location that enlarges with

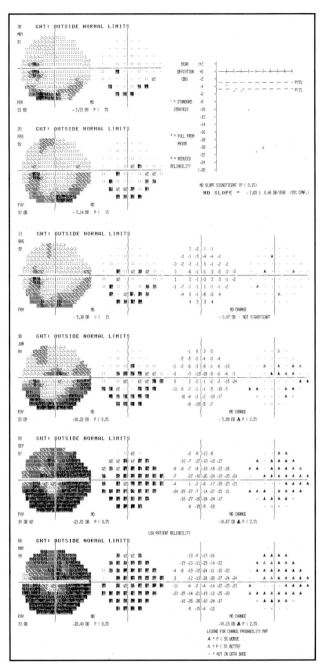

Figure 8-20. Glaucoma change probability analysis printout of the same patient in Figures 8-18a and b. FASTPAC determinations are not included in the STATPAC 2 analysis. The first two fields serve as the baseline. The cluster of black triangles in the most recent visual fields identifies the area where progressive field loss is occurring compared to the baseline.

time. It should again be emphasized that none of these displays allows the clinician to detect progression reliably with fewer than six visual fields.

This chapter has emphasized the Humphrey system for automated perimetry because this is the most widely used system in North America and is the one available to me. It should be noted that equally sophisticated testing procedures and analysis programs are available from Octopus and other manufacturers. When patients cannot perform automated perimetry or where automated perimetry is unavailable, manual quantitative perimetry with the Goldmann perimeter is a useful alternative.

Newer types of perimetry utilizing targets more complex than simple white light are now undergoing development. Although none has come into widespread clinical use, there is considerable potential for their use in the future.

The use of a blue test object on a yellow background is called short-wavelength automated perimetry (SWAP). This test is commercially available. There is some evidence that SWAP is more sensitive that white-light perimetry for detecting early glaucomatous damage.

Other types of perimetry that show promise in glaucoma include high-pass resolution perimetry, which utilizes ring-shaped targets, and motion-detection perimetry, which uses moving spots within a target.

BIBLIOGRAPHY

American Academy of Ophthalmology. Ophthalmic procedures assessment automated perimetry. *Ophthalmology.* 1996;103: 1144-1151.

American Academy of Ophthalmology. *Preferred Practice Pattern Primary Open-angle Glaucoma.* San Francisco, Calif, 1996.

Anderson DR. *Automated Static Perimetry.* St. Louis, Mo: Mosby Year Book; 1992.

Budenz DL. *Atlas of Visual Fields.* Philadelphia, Pa: Lippincott-Raven; 1997.

Drake MV. *A Primer on Automated Perimetry. Focal Points Clinical Modules for Ophthalmologists.* San Francisco, Calif: American Academy of Ophthalmology; 1993:11(8).

Heijl A, Lindgren G, Lindgren A, et al. Extended empirical statistical package for evaluation of single and multiple fields in glaucoma: Statpac 2. In: Mills RP, Heijl A, eds. *Perimetry Update* 1990/91. Amstelveen, the Netherlands: Kugler & Ghedini; 1991:303-315.

Heijl A, Lindgren G, Olsson J. A package for the statistical analysis of visual fields. In: Heijl A, ed. *Seventh International Visual Field Symposium.* Dodrecht, Netherlands: Dr W Junk; 1987: 153-168.

Lieberman MF. *Glaucoma and automated perimetry. Focal Points Clinical Modules for Ophthalmologists.* San Francisco, Calif: American Academy of Ophthalmology; 1993:11(9).

Lynn JR, Fellman RL, Starita RJ. Principles of perimetry. In: Ritch R, Shields MB, Krupin T, eds. *The Glaucomas.* 2nd ed. St Louis, Mo: Mosby; 1996:491-521.

Stewart WC, Hunt HH. Threshold variation in automated perimetry. *Surv Ophthalmol.* 1993;37:353-361.

Werner EB. *Manual of Visual Fields.* New York, NY: Churchill Livingstone; 1991.

Chapter Nine

Clinical Features of the Primary and Secondary Glaucomas

Joseph W. Sassani, MD

There are many disease processes that produce the characteristic optic nerve cupping and visual field loss, which are the hallmarks of the clinical syndrome known as *glaucoma*. Figures 9-1a and b illustrate the clinical and histologic appearance of advanced glaucomatous optic nerve injury. The goal of glaucoma therapy is to prevent progression to this advanced stage. Early diagnosis of glaucoma, however, is dependent on consensus as to the criteria for the diagnosis. Unfortunately, the published literature is far from unanimous in its definition of glaucoma. Recently, Bathija and colleagues reviewed several prominent ophthalmic journals regarding the definition of glaucoma as stated in articles from representative years. Approximately 36% used both optic disc and visual field criteria, 13% used optic disc or visual field criteria, 26% used only visual field criteria, 20% used only intraocular pressure (IOP), and 5% used only optic disc criteria.[1] The present chapter provides an overview of the most important of these disease processes or syndromes resulting in glaucoma.

Most of the pathways to glaucoma are accompanied by an IOP above the statistically normal range. Nevertheless, one must not lose sight of the fact that approximately 30% of individuals classified as having glaucoma display an IOP that is within the normal range.[2,3,4] These patients are said to have *normal pressure glaucoma* (low pressure glaucoma) and are discussed later in this chapter and in the chapter focusing on the optic nerve. Most of the present chapter discusses the majority of glaucoma patients, those displaying elevated IOP.

It also must be noted that most individuals having an IOP above the statistically normal range do not display characteristic glaucomatous optic nerve cupping and field loss that would be diagnostic of glaucoma. These patients are classified as *ocular hypertensive, glaucoma suspects, or pre-glaucoma*. The fact that they do not give evidence of glaucomatous damage may reflect the limitations on our ability to fully analyze the optic nerve or to limitations of currently utilized psychophysical tests for glaucomatous

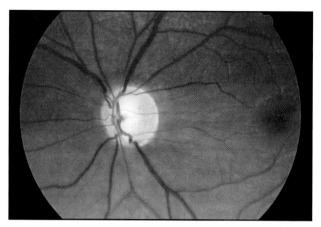

Figure 9-1a. Clinical photograph of advanced glaucomatous optic nerve cupping.

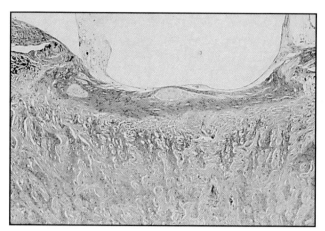

Figure 9-1b. Photomicrograph of extensive optic nerve cupping illustrating extreme loss of optic nerve fibers.

visual loss. As our examination and testing techniques become more sensitive, the author suspects that fewer patients will be categorized as ocular hypertensive.

CLASSIFICATION OF GLAUCOMA

The following outline summarizes and classifies the forms of glaucoma according to a mixed anatomic and pathophysiologic scheme. I believe it is critical that the student of glaucoma be able to visualize the normal architecture of the anterior chamber angle (Figure 9-2). Moreover, such an understanding is necessary in order to delineate the mechanisms leading to a particular glaucomatous state because the therapy for glaucoma hinges on such an understanding. This chapter includes histolopathologic illustrations of some forms of glaucoma in order to assist the reader in visualizing the pathophysiology of these entities.

I.   Normal outflow
II. Impaired outflow
   A. Congenital glaucoma
   B. Primary glaucoma
     1. Angle closure
       a. With pupillary block
       b. Without pupillary block
     2. Open-angle
   C. Secondary glaucoma
     1. Angle-closure
       a. With pupillary block
       b. Without pupillary block
     2. Open-angle

As stated previously, the above classification system depends on a thorough understanding of the examination of the anterior chamber angle through gonioscopy. Although various means have been proposed to estimate anterior chamber angle depth including the flashlight test and van Herick's test,[5] these methods are inadequate for examination of the patient suspected of having glaucoma.[6,7] For this reason, the reader is strongly encouraged to read the chapter on gonioscopy before attempting an understanding of the various forms of glaucoma.

NORMAL OUTFLOW
Hypersecretion Glaucoma

Hypersecretion glaucoma was described by Becker and associates in 1956.[8] Patients are said to be mostly middle-aged women who exhibit elevated IOP accompanied by a normal outflow facility. This is probably an extremely rare entity and some individuals even question its existence.

IMPAIRED OUTFLOW
Congenital Glaucoma

Congenital glaucoma is discussed in Chapter 10 and will not be discussed in detail in this chapter. Individuals with congenital glaucoma have a characteristic histologic appearance to the chamber angle illustrated in Figure 9-3 and characterized by deLuise and Anderson[9]:

1. An anterior insertion of the iris on the ciliary body but an open angle.
2. The presence of a perforate trabecular meshwork with thicker than normal trabecular beams.

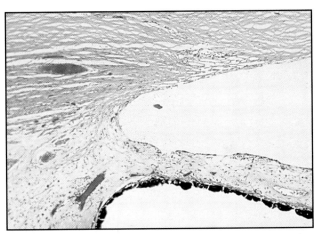

Figure 9-2. Photomicrograph of normal open anterior chamber angle. Blood is present in Schlemm's canal.

3. Internally patent intertrabecular spaces with compression and lack of intertrabecular space of the more externally located trabecular sheets.
4. An amorphous material in the subendothelial region of Schlemm's canal.
5. Decreased numbers of Holmberg vacuoles on the endothelium of Schlemm's canal.
6. The presence of iris processes (pectinate ligaments).
7. A poorly developed scleral spur resulting in longitudinal fibers of ciliary muscle passing through to insert directly onto the trabecular meshwork.
8. Anteriorly displaced ciliary processes, which are pulled inward secondary to an enlarging globe but a static sized lens.
9. Finally, a compact mass of compressed trabecular tissue is found near the anterior chamber surface of the trabecular meshwork, which tends to give the appearance of being imperforate on light microscopy.

It should be understood, however, that the embryologic considerations related to congenital glaucoma have importance relative to other forms of glaucoma, particularly secondary glaucoma. We will refer to them again as these types of glaucoma are discussed.

Primary Glaucoma

Primary Angle-Closure Glaucoma (PACG)

In PACG, the iris contacts the filtering trabecular meshwork obstructing the egress of aqueous through

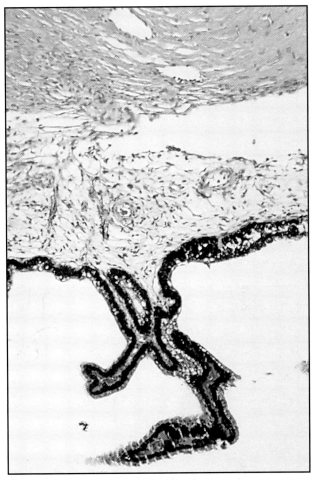

Figure 9-3. Photomicrograph of "embryologic" configuration of the anterior chamber angle. Note anteriorly placed ciliary processes, tissue in the chamber angle, and anomalous insertion of ciliary muscle.

the trabeculum (a recent review presents an historical overview of angle-closure glaucoma).[10] The process can be likened to bringing one's hand closer and closer to a drain through which water is leaving a sink or bathtub. Although the hand may start at a variable distance from the drain opening, at some distance a breakpoint is reached at which the flowing water rapidly draws the hand downward, thereby occluding the outflow of water. A similar mechanism pertains in PACG. In the latter, the iris comes in close approximation to the trabecular meshwork where it finally is drawn in tight opposition thereby obstructing aqueous outflow and resulting in a precipitous rise in IOP (Figure 9-4).

PACG can be further subclassified depending upon whether the underlying mechanism involves pupillary block or whether it is on the basis of a

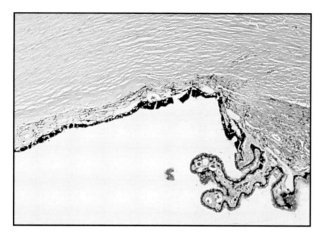

Figure 9-4. Histologic appearance of angle-closure. Note diffuse approximation of the iris to the posterior cornea in this example of chronic angle-closure.

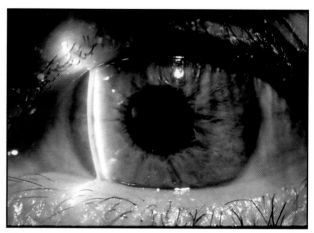

Figure 9-5. Slit-lamp photograph illustrates diffuse shallowing of the anterior chamber secondary to typical pupillary block.

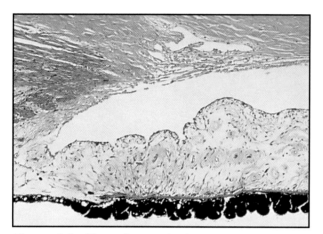

Figure 9-6. Photomicrograph demonstrates histologic appearance of uniformly narrowed angle secondary to pupillary block.

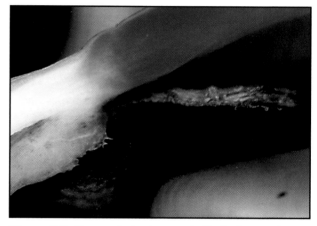

Figure 9-7. Gross photomicrograph illustrating a plateau configuration to the peripheral iris.

plateau iris configuration. In the former case, relative resistance to the passage of aqueous humor between the iris and lens results in a uniform anterior bowing of the iris as a result of increased posterior chamber aqueous pressure secondary to this relative pupillary block (Figure 9-5). Affected patients tend to have a uniformly anteriorly bowed iris contour resulting in a uniformly shallow anterior chamber (Figure 9-6). In contrast, individuals with plateau iris syndrome have an odd iris contour resembling a horizontally oriented hockey stick (Figure 9-7). The anterior chamber appears deep centrally on slit lamp examination, however, the peripheral chamber abruptly shallows near the inlet to the anterior chamber angle (Figure 9-8). In these patients, the iris contour draws it against the trabecular meshwork when the pupil dilates even though

there is no extensive pupillary block. In these individuals, angle-closure may occur on pupillary dilation even in the presence of a patent iridectomy/iridotomy. [11,12] This characteristic is not surprising because iridotomy eliminates pupillary block, which is not the primary mechanism in these individuals. Wand and associates have distinguished the syndrome from the similar-appearing plateau configuration. They state that the latter entity responds favorably to iridotomy. [13] Ultrasound biomicroscopy is discussed in more detail in Chapter 5. It has demonstrated that eyes with plateau iris syndrome have anteriorly placed ciliary processes, which support the peripheral iris in an anteriorly displaced location even after iridotomy is performed (Figure 9-9). [14,15]

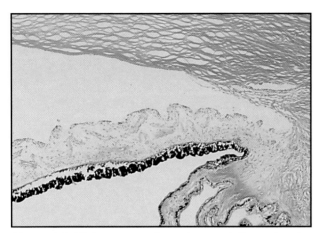

Figure 9-8. Higher power photomicrograph illustrating the histologic appearance of plateau iris configuration. The anterior chamber is relatively deep but narrows significantly at the chamber angle.

Pupillary block is the most common mechanism for PACG in white patients. Nevertheless, plateau iris may be of particular significance in blacks who develop chronic angle-closure, which may be misdiagnosed as chronic open-angle glaucoma.[16]

The ultrasound biomicroscope also has been shown to be useful in delineating the pathophysiology of pupillary block PACG (see Chapter 5).[17] The initial stage of angle-closure appears to be secondary to increased pressure in the posterior chamber resulting in iris bombe. Kondo and colleagues performed ultrasound biomicroscopic examination on the anterior segments of 32 individuals with narrow anterior chamber angles who were subjected to a prone provocative test.[18] Ten eyes of six patients exhibited elevated IOP during the test. The ultrasound biomicroscope, however, demonstrated that their irises exhibited a markedly convex configuration although their anterior chamber angles initially remained open. Thus, no angle-closure could be demonstrated at the time of initial IOP rise accompanying the prone provocative test implying that the pressure rise was on the basis of elevated pressure in the posterior chamber. The dark-room prone-position test has been recommended by some authors as a useful means of estimating the contribution of pupillary block component in angle-closure eyes prior to laser iridotomy.[19]

The sudden rise in IOP accompanying PACG presents a striking clinical picture (Figure 9-10). Patients typically complain of severe ocular pain. The eye is markedly injected, the cornea is hazy secondary to corneal edema, and the pupil is fixed and mid-dilat-

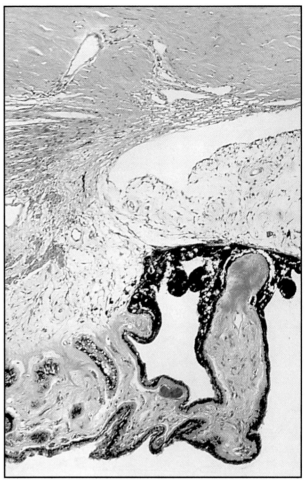

Figure 9-9. Photomicrograph reveals aberrant anterior ciliary processes closely approximated to the posterior peripheral iris. Such ciliary processes may contribute to plateau iris configuration.

ed as a result of sphincter ischemia. Secondary iris atrophy may be seen after the acute attack (Figure 9-11). Lens damage resulting from the attack is reflected in anterior lens opacities, glaukomflecken (Figure 9-12).[20] There may be severe systemic symptoms mimicking an abdominal or even a cardiac emergency.[21] In the latter instances, PACG may present with symptoms that distract the clinician from the primary diagnosis. Conversely, the presence of a severe systemic illness, particularly one requiring general anesthesia and intensive care, may mask the presence of PACG.[22]

Siriwardena and associates found that in only 39.5% of cases of PACG was the diagnosis correctly made by the referring clinician resulting in a mean delay in diagnosis of 5.8 days.[23] These authors noted that general practitioners were most likely to have dif-

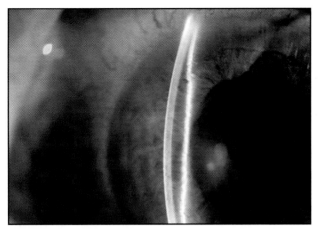

Figure 9-10. Clinical photograph of angle-closure attack. Iris is bowed anteriorly by pupillary block. Ocular and systemic symptoms typically are seen. Courtesy of Ali Aminlari, MD, FACS.

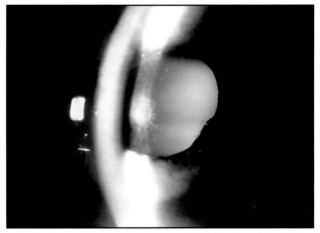

Figure 9-11. Clinical photograph of iris atrophy secondary to angle-closure. Courtesy of Ali Aminlari, MD, FACS.

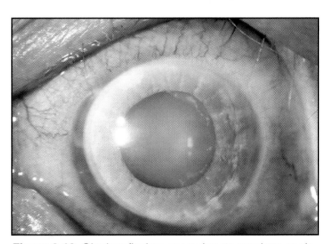

Figure 9-12. Glaukomflecken secondary to previous angle-closure attack. Courtesy of Ali Aminlari, MD, FACS.

ficulty in making the diagnosis. The importance of timely referral to a vision specialist for any patients with a subjective reduction in vision and a red eye also has been emphasized.[24]

In their extensive review of the epidemiology of PACG, Congdon and colleagues pointed out that PACG comprises approximately the same percentage of glaucoma among Asians and Inuits as does primary open-angle glaucoma (POAG) among white populations (75% to 95%).[25] The prevalence of PACG among Inuits has been reported as 2% to 8% compared to 0.1% among whites.[25] An increased prevalence of angle-closure among Inuits is associated with female sex and advancing age.[26,27] Similarly, an incidence of angle-closure of 12.2 per 100,000 per year among individuals aged 30 or more years was detected in a prospective, island-wide incidence study in Singapore.[28] Chinese ethnic origin, age of 60 years or more, and female sex all were associated with an increased risk of angle-closure.

An incidence of PACG of 8.3 per 100,000 individuals aged 40 years or older was noted in a retrospective study in Olmstead County, Minnesota.[29] The probability of monocular blindness was 14% at the time of diagnosis and had a 5-year probability of 4% for those not monocularly blind at diagnosis. The prevalence of PACG is particularly high among individuals in Mongolia who had a prevalence of 1.4% of PACG (approximately one third the prevalence of POAG) and of 6.4% of occludable angles.[30] A similar high prevalence of occludable angles has been found in Vietnamese individuals. In one study, 47.8% of

those 55 years of older had grade 0 to 2 angles and 8.5% had grade 0 to 1 angles.[31]

In a non-selected white population aged 55 years or older subjected to a screening examination involving mydriasis with 0.5% tropicamide and 5% phenylephrine, Wolfe and associates detected a prevalence of narrow angles of 2.2%. Only two individuals (0.03%) developed angle-closure glaucoma; however, 0.5% thymoxamine drops were administered after the examinations to reverse mydriasis.[32] Similarly, Patel and associates emphasized the extremely low rate of PACG immediately following ocular screening examinations.[33] The prevalence of narrow angles was twice as high in women as men. Others, however, have criticized various aspects of the report, and have questioned the relationship between screening and even gonioscopic angle examination and the prediction of subsequent angle-closure attacks.[34,35] Rarely, PACG has been reported in children.[36]

PACG can be associated particularly with the use of parasympatholytic medications and with sympathomimetics. These medications need not be topically applied ocular medications. Other medications also have been associated with PACG.[37-43] As an example, angle-closure accompanying systemic administration of atropine during cardiac catheterization has been reported.[44] angle-closure also has been associated with substance abuse of cocaine, which can cause mydriasis.[45]

Individuals with a predisposition to acute angle-closure from a pupillary block mechanism have been described as having a characteristic configuration to their ocular anterior segments. Such eyes tend to have smaller corneal diameters, a smaller corneal radius of curvature, shorter axial length, and decreased anterior chamber depth compared to normal eyes.[46-52] It must be remembered that these are not independent variables and are interrelated. The ratio of lens thickness to ocular axial length is one way to express the relationship between these two variables.[52-54] An increased lens thickness/ocular axial length ratio is found in angle-closure patients.[52-54]

When axial length and anterior chamber depth (including corneal thickness) were compared between patients who had experienced angle-closure and a control group, anterior chamber depth of less than 2.70 mm was found to be the most sensitive (94%) and specific (93%) parameter differentiating acute PACG patients from nonglaucomatous controls.[55] Similarly, Congdon and associates have performed biometry on Chinese, white, and black populations to test the hypothesis that Chinese have shallower anterior chambers than do whites.[56] Surprisingly, mean anterior chamber depth and axial length did not differ significantly among the three groups examined. Sawada and colleagues have suggested that there are differences in topological features between the fellow eyes of individuals with a history of angle-closure and anatomically narrow angles of individuals who have not had angle-closure in either eye.[57,58] The pathophysiologic relationships of these narrow angle configurations to the development of PACG have not yet been determined.

Talluto and colleagues reported elderly identical twins with simultaneous angle-closure.[59] The authors emphasized the increased risk of angle-closure in individuals having a first-degree relative with acute angle-closure and suggested screening of these individuals for occludable angles.

The strong association between PACG and pseudoexfoliation (PXE) syndrome recently has been reviewed extensively.[60] Occludable angles have been found in 9% to over 21% of patients with PXE.[61,62] Abnormal lens mobility may be one mechanism predisposing to angle-closure in individuals with PXE.[63] As Ritch has emphasized, it is most important that gonioscopy be performed in all patients with elevated IOP, particularly in the presence of PXE, because patients with PXE may present with extremely high pressures even in the absence of angle-closure. Conversely, as already noted, these patients have an increased incidence of angle-closure. Only careful gonioscopy can properly discern the mechanism and appropriate treatment for these patients.[60]

Angle-closure has been associated with childhood cystinosis in which the typical crystals may thicken the iris and, presumably, precipitate the attack in that manner.[64] Iridoschisis[65] and Fuchs dystrophy also are associated with angle-closure.[66,67]

The treatment of PACG is discussed further in Chapter 12, which includes laser therapy for glaucoma. It suffices to say here that Nd:YAG laser iridotomy has become the standard treatment for this entity[68] and is equally successful as surgical iridectomy.[69,70] Prophylactic laser iridotomy also is the preferred treatment for the fellow eye following an initial attack of PACG, although topical pilocarpine may be used as a temporizing treatment if iridotomy must be delayed.[71-73] Prophylactic iridotomy also should be considered for individuals with dangerously narrow angles who have not yet had an acute attack.[74,75] Laser iridotomy should never be performed hastily as significant complications, including malignant glaucoma,[76] have been reported from the procedure.[68] The reader is referred to the discussion by Wilensky and associates on the risks and benefits of prophylactic laser iridectomy.[77] Argon laser peripheral iridoplasty may be helpful in special situations involving angle-closure.[78]

Primary Open-Angle Glaucoma (POAG)

Overall, POAG is present in 2% to 3% of Americans, however, the prevalence increases with age so that 5% of individuals 75 years of age or older have POAG.[4] It usually is bilateral, although involvement may be asymmetric. POAG is the most frequently encountered form of glaucoma in whites (75% to 95%), however, it is much less common among Inuits and Asians in whom PACG comprises 80% to 90% of the glaucoma.[25] Considerable racial variability exists regarding the prevalence of POAG even within the United States. Black Americans have been found to have a four to five times greater prevalence of POAG than whites in the Baltimore Eye Survey.[79] In that study, over 11% of black individuals were affected by glaucoma by age 80 years.[79]

Once the presence of characteristic glaucomatous optic nerve cupping and visual field loss have confirmed the presence of glaucoma, the specific diagnosis of POAG is one of exclusion that requires a complete ocular examination to exclude angle-closure or findings suggestive of secondary glaucoma. Such an examination should include:

- Slit-lamp evaluation for the presence of pigment dispersion syndrome, pseudoexfoliation, etc
- Gonioscopic examination to document that the anterior chamber angle is open and free of neovascularization, recession, or other findings suggesting secondary glaucoma
- A thorough posterior segment examination to exclude retinal detachment, debris in the vitreous, etc.

One also must be aware that there is considerable diurnal IOP fluctuation, particularly in individuals with POAG and ocular hypertension.[80,81] Thus, POAG patients in whom the IOP is measured later in the day may erroneously be classified as normal pressure glaucoma, particularly if the pressure is measured in the early afternoon.[80] The early morning rise in IOP seen in some POAG patients may be extremely brief in duration.[82] Moreover, ocular hypertension and POAG patients are more likely to display erratic IOP diurnal pressure curves without a diurnal rhythm.[81,83]

Systemic abnormalities including arterial hypertension[84] and coagulation disorders[85,86] have been associated with POAG. Nevertheless, progression of POAG has been associated with lower systolic blood pressure both during the day and at night.[87]

POAG is a familial disease. Positive family history is present in 50% of patients with POAG.[88] Georopoulos and associates followed 345 untreated glaucoma suspects with ocular hypertension for a period of 6 to 8 years.[84] They found that progression to glaucoma was significantly associated with a family history of glaucoma. Recently, research in the field of molecular genetics has yielded exciting results on the genetic basis of glaucoma. Damji and Allingham have suggested that future classification schemes for glaucoma will be by a system based on genetic causes.[89] The reader is referred to Chapter 2 for additional information on the genetic aspects of glaucoma.

The pathophysiology leading to decreased aqueous outflow is not certain in POAG; however, the area of the obstruction has been localized to the region of the trabecular juxtacanalicular tissue adjacent to Schlemm's canal.[90-95] Alvarado and Murphy also have postulated that abnormalities in the cul-de-sac area of the trabecular meshwork is correlated with increases resistance to aqueous outflow in POAG.[96] Various substances including plasma-derived proteins and glycosaminoglycans have been demonstrated in the aqueous outflow pathway. Their role in the functioning of that system in the normal state and in POAG has not been determined.[97-100]

Some authors have viewed the changes in the trabecular region in POAG as an accentuation of normal aging changes in this region.[101,102] One example of such a change is a decrease in the number of trabecular endothelial cells compared to similar-aged individuals.[102,103] Similarly, there is a disproportionate hyalinization and sclerosis of the scleral spur region and compaction of the uveal meshwork in POAG patients compared to age-matched individuals.[101]

In normal aging individuals, a progressive decrease in aqueous outflow facility is accompanied by a parallel reduction in aqueous production. A disproportionate decrease in aqueous outflow facility secondary to the above described premature aging changes in the trabecular region would be expected to result in increased IOP. It is, perhaps, reasonable to speculate that premature aging changes in the region of the lamina cribrosa in some individuals might predispose them to optic nerve damage, particularly in the presence of increased IOP. Further research involving tissue from individuals in the earlier stages of POAG will be required to further illuminate the pathophysiologic mechanisms in POAG.

Chapter 11 presents the decision process and drug preparations available for the medical therapy of POAG. Chapters 12 and 13 discuss the non-incisional and incisional therapies, respectively.

Secondary Glaucoma

Secondary Angle-Closure Glaucoma (SACG)

SACG can be categorized using the same mixed anatomic pathophysiologic scheme as PACG as follows:

I. SACG with pupillary block
    A. Untreated PACG
    B. Phacogenic
        1. Phacomorphic
        2. Secondary to lens subluxation or dislocation
    C. Posterior synechia induced
        1. Inflammatory
        2. Aphakic or pseudophakic pupillary block
        3. Ciliary block (malignant glaucoma)
II. SACG without pupillary block
    A. Secondary to sheet-like cellular or vascular proliferations within the anterior segment
        1. Neovascular glaucoma (rubeosis iridis)
        2. Iridocorneal endothelial (ICE) syndrome
        3. Endothelialization of the anterior chamber angle
        4. Epithelial downgrowth
        5. Stromal ingrowth
    B. Secondary to anterior displacement of anterior segment structures
        1. Postoperative failure of formation of the anterior chamber
        2. Tumor or cyst related
        3. Retinopathy of prematurity
        4. Persistent hyperplastic primary vitreous
    C. Miscellaneous
        1. Iridoschisis

Untreated PACG

Previous attacks of PACG may result in the formation of peripheral anterior synechias (see Figures 9-4 and 9-13). As noted previously, progressive synechia formation and chronic angle-closure is more frequently seen in black patients than in whites. Additionally, repeated attacks of angle-closure may damage the trabecular meshwork resulting in reduced aqueous outflow even without synechia formation.

Phacogenic

Phacomorphic Glaucoma

The gradual lens enlargement that results from the progressive addition of lens fibers with age probably plays a role in most cases of primary pupillary block angle-closure glaucoma. Additionally, sudden lens cortical swelling may accompany cortical hydration in the final stages of cortical cataract formation (Figure 9-14). In this setting, the iris is displaced anteriorly and the lens swelling also increases pupillary block. The treatment is cataract removal once the acute pressure rise is controlled. A clue to the phacomorphic component of the problem may be found in the difference in anterior chamber depth on comparing the two eyes.

Phacogenic Glaucoma Secondary to Lens Subluxation or Dislocation

In the normal anatomic situation, the lens is tethered in the posterior chamber by zonules, which limit its anterior movement. Laxity or breakage of zonules (including form trauma) permits lens movement, which in its extreme case can result in dislocation of the lens into the anterior chamber producing an inverse form of pupillary block as the pupil becomes occluded as it bows forward in contact with the posterior lens surface. In the more typical case, anterior movement of the lens occludes the pupil producing pupillary block and secondary angle-closure. Syndromes associated with such abnormal lens mobility include Marfan's and Weill-Marchesani syndromes, and homocystinuria.[104-116] As noted previously, zonular weakness and abnormal lens movement is more commonly seen in office practice in the setting of PXE syndrome. PXE syndrome may present a particularly confusing picture to the clinician because such patients may develop extremely elevated IOPs even in the absence of angle-closure.[60] Nevertheless, an occludable angle has been reported in 9.3% of PXE patients.[61] Thus, it is extremely important that the clinician be confident in the gonioscopic examination of these patients before attempting to treat the patient with PXE.

Lens subluxation is commonly associated with aniridia and may be present in 56% of such patients (Figures 9-15a and b).[117]

The individual with an abnormally mobile lens may consult the clinician because of fluctuating

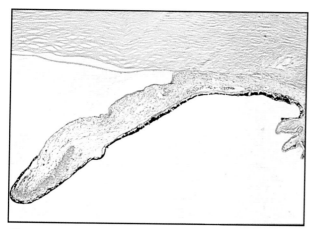

Figure 9-13. Photomicrograph illustrates peripheral anterior synechia secondary to chronic angle-closure.

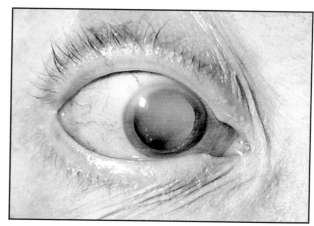

Figure 9-14. Advanced cataract such as illustrated in this clinical photograph may result in anterior iris displacement and precipitate angle-closure, particularly when such lenses become intumescent. Courtesy of Ali Aminlari, MD,

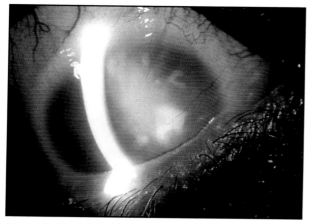

Figure 9-15a. Clinical photograph of aniridia. Lens subluxation and angle-closure frequently accompany this disorder.

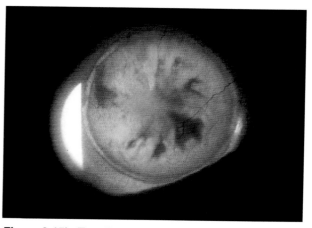

Figure 9-15b. Transillumination photograph of aniridia.

refractive error. The ocular clinician, therefore, may be helpful in making the diagnosis of these syndromes. It is particularly important that homocystinuria be recognized preoperatively in order to avoid serious and even fatal complications that may accompany anesthesia and surgery on these patients.[118-122] Early diagnosis in infancy also permits therapy of the disorder with vitamins and dietary measures, which can be helpful in reducing complications.[123]

Posterior Synechia Induced Angle-Closure Glaucoma

Posterior synechias usually are adhesions between the iris and the lens, although such adhesions may also form between the iris and vitreous face as is seen in aphakic pupillary block glaucoma. Most posterior synechias are secondary to inflammation, such as is seen in iritis, particularly that secondary to sarcoidosis. Posterior synechias also result from chronic miotic therapy, making cataract surgery particularly difficult in such patients.

The pupillary block that results from posterior synechias produces anterior bowing of the iris with resulting angle-closure. The situation produced is particularly dangerous because the underlying inflammation may contribute to the rapid formation of peripheral anterior synechias once angle-closure has occurred. Treatment, in the absence of an iris plane intraocular lens, is forceful pupillary dilation in an attempt to break the posterior synechias. Pharmacologic dilation may be supplemented by iridoplasty. Although the latter therapy risks increasing inflammation, it may be particularly helpful in the presence of an extremely shallow anterior chamber in which iridotomy risks damage to the corneal endothelium. Alternatively, laser iridotomy may be employed as the laser surgical procedure (see Chapter 12).

Ciliary Block Glaucoma (Malignant Glaucoma)

The term *malignant glaucoma* refers to the frustration experienced by earlier clinicians as they attempted to treat this difficult condition and does not indicate a neoplastic process. The correct pathophysiologically oriented name for the entity is *ciliary block glaucoma*. As the name implies, the obstruction to passage of aqueous in this disorder is at the level of the iris-ciliary body plane. It has been the subject of extensive reviews.[124-126]

The term actually refers to a process that may be precipitated by a variety of surgical procedures including cataract extraction, filtration surgery, iridectomy, and laser iridotomy. It may occur immediately following the procedure or may be delayed for many years.[127] Apparently spontaneous cases have been reported.[128-130]

The relatively minimal ocular disturbance afforded by laser iridotomy initially was hoped to be protective against malignant glaucoma; however, it has been reported following laser iridotomy, including bilateral cases.[76,131,132] Other reported precipitating events have included YAG laser posterior capsulotomy,[133] laser suture lysis accompanying filtration surgery,[134,135] and glaucoma seton surgery.[136] An unusual form of malignant glaucoma has been reported to accompany fungal corneal infections.[137-139]

The common feature in the various precipitating events for malignant glaucoma appears to be an initial shift of the anatomic relationship of the vitreous face relative to the ciliary body and the lens (if phakic). Such a shift may be precipitated by even a transient differential in the pressure relationship between the anterior and posterior chambers. Subsequently, the vitreous face obstructs the flow of aqueous between it, the lens, and the ciliary body face. As a result of this obstruction, aqueous collects within the vitreous compartment compounding the "ciliary block" by further compressing the vitreous face or lens against ciliary ring trapping additional aqueous in the vitreous compartment.[140,141]

Ultrasound biomicroscopy has confirmed the pathophysiology of this entity[142-144]; however, changes in or abnormalities in vitreous permeability may play some role in its pathogenesis.[145]

The treatment of malignant glaucoma requires reestablishing the flow of aqueous into the anterior chamber by removing the obstruction at the level of the ciliary ring. In a manner similar to the treatment for posterior synechia induced pupillary block, the initial medical therapy is cycloplegia to widen the ciliary ring, and systemic hyperosmolar agents to permit reduction in vitreous compartment volume. Ultimately, vitreous face disruption treats and prevents aqueous flow obstruction at that level. Vitreous face disruption may be accomplished in a variety of ways including YAG capsulotomy in pseudophakic patients.[146-149] Pars plana vitrectomy may be necessary if these other, less invasive measures, are unsuccessful.[150-152]

SACG Secondary to Cellular Proliferations Onto Anterior Segment Structures

Numerous cell types may proliferate on the anterior surface of the iris eventually resulting in peripheral anterior synechia formation. Ectropion uvea (displacement of the posterior pigment epithelium onto the anterior iris surface) may be a clinical indication of the proliferation the presence of such a membrane (Figures 9-16 and 9-17).

Neovascular Glaucoma (Rubeosis Iridis)

The final common pathway for aqueous outflow obstruction in neovascular glaucoma (NVG) is the proliferation of a fibrovascular membrane on the anterior iris face (see Figure 9-17) and the subsequent contraction of myofibroblastic elements within that membrane resulting in peripheral anterior synechia formation (Figure 9-18).[153] In its initial stages, prior to synechia formation, the pressure rise in NVG is secondary to an open-angle mechanism as the components of the membrane grow over and through the trabecular meshwork, although the iris is not in contact with the trabecular surface.

The common pathophysiologic inciting mechanism for the entities producing NVG is retinal ischemia (Figure 9-19). Brown and associates reviewed 208 patients with NVG.[154] Retinal venous obstructive disease was present in 36.1%, diabetic

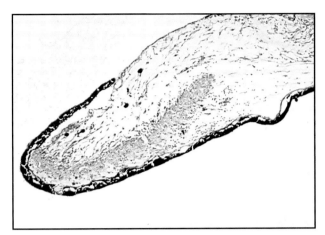

Figure 9-16. Photomicrograph of an endothelialized anterior iris membrane resulting in ectropion uveae.

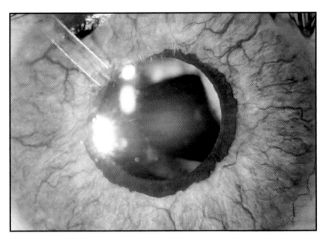

Figure 9-17. Neovascular membrane on the anterior iris surface has resulted in ectropion uveae. Note vessels on the iris surface. The accompanying fibroblastic component of the membrane often is relatively transparent but can be demonstrated by oblique illumination by the beam of the slit-lamp.

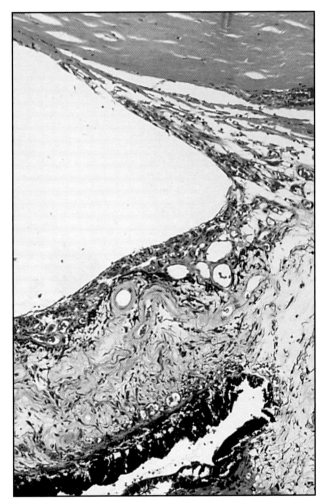

Figure 9-18. Photomicrograph of angle-closure resulting from a neovascular membrane. The synechia has broken as a fixation artifact.

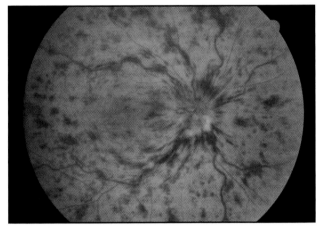

Figure 9-19. Fundus photograph of central retinal vein occlusion, a common cause of retinal ischemia resulting in neovascular glaucoma. Courtesy of David A. Quillen, MD.

retinopathy in 32.2%, and carotid artery obstructive disease in 12.9%. Systemic arterial hypertension was present in 51% and diabetes mellitus was noted in 46% of all patients. All but one of the 25 bilateral cases of NVG occurred in patients with diabetic retinopathy. Women comprised 65% of patients with NVG secondary to diabetes and 57% of the venous obstruction group, while men accounted for 74% of cases in which NVG occurred secondary to carotid artery obstructive disease. They concluded that extensive retinal ischemia was present in 97% of involved eyes. The ischemic retina is believed to produce a vasoproliferative substance that stimulates and supports vascular proliferation. Recently, this topic has been reviewed.[155-157] Other causes of NVG include chronic retinal disease, uveal melanoma, long-standing retinal detachment, previous ocular injury, and Fuchs heterochromic iridocyclitis.

A factor compounding trabecular region effects of iris neovascularization is the fact that these "new" blood vessels are extremely fragile and bleed easily. Thus, an outflow mechanism already compromised by membrane overgrowth or synechia formation may be further stressed by hyphema formation. The association of spontaneous hyphema and iris neovascularization is of particular importance in children in whom iris neovascularization is associated with retinoblastoma.[158,159] Any child presenting with "spontaneous" hyphema must be suspected of harboring an intraocular tumor until it is excluded by a thorough examination. Additionally, a more common cause of "spontaneous" hyphema in children is child abuse.[160] Other causes for such hyphemas include medulloepithelioma, iris juvenile xanthogranuloma, pseudogliomas, and blood dyscrasia.[161-166]

Iridocorneal Endothelial (ICE) Syndrome

ICE syndrome (Figure 9-20) refers to three entities—Chandler's syndrome, iris-nevus (Cogan-Reese) syndrome, and essential iris atrophy.[167-171] Each of these entities may occur with its characteristic presentation in an individual patient; however, other individuals may display significant overlap in the presentation.[167-174]

I believe that the classification by Bahn of abnormalities relating to tissues derived from neural crest is most helpful in analyzing several anterior segment glaucoma syndromes.[175] In this scheme, the ICE syndrome entities represent abnormalities of neural crest cell proliferation. The etiology for this proliferation need not be on a congenital basis. For example, some authors have suggested that herpes simplex virus infection plays an important role in pathogenesis of the endothelial proliferation noted in the ICE syndrome disorders.[176-179]

The ICE syndrome components have features in common with Axenfeld-Rieger syndrome and posterior polymorphous dystrophy (PPMD). PPMD shares the features of endothelial abnormalities on specular microscopy, corneal edema, iridocorneal adhesions, endothelialization of the anterior chamber angle, and glaucoma with the ICE syndrome. Although some authors have suggested epithelial characteristics for the cells in Chandler's syndrome,[180,181] generally, the endothelium in the ICE syndrome does not display epithelial-like characteristics, which are found in PPMD.[182] PPMD usually is familial, bilateral, and tends not to be progressive, unlike the ICE syndrome.[182]

In its pure form, the most characteristic finding in Chandler's syndrome is corneal dystrophy that may be evident even with modest IOP elevation.[183-185] Patients usually do not exhibit the iris surface nodules, iris stromal thinning, and pupillary distortion typical of other ICE syndrome entities.

In their study of 82 cases of essential iris atrophy, Shields and colleagues noted that a corneal abnormality appeared early. A corneal endothelial disturbance was present in 55% of cases, and corneal edema was present in 50%.[168] They found peripheral anterior synechias in all but one of the cases. The pupil was distorted in 71% of the cases usually in the direction of the most prominent synechia. Stromal atrophy was noted in 71%, and iris holes occurred in 33%. They concluded that the prognosis for most patients was slow progression with eventual involvement of vision because of corneal edema, secondary glaucoma, or both. In their study, treatment of increased IOP was required in 77% of the cases, and 44% required surgical intervention.

In essential iris atrophy, the initially noted clinical event is the formation of a focal peripheral anterior synechia, which may simulate an unsuspected perforating injury. Later, a full-thickness stromal hole may develop, usually in the quadrant opposite the initial peripheral anterior synechia in an area not covered by the proliferating endothelial membrane.[186] The cause for the iris stromal hole formation is not known; however, it probably is not simple traction. A vascular cause for the stromal atrophy has been supported by some[187] and disputed by others.[188,189]

Ultimately, progression of the initial peripheral anterior synechia may result in extensive angle-closure and severe glaucoma, which may require filtration surgery. Corneal transplantation also may be required and has been give a variable prognosis.[190,191]

Iris nevus (Cogan-Reese) syndrome displays synechia formation and iris stromal thinning to a much less severe degree than are noted in essential iris atrophy. The characteristic feature, however, is the presence of iris nodules and a matted or whorl-like pattern to the anterior iris surface (Figure 9-21).[174,192,193] On slit lamp examination, the iris surface is effaced and the iris nodules appear to bulge through

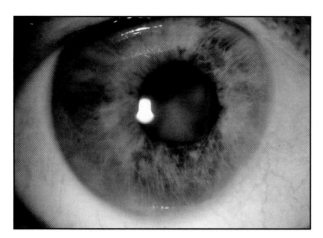

Figure 9-20. Clinical photograph of iris effacement and pupillary distortion characteristically found in ICE syndrome. Courtesy of Ali Aminlari, MD, FACS.

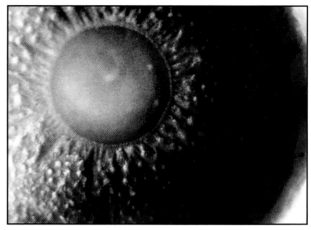

Figure 9-21. Clinical photograph of iris nodules, which are found characteristically in iris-nevus syndrome. Courtesy of Ali Aminlari, MD, FACS.

holes in the surface endothelial membrane. The changes in the iris surface may lead to a mistaken diagnosis of melanoma.

Endothelialization of the Anterior Chamber Angle

As noted previously, normal adult human corneal endothelium does not proliferate. The ICE syndrome, which already has been discussed, represents a pathologic proliferation of corneal endothelium. Endothelium also may proliferate as a reactive process most frequently seen following trauma or iris neovascularization (Figures 9-22a and b). In the latter cases, the endothelial cells may exhibit myoblastic features. [194]

Colosi and Yanoff found endothelial proliferation involving the anterior chamber angle (Figure 9-23) in 20% of enucleated globes they reviewed and noted that the process had frequently been overlooked at the time of initial histopathologic examination. [195]

Epithelial Downgrowth

Epithelial downgrowth is a very uncommon complication of ocular surgery. Its incidence was reported as 0.06% to 0.08% in two large series, with decreased vision, red eye, and pain being the most common presenting complaints. [196,197] There is probably a greater incidence of epithelial downgrowth following keratoplasty (0.27%) than following cataract surgery (0.091% to 0.11%). [198]

The epithelium usually gains access to the anterior chamber at the margin of an anterior segment surgical wound. Classically, most wounds for cataract

surgery have been made superiorly. Thus, in a typical case of epithelial downgrowth, a horizontally oriented area of endothelial haze is noted clinically to progressively migrate inferiorly on the posterior cornea. [199] These posterior corneal changes may be accompanied by chronic inflammation and, initially, by ocular hypotony. Later, severe glaucoma may develop. Corneal striae and stromal vascularization may be seen overlying the area of corneal involvement.

Epithelium can proliferate much more luxuriantly on the anterior iris than on the posterior cornea. Thus, as in the ICE syndrome and in iris neovascularization, it may initially be visualized as iris surface effacement before it is visible elsewhere. [200]

The histological counterpart of the clinical findings is a multilayered epithelial sheet proliferating on the posterior cornea, angle structures, and iris surface (Figure 9-24), and may even involve posterior segment structures. [201-203]

Factors that have been cited as predisposing to epithelial downgrowth include poor wound apposition, fistulas, postoperative hypotony, and surgical complications, such as inflammation and hemorrhage. [196,204-206]

The glaucoma in epithelial downgrowth may result from several mechanisms. Epithelial cell debris may plug the trabecular meshwork resulting in secondary open-angle glaucoma. [196] Pupillary block angle-closure glaucoma can be produced by posterior synechias formed as the epithelial sheet overgrows the pupillary margin. Ultimately, secondary angle-closure without pupillary block results from progressive

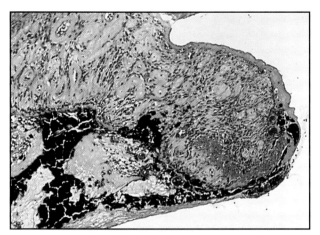

Figure 9-22a. Photomicrographs illustrate endothelialization superimposed on angle-closure secondary to a neovascular membrane.

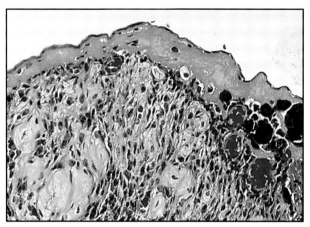

Figure 9-22b. Higher magnification of endothelialized iris neovascular membrane.

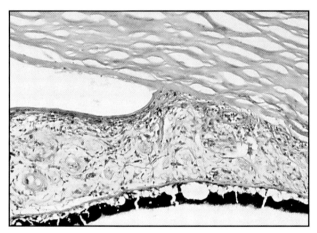

Figure 9-23. Photograph of endothelial membrane and closed angle.

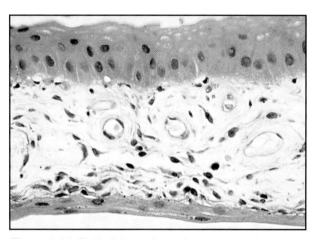

Figure 9-24. Epithelial membrane is present on the anterior iris surface in this photomicrograph of epithelial downgrowth.

peripheral anterior synechias formed by the proliferating epithelial sheet.[197]

Laser photocoagulation of the anterior iris surface may be helpful in delineating the extent of the iris sheet on the anterior iris surface. Specular microscopy also can be of assistance in the diagnosis of epithelial downgrowth.[207,208] Cytologic examination of material obtained from scraping of the inner surface of Descemet's membrane or from aspirate of aqueous humor may be helpful in substantiating the diagnosis.

The clinical progression of the glaucoma secondary to epithelial downgrowth may be variable in its course. Thus, the risks of radical surgery required to extirpate the intraocular foci of epithelium must be weighed against the benefits to be accrued to the patient.

Stromal Ingrowth

Stromal ingrowth (Figure 9-25) most frequently accompanies unsuccessful corneal transplants.[209,210] Nevertheless, it may result from other surgical procedures particularly if they have been complicated by vitreous loss and incarceration.[211,212] These membranes usually appear to represent direct proliferation of keratocytes through a dehiscence in Descemet's membrane; however, some retrocorneal fibrous membranes have been postulated to represent fibrous metaplasia of corneal endothelium.[213,214] Proliferation of this fibrous tissue over anterior segment structures may result in peripheral anterior synechias and secondary angle-closure glaucoma (Figure 9-26).

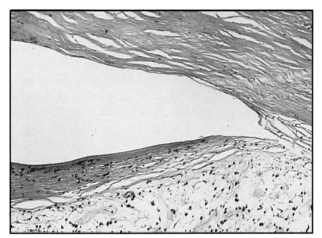

Figure 9-25. Photomicrograph demonstrates stromal ingrowth, which has separated into two component parts secondary to fixation artifact. Such membranes frequently are present in the clinical setting of a failed corneal transplant.

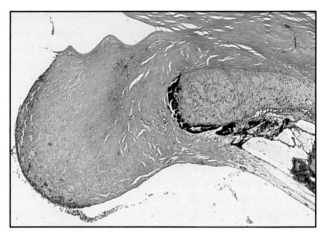

Figure 9-26. Massive stromal ingrowth has closed anterior chamber angle and has proliferated over more posterior structures.

SACG Secondary to Anterior Displacement of Anterior Segment Structures

Postoperative Failure of Anterior Chamber Reformation

Failure of the anterior chamber to reform most frequently results from glaucoma surgery either filtration procedures[215] or seton operations.[216,217] This surgical complication is particularly likely to occur if adjunctive antimetabolites are employed at the time of surgery.[218-220] The common feature of these procedures is the presence of overfiltration or wound leaks.[215-217,221] Viscoelastic agents and releasable sutures help prevent overfiltration in the immediate postoperative period and have helped decrease the incidence of flat or delayed anterior chamber reformation.[222-227] The clinician must be cognizant of the fact that anterior chamber shallowing following intraocular surgery may be secondary to aqueous misdirection and resulting malignant glaucoma.[228-231]

If delayed anterior chamber reformation is not corrected promptly, peripheral anterior synechias usually are produced (see Figure 9-4). Additionally, hypotony may result in cilio-choroidal "detachment" (actually an effusion).[232] The decreased posterior segment volume secondary to the cilio-choroidal detachment results in anterior displacement of the iris-lens diaphragm thereby compounding the anterior chamber shallowing. The cilio-choroidal detachment may require surgical drainage if it fails to resolve in a reasonable period of time or if it contributes to other

complications. Similarly, corneal-lens contact secondary to anterior chamber shallowing usually requires immediate surgical correction to prevent cataract formation.[233,234]

Iris and Ciliary Body Cysts

The iris-lens diaphragm may be displaced anteriorly by cysts of the iris and anterior ciliary body thereby shallowing or closing the anterior chamber angle (Figure 9-27). This complication is particularly likely to occur if the cysts are multiple.[235] The cysts may be idiopathic or may be secondary to entities such as trauma or late syphilitic interstitial keratitis.[236-238] Primary cysts tend to be stationary; however, this is not universally true.[238,239] The ultrasound biomicroscope is useful in delineating these cysts,[240] which frequently are misdiagnosed as anterior segment melanomas.[241]

In addition to angle-closure secondary to cyst formation, late syphilitic interstitial keratitis also may be associated with angle-closure secondary to peripheral anterior synechia formation.[236,242,243]

Intraocular Tumors

Yanoff has demonstrated that intraocular tumors, if large, may displace the iris-lens diaphragm anteriorly in a manner similar to that of iris and ciliary body cysts.[244] Any other accompanying abnormality, such as a retinal detachment, that decreases the volume of the ocular posterior compartment further compounds the anterior chamber shallowing. The presence of

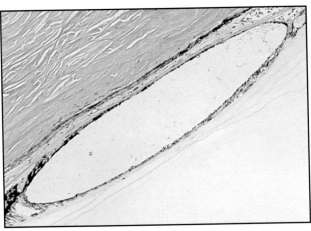

Figure 9-27. Photomicrograph of a relatively small cyst of the pars plana. When very large, such cysts may displace the iris-lens diaphragm anteriorly resulting in angle-closure.

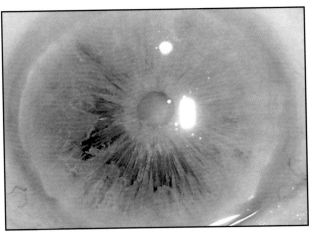

Figure 9-28. Clinical photograph of deterioration of anterior iris in iridoschisis.

inflammation, iris neovascularization, etc, may result in posterior synechias and secondary pupillary block angle-closure. Large tumors also may be associated with angle-closure secondary to rubeosis iridis or on a phacomorphic basis secondary to cataract formation. Iris thickening from lesions that diffusely infiltrate the iris may thicken the peripheral iris enough to close the angle.

Retinopathy of Prematurity (ROP) and Persistent Hyperplastic Primary Vitreous

ROP may be associated with progressive anterior segment crowding resulting in secondary angle-closure.[245] In a small series, significant peripheral anterior synechias were found in 12% of eyes with stage IV or V ROP.[246] Unsuspected glaucoma may be a cause of decreased vision in severe ROP.[247]

Anterior segment crowding may be progressive with age in ROP. Thus, adult individuals with a history of ROP should have periodic examinations for glaucoma.[245]

Persistent hyperplastic primary vitreous (PHPV) is a congenital ocular disorder. It is characterized by microphthalmos, cataract, and leukocoria.[248] Progressive cataract formation may contribute to angle-closure. Lensectomy may help prevent glaucoma in PHPV.[249] Organization of intraocular hemorrhages may involve anterior segment structures and secondary iridocorneal adhesions.

Miscellaneous

Iridoschisis

Iridoschisis is a bilateral condition involving elderly men and women (Figure 9-28). It is characterized by the formation of a cleft within the iris stroma, particularly involving the inferior one half of the iris. Initially, the stromal fibers remain attached at the pupil and iris periphery. Later, the fibers become detached at one end, which is seen to float free in the anterior chamber. Pupillary distortion is not a prominent feature, unlike the ICE syndrome. Glaucoma develops in 50% of patients secondary to peripheral anterior synechia formation.

The iridoschisis has been associated with primary angle-closure glaucoma.[65] Familial cases have been reported and it may be associated with trauma, keratoconus, syphilitic interstitial keratitis, and microphthalmos.[250-255]

No vascular or neural abnormalities have been demonstrated on histopathologic examination of affected tissue, however, stromal atrophy has been noted.[256]

Secondary Open-Angle Glaucoma (SOAG)

SOAG is characterized by the presence of an angle that is open on gonioscopic examination. There is decreased aqueous outflow as a result of pathophysiologic mechanisms other than POAG. This chapter discusses selected entities causing SOAG and, for the sake of clarity, they will be illustrated in their pure forms. The classification scheme utilized for SOAG attempts to cluster entities with similar pathophysiologic mechanisms.

SOAG can be classified as follows:

I. SOAG caused by cells or debris in the anterior chamber angle
    A. Hyphema
    B. Uveitis
        1. Glaucomatocyclitic crisis (Posner-Schlossman syndrome)
        2. Fuchs heterochromic iridocyclitis
    C. Pigment dispersion syndrome (PDS) and pigmentary glaucoma
    D. Pseudoexfoliation glaucoma
    E. Hemolytic and "ghost cell" glaucoma
    F. Phacolytic glaucoma
    G. Nondenatured lens material-induced glaucoma
    H. Melanomalytic or melanocytomalytic glaucoma
    I. Tumor seeding of the trabecular meshwork
    J. Schwartz-Matsuo syndrome
II. SOAG caused by damaged outflow channels
    A. Previous uveitis
    B. Blunt trauma
    C. Repeated hyphema
    D. Siderosis and hemosiderosis oculi
    E. Repeated attacks of acute angle-closure glaucoma
    F. Early rubeosis or other anterior segment cellular proliferative disorder
III. SOAG caused by corneoscleral and extraocular disease
    A. Interstitial keratitis
    B. Orbital venous thrombosis
    C. Encircling element following retinal disease
    D. Retrobulbar mass
    E. Leukemia
    F. Mediastinal mass
IV. SOAG secondary to miscellaneous causes
    A. Steroid-induced glaucoma
    B. Alpha-chymotrypsin glaucoma

Hyphema

Hyphema refers to blood within the anterior chamber (Figure 9-29). Hypopyon is inflammatory debris (pus) in the anterior chamber. Hyphema most frequent-

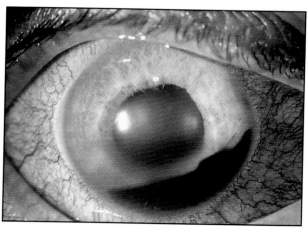

Figure 9-29. Clinical photograph of hyphema, blood in the anterior chamber.

ly is found secondary to trauma or iris neovascularization. In its early stages, iris neovascularization produces SOAG due to membrane overgrowth of angle structures without causing iris-trabecular apposition. Later, however, the myofibroblasts within the fibrovascular membrane found in rubeosis iridis cause mechanical distortion of anterior segment structures and SACG with peripheral anterior synechias.[153] Posterior synechias, such as to the anterior lens, also may result in SACG from a pupillary block mechanism.

In order to understand the mechanism for ocular damage from blunt trauma, and particularly the mechanism for hyphema formation, one must recall that the eye is a fluid-filled sphere. Compression of the cornea at the instant of blunt trauma sets up a shock wave the propagates throughout the eye. We already have discussed its possible effect of lens dislocation as contributing to SACG. One of its initial points of impact is in the anterior chamber angle. The force may cause scarring within the trabecular meshwork resulting in SOAG. If sufficiently forceful, the shock wave lacerates into the anterior face of the ciliary body tearing the anterior arterial circle (recession of the anterior chamber angle is a marker for such severe trauma). Thus, blood under arterial pressure is released into the anterior chamber. Initially, the blood may obstruct the trabecular meshwork severely compromising aqueous outflow (Figure 9-30). Later, as the clot undergoes dissolution, red blood cell debris and the macrophages that engulf it also may plug the trabeculum resulting in hemolytic glaucoma. Similarly, "ghost" degenerated red blood cells from a vitreous hemorrhage may obstruct the trabecular meshwork after they gain

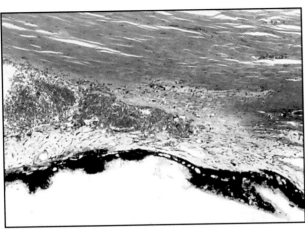

Figure 9-30. Photograph of blood filling the anterior chamber angle.

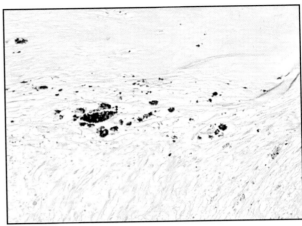

Figure 9-31. Prussian blue stain demonstrates iron, which is toxic to trabecular structures and may result in SOAG.

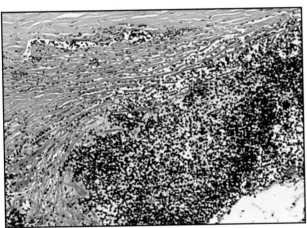

Figure 9-32. Red blood cells and their debris fill the trabecular meshwork in this photomicrograph.

access to the anterior chamber through a disrupted vitreous face.[257,258] Iron released by the hemoglobin acts as an enzymatic poison to anterior segment structures including the trabecular meshwork, thereby providing another compromise to aqueous outflow (Figure 9-31). Finally, organization of the hyphema may result in SACG.

Several days following the initial injury, spontaneous rebleeding, which may occur more frequently in black individuals,[259-264] may repeat the cycle leading to further trabecular compromise.[265-268] Rebleeding has a poorer visual prognosis, particularly in children.[269] Trabecular scarring may follow recurrent hyphema.

Black patients with sickle cell disease are at particular risk to develop visual loss secondary to ischemic optic neuropathy during IOP rise in hyphema.[270] Moreover, such patients are more likely to experience elevated IOP associated with hyphema, because sickled red blood cells pass poorly through the trabecular meshwork (Figure 9-32).[271-273]

Apparent spontaneous hyphema in children must be viewed with great skepticism as, most frequently, such cases represent occult trauma, particularly child abuse.[160,274] Other important causes of spontaneous hyphema in children include juvenile xanthogranuloma,[275] retinoblastoma,[158,276,277] and medulloepithelioma.[165,278]

The most severe form of hyphema is the "black ball," the clot of which is composed of concentric layers of fibrin lacking fibroblastic or neovascular proliferations.[279]

Elevated IOP at the time of hyphema may result in corneal "blood staining." The key factor in corneal susceptibility to this complication, however, is the health of the endothelium. Thus, blood staining has been reported in the presence of relatively low IOP if the endothelium is compromised.[280] Corneal blood staining is caused by the passage of red blood cell debris and hemoglobin through the endothelial barrier into the stroma (Figure 9-33).[281,282] The presence of porphyrins accompanying corneal blood staining has been postulated to sensitize the tissues to photic damage thereby contributing to keratocyte and endothelial damage.[283,284]

Uveitis

Uveitis may result in glaucoma through several mechanisms. We have discussed SACG as a result posterior synechias causing iris bombe. Inflammatory

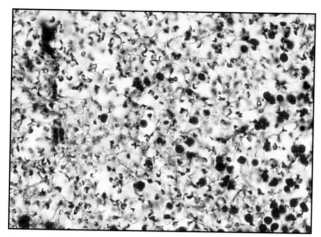

Figure 9-33. Photomicrograph compares the relative sizes of whole red blood cells, and degenerated cells and hemoglobin debris. It is the fragments of red blood cells and hemoglobin that result in corneal blood staining.

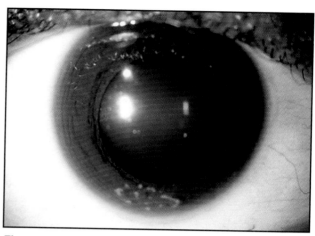

Figure 9-34a. Clinical photograph demonstrates inflammatory precipitates on the inferior cornea.

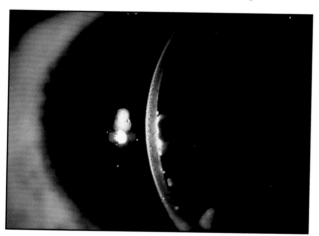

Figure 9-34b. Clinical photograph demonstrates inflammatory precipitates on the inferior cornea.

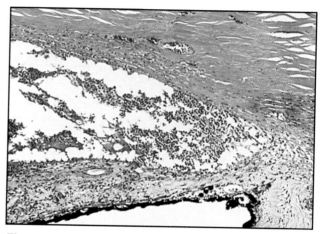

Figure 9-34c. Photomicrograph of inflammatory cells in the anterior chamber angle. Such inflammatory debris may obstruct the trabecular meshwork.

cells and debris may plug the trabecular meshwork (Figure 9-34, a-c). Moreover, trabeculitis, such as that in sarcoidosis, may decrease trabecular function resulting in SOAG. Chronic or recurrent inflammation may cause trabecular scarring thereby decreasing aqueous outflow.[285] Finally, topical or systemic steroids for the treatment of uveitis may cause SOAG in "steroid responders."

The clinician must be aware that aqueous production usually is decreased secondary to intraocular inflammation. Thus, IOP may be normal or even decreased even if aqueous outflow is decreased. Later, recovery of aqueous production following the reversal of the inflammatory process may result in increased IOP reflecting damage to the aqueous drainage mechanism.[285]

SOAG may be seen as a result of low-grade chronic anterior uveitis in oculodermal melanocytosis. The melanocytosis also may contribute to aqueous outflow obstruction.

Two specific inflammatory syndromes associated with SOAG will be discussed—glaucomatocyclitic crisis and Fuchs heterochromic iridocyclitis.

Glaucomatocyclitic Crisis (Posner-Schlossman Syndrome)

This syndrome originally was designated the "syndrome of glaucomatocyclitic crises" thereby emphasizing the recurrent nature of the entity.[286,287] It usually is unilateral, in adults, in the third through fifth decades. During attacks, which may be hours to weeks in duration, IOP may rise to 40 to 60 mmHg. As a result, patients may note halos around lights and may experience decreased vision from corneal edema. The pupil may be mildly dilated during the attack.

During the attack, discomfort usually is minimal as is the inflammatory reaction, which may consist of a few fine keratic precipitates on slit-lamp examination. Later, the precipitates can become "mutton fat" in appearance. The angle appears normal to gonioscopic examination. Aqueous outflow facility is decreased and aqueous production has been reported to be elevated during attacks. Following these acute episodes, the IOP may decrease to below normal levels. There may be a persistent elevation of IOP and decreased outflow facility following the resolution of the acute episode. Glaucomatous optic nerve damage is not characteristic; nevertheless, cupping may occur and has required filtration surgery.

Posner-Schlossman syndrome has been associated with POAG.[288,289] Theories as to the cause of the entity include a developmental anomaly of the anterior chamber angle, abnormal prostaglandin production, and herpes simplex virus infection.[290-294]

Decreased corneal endothelial cell count has been demonstrated in individuals with recurrent attacks of Posner-Schlossman syndrome.[295]

Fuchs Heterochromic Iridocyclitis (FHI)

In 1906, Fuchs described 38 cases and summarized previously reported patients characterized by heterochromia (difference in iris color on comparing each eye) and cataract.[296] This syndrome is known as FHI.[297-299] Other characteristic features include stromal atrophy with the involved eye tending to be hypochromic relative to the fellow eye. Later, increased visibility of the iris pigment epithelium may result in the involved iris appearing darker than the fellow eye. Mild iritis with fine keratic precipitates, iris muscle atrophy, and mydriasis also may be observed. Iris crystals and a possible increased frequency of subconjunctival hemorrhage also have been reported in the syndrome.[300,301] Goble and Murray have suggested an association between FHI and sarcoidosis.[302]

The most frequent presenting complaint in one study was decreased vision (96.1%).[303] Only 18.2% complained of pain. FHI was the initial diagnosis in 50.6% at presentation. Heterochromia was noted in

70.1% and was bilateral in 15.6% of patients. Cataract was present in 73% and 40.4% had cataract surgery by the time of presentation (Figure 9-35). Glaucoma was diagnosed in 15.7% at presentation and in 21.3% at review, by which time 9% of the total had required filtration surgery.[303]

The high prevalence of filtration surgery in the above study supports the commonly held belief that glaucoma is particularly difficult to control in FHI. Further support for this belief was found by La Hey and associates who found that 27% of those with FHI in their study had glaucoma, and filtration surgery was required in 73% of those with glaucoma.[304]

The cause of FHI has not been established. Iris perfusion defects and leakage of iris vessels on fluorescein angiography are among the iris vascular anomalies that have been noted in FHI.[305] As a result of these findings, anterior segment ischemia has been suggested as one cause of FHI.[305] Norrsell and colleagues confirmed that leaking iris blood vessels rather than iris atrophy was the probable source of the anterior chamber flare.[306] Immunological studies on samples of aqueous humor have confirmed the presence of abnormalities in these patients.[307,308]

Iris neovascularization may be present and may give rise to the filiform hemorrhage seen during cataract surgery in these patients. Unlike the forms of iris neovascularization previously described in this chapter, that associated with FHI tends to be non-progressive and does not tend to result in extensive PAS formation. Nevertheless, it may give rise to the filiform hemorrhage characteristic of the disorder, and frequently precipitated by intraocular surgery. Such hemorrhage usually is self-limited and of no clinical significance. Iris and filtering angle neovascularization combined with trabeculitis are thought to result in the associated glaucoma.[309]

Intractable glaucoma has been reported secondary to posterior capsulotomy in one patient with this disorder.[310] The eye had been free of inflammation and glaucoma for 27 years prior to the procedure.

Pigment Dispersion Syndrome (PDS) and Pigmentary Glaucoma (PG)

PDS classically is found in young adult, male myopes.[311,312] It was noted in 10% of white and black subjects with and without glaucoma.[313] PDS is the subject of a recent review.[314]

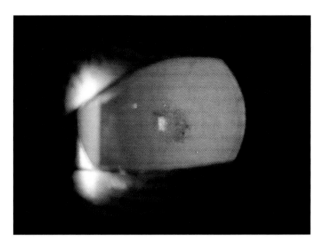

Figure 9-35. Clinical photograph of cataract, which is a frequent finding in Fuchs heterochromic iridocyclitis.

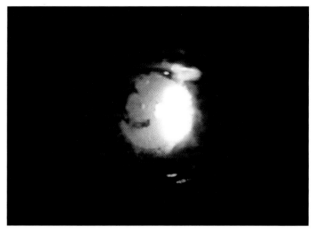

Figure 9-36. Iris transillumination is present in pigmentary glaucoma. Courtesy of Ali Aminlari, MD, FACS.

PDS is characterized by disruption of iris pigment epithelium resulting in typical iris transillumination at the junction of the inner two thirds with the outer one third of the iris, which is demonstrable on slit-lamp examination (Figure 9-36). A band of increased granular iris pigmentation overlies the ring of increased iris transillumination and is believed to be caused by many pigment-laden macrophages within this area of iris stroma. Iridodonesis may be present. The trabecular meshwork is heavily pigmented on gonioscopic examination (Figure 9-37). The presence of zonular and peripheral lenticular pigmentation have been cited as helpful diagnostic findings for PDS in blacks, particularly when classic findings are absent.[315]

Another typical finding in PDS is the presence of a Krukenberg's spindle, which is a vertically oriented column of pigment on and in central and inferior corneal endothelium (Figure 9-38). Significant deposits of pigment also are found on the iris surface, lens, zonules, and within the trabecular meshwork (Figure 9-39).

The pathophysiology of pigment release in PDS may be secondary to an inverse pupillary block mechanism in which posterior bowing of the iris results in rubbing of the pigment epithelium against bundles of zonules or on ciliary processes thereby releasing pigment,[316-321] although some have questioned this mechanism.[322] The posterior bowing of the iris in PDS may be accentuated by accommodation.[323] It can be prevented temporarily by refraining from blinking.[324] Ultrasound biomicroscope examination supported this mechanism in patients who exhibit the characteristic concave iris contour.[321,324-327] A more posterior iris

insertion has been noted in PDS, and may contribute to increased iris chafing in the syndrome.[328]

In some black patients, the syndrome is atypical and may involve older, female, hyperopic individuals who may not demonstrate iris transillumination.[329] The black individuals also tend to have a flatter iris insertion into the ciliary body.[329]

Pigmentary glaucoma (PG) is pigment dispersion syndrome accompanied by glaucoma. Migliazzo and colleagues noted progression to glaucoma in 35% of their series of PDS patients with ocular hypertension over a mean follow-up period of 17 years.[330]

A pigment "shower" may be found within the aqueous after pupillary dilation or after exercise. Increased IOP in some PDS patients caused by such pigment release during exercise is well recognized but not universally accepted.[331,332] Posterior iris concavity also tends to increase with exercise in some patients.[333] Pigment dispersion may be increased secondary to cataract formation,[334] and has been reported in pseudophakia.[335-337]

Prophylactic or therapeutic iridotomy has been suggested for those patients who demonstrate posterior iris bowing.[319-321,327] Such therapy may be particularly useful in younger patients.[338] Restitution of a normal iris configuration after laser iridotomy has been documented by ultrasound biomicroscope examination.[339] Nevertheless, the value of the procedure in pigmentary glaucoma has been questioned.[340] It has been suggested that laser iridotomy may not completely eliminate exercise-induced pigment dispersion in PDS.[341]

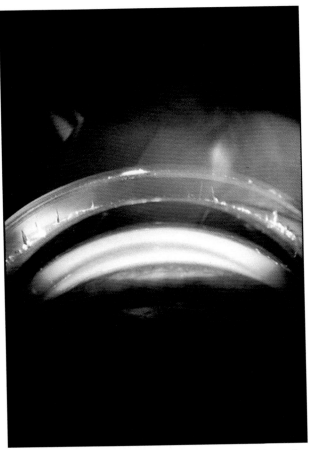

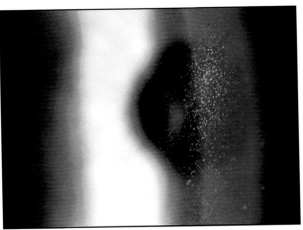

Figure 9-38. Slit-lamp photograph reveals Krukenberg spindle on the posterior cornea in pigmentary glaucoma.

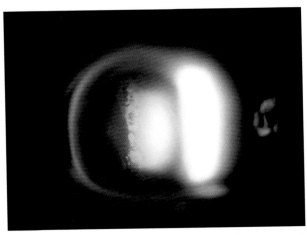

Figure 9-37. Heavy iris pigmentation is found in this gonio-photograph in pigmentary glaucoma.

Figure 9-39. Pigment is found on the posterior surface of the lens in pigmentary glaucoma. Courtesy of Ali Aminlari, MD, FACS.

Some authors have cited the frequent occurrence of anomalous iris processes in PG as evidence for a congenitally anomalous anterior chamber angle as the cause for the glaucoma.[321] Such processes have been demonstrated to be present in 75% of untreated PDS patients based on ultrasound biomicroscopic examination.[321] Other authors believe that the PDS gene may merely be located close to a gene for POAG so that they tend to be inherited together.

Argon laser trabeculoplasty has a high success rate in PG. Life-table analysis demonstrates a success rate of 80% at 1 year, 62% at 2 years, and 45% at 6 years after treatment in one study.[342]

The incidence of retinal detachment is increased in PDS.[343] Additionally, lattice retinal degeneration was found in 20%, full-thickness retinal breaks were present in 11.7%, and asymptomatic retinal detachments were found in 3.3% of PDS patients.[344] Similar findings have been noted by others.[345] Abnormal retinal pigment

epithelium has been demonstrated in PDS by electro-oculography.[346]

The mechanism for the pressure rise found in PG is not known. Differences in trabecular cellularity or morphology were unable to be found in nine normal human eye anterior segments examined for pigment-associated differences in trabecular cellularity or morphology (Figure 9-40).[347] Furthermore, long-term IOP elevation was not able to be produced by infusing melanin granules into monkey eyes.[348] The authors concluded that factors other than, or in addition to, pigment particle accumulation in the trabecular meshwork must be involved in the mechanism of human pigmentary glaucoma.[348] Similarly, most of the pigment in PDS is not in the juxtacanalicular connective tissue.

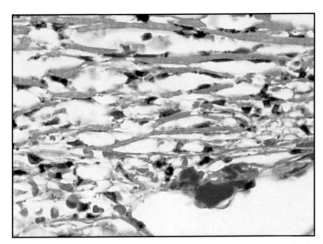

Figure 9-40. Pigmentation of the anterior chamber angle is found in pigmentary glaucoma. The relationship of such pigmentation to the pathogenesis of the glaucoma is not clearly understood.

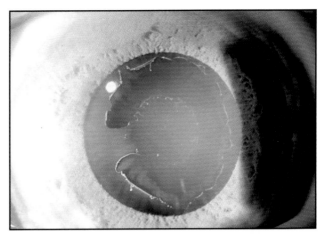

Figure 9-41. Typical deposits of "frosting" are noted in this slit-lamp photograph of pseudoexfoliation syndrome.

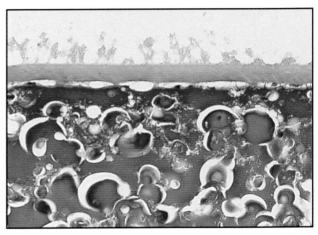

Figure 9-42. Histopathologic appearance of pseudoexfoliation material on the lens capsule.

One study reported that only 3.5% of the pigment in PDS was in the juxtacanalicular tissue, and 96.5% in the corneoscleral and uveoscleral tissue on histologic examination.[349] These authors also concluded that the glaucoma in PDS cannot be directly attributed to pigment accumulation in the juxtacanalicular tissue. Clinically, however, worsening of glaucoma is associated with increased pigment dispersion.[350]

Alvarado and Murphy have postulated that reduction in trabecular cul-de-sac area accounts for a major portion of the increase in aqueous outflow resistance in PDS.[96]

The presence of ring melanoma must be excluded in any atypical cases of PDS or pigmentary glaucoma.[351]

Pseudoexfoliation Glaucoma (PXE)

PXE is the subject of a recent extensive review.[352] Initially PXE referred to granular or "frost-like" material deposited on the lens surface (Figure 9-41). The term *pseudoexfoliation* was intended to contrast this entity from *true exfoliation*, which is a separation within the lens capsule that most frequently results from occupational exposure to infrared irradiation.[353] Although the initial description of pseudoexfoliation called attention to characteristic deposits on the anterior lens capsule (Figure 9-42), PXE material has been found in the conjunctiva of individuals with "preclinical" PXE[354] and in PXE patients.[355,356] Other locations at which the material has been identified include the wall of a short posterior ciliary artery in the orbit,[357] in eyelid skin,[358] and in other extraocular structures such as extraocular rectus and oblique muscles, vortex veins, and the optic nerve sheaths of PXE patients.[359,360]

The systemic nature of PXE is evidenced by the finding of typical material in skin biopsy specimens,[361] and in skin, heart, lung, liver, kidney, and meninges at autopsy.[362,363] Mitchell and associates noted an association between PXE and history of angina, acute myocardial infarction, or stroke.[364] The prevalence of PXE is increased in individuals who have had a transient ischemic attack further suggesting a circulatory abnormality in the eyes of these patients.[365]

One of the other characteristic clinical findings in PXE is increased anterior chamber angle pigmentation.[366] Moreover, Sampaolesi's line, a linear deposit of pigment anterior to Schwalbe's line, characteristically is present in PXE.[367] It may cause errors in estimation of the width of the anterior chamber angle on gonioscopic examination.

Earlier we discussed the increased incidence of angle-closure in PXE. It is important to gonioscopically discern the anterior chamber angle anatomy in PXE, because such patients may present with extremely elevated IOP even in the absence of angle-closure.[60,368-370] An occludable angle has been reported in 9.3% of PXE patients.[61] Obviously, the treatment of increased IOP associated with PXE differs tremendously depending upon the mechanism underlying the pressure elevation in PXE.

Peripheral and generalized iris transillumination is typical of PXE and has been proposed as evidence for iris vascular insufficiency.[371,372] Asano and colleagues have suggested that abnormal extracellular matrix production and/or vascular abnormalities result in tissue hypoxia in PXE and cause degenerative tissue changes.[373] They further postulate that muscle cell atrophy potentiates the poor pupillary dilation in the syndrome. Other iris findings reported in PXE include pupillary ruff defects, iris sphincter transillumination, a whorl-like pattern of particulate pigment deposition on the iris sphincter, pigment deposition on the peripheral iris and trabecular meshwork, and the accumulation of PXE material on the zonules and ciliary body.[374,375] Degenerative changes in the iris stroma and muscular layers of the iris have been noted on electron microscopic examination.[376]

There is considerable racial and ethnic variation in the incidence of PXE, which worldwide varies from 0% in Eskimos to 21% in Finns over 60 years of age.[377-383] There is an increased incidence of cataract and glaucoma among PXE patients in the Eastern Mediterranean area of Turkey where glaucoma in PXE individuals was 34.3%, and the prevalence of PXE in glaucoma patients was 46.9%.[384]

There is a particularly high incidence of PXE in African Bantus in whom there is a 6.4% prevalence in the age group 30 to 39.[385] There also is an increased prevalence among Navajo Indians,[386] and among the male Spanish-American population of New Mexico.[387] Jones and colleagues noted a 22 times increased incidence of glaucoma associated with PXE in New Mexico.[387] In contrast, the Framingham Eye Study noted a prevalence of only 0.6% for the 52 to 64 age group.[388]

PXE may be found in association with PDS.[389] The prevalence of PXE is decreased in individuals with diabetic retinopathy, particularly proliferative diabetic retinopathy.[390] There appears to be an increased prevalence with age up to 75 to 80 years, after which it may decline in prevalence.[391]

In a study of 100 consecutive patients in whom PXE was an incidental finding, 78% had normal IOP, 15% were ocular hypertensives, and 7% had glaucoma.[392,393] If such individuals are followed for prolonged periods, one finds an increased incidence of elevated IOP. In a study of PXE patients followed from 1940 to 1980, elevated IOP developed in 5.3% in 5 years in those who initially had normal IOP, and increased to 15.4% in 10 years.[394] A retrospective study of 164 patients with PXE found that 34.5% of initially normotensive eyes developed ocular hypertension or glaucoma.[395]

It has been stated that glaucoma is more difficult to control in PXE and may be associated with more severe optic nerve damage than typical POAG.[377,387,396,397] PXE was found in 87.8% of those undergoing trabeculectomy in a Greek population.[398] PXE also may increase the chances of eventual enucleation. Henke and Naumann found a prevalence of PXE of 3.4% among 455 enucleated eyes.[399] Elastosis of the optic nerve head has been reported in PXE compared to POAG.[400] Gottanka and colleagues found that the severity of glaucoma in PXE is related to the amount of the material in the cribriform region and to the location of PXE material near the inner wall of Schlemm's canal.[401] One might postulate that such structural changes in the optic nerve head could contribute to poor structural support in this region and secondary increased IOP sensitivity to glaucomatous damage in these patients. Nevertheless, utilizing color stereo photographs, Jonas and Papastathopoulos were unable to find features characteristic of PXE optic discs except for slightly smaller discs in the PXE patients.[402] HLA antigens are associated with PXE suggesting a genetic component to the disorder[403]; moreover, the severity of glaucoma in PXE may be associated with blood group.[404]

The mechanism by which glaucoma results in PXE is not known with certainty. It has been suggested that obstruction to aqueous outflow results from PXE material or by pigment released from the iris pigment epithelium.[367,405-408] The trabecular meshwork and its endothelium may undergo secondary and degenerative changes, which are additive to the obstructive effects of the material deposited within it.[409,410] A congenitally anomalous anterior chamber angle (goniodysgenesis) has been suggested to contribute to the glaucoma in PXE.[411] The gene for PXE also may be closely associated with a gene for POAG.[412] Thus, PXE may not be directly responsible for the glaucoma associated with the disorder. Rather, it may be a marker for the associated glaucoma gene.

Zonular abnormalities have reported in association with PXE.[413,414] Such abnormalities in PXE can be demonstrated using the ultrasound biomicroscope.[415] Therefore, it is not surprising that at an increased incidence of cataract surgery complications has been found in PXE.[416-421] For example, vitreous loss has been reported in 1.8% of those without PXE and in 9% of those with PXE among 1205 cataract extractions.[417] Scorolli and associates noted an odds ratio of 5.1 for cataract surgical complications in the presence of PXE compared to when it was absent.[422] A contributing factor to such vitreous loss is the fact that poor pupillary dilation frequently is encountered in PXE patients.[417] An additional difficulty of PXE patients relative to cataract surgery is that an increased incidence of secondary cataract following cataract surgery has been noted in PXE.[423]

PXE material has been characterized as similar to an elastic substance.[424-432] The fibrils are 20 to 30 nm thick with 10 nm subunits. They may be 800 to 900 nm long and have a characteristic 50 nm periodicity. The material has been produced in cultured tissues from PXE patients.[433] A precapsular layer composed of microfibrils, amorphous material, and granular inclusions has been cited as a possible precursor to PXE.[434] Fibrillin is said to be an intrinsic component of PXE material.[435] The possibility exists that enhanced fibrillin expression or abnormal aggregation of microfibrils containing fibrillin may be related to the pathogenesis of PXE.[435] Hyaluronan also has been demonstrated to coat fibrillar material in PXE.[436] Kuchle and associates noted abnormal blood-aqueous barrier in PXE and localized the abnormality primarily to the iris.[437,438] Dotsenko and colleagues also have postulated an abnormality in blood-ocular barrier in PXE, and that the plasma kallikrein-kinin system participates in that disturbance.[439] Blood-ocular barrier abnormalities have been suggested in PXE.[440]

Other authors have added to our knowledge of the nature of PXE material. Morrison and Green noted that glycosaminoglycans, which may comprise the interfibrillar portion of the material, have been found in PXE.[409] They found the material to be loosely adherent to most anterior segment structures, firmly adherent to the equatorial lens capsule, posterior epithelium of the iris, and the nonpigmented ciliary epithelium. In this region the material is present within epithelial cells and associated with a disorganized, reduplicated basement membrane.[409] They also noted that other studies have demonstrated the similarities between PXE material and zonules, and that the fibrils are related to the microfibrillar portion of elastin, which has the staining properties of oxytalan, the microfibrillar component of elastic tissue.[441,442] It even has been proposed that PXE material may represent degenerated zonular fibers.[413]

Various other observations of PXE material have identified and characterized glycoconjugates of the material.[443] A similarity of PXE material to amyloid has been debated.[409,444] Immunohistochemical studies have caused some authors to conclude that PXE material is a multicomponent expression of a disordered extracellular matrix synthesis including the incorporation of the major non-collagenous basement membrane components.[445] Kubota and colleagues have postulated that proteoglycans and the HNK-1 epitope may play an important role in the formation of PXE material through their adhesive properties.[446,447] Other biochemical abnormalities have been demonstrated in cultured fibroblasts from the iris and corneal stroma in patients with PXE.[448]

Phacogenic SOAG

We already have discussed several mechanisms through which the lens may contribute to angle-closure glaucoma. Similarly, the lens may help produce SOAG through several mechanisms. Leaking lens protein from a Morgagnian cataract may incite a marked macrophage (histiocytic) response (Figure 9-43a and b). Examination of eyes enucleated following glaucoma resulting from hypermature cataracts has confirmed this mechanism.[449] The authors noted that swollen macrophages, which have phagocytosed lens material, may obstruct the trabecular meshwork resulting in aqueous outflow obstruction. They coined the term *phacolytic glaucoma* to designate the severe rise in IOP that is characteristic of the entity. Similar findings were reported by Yanoff and Scheie based on

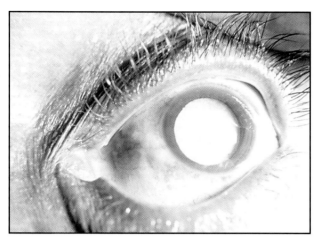

Figure 9-43a. Mature cataract may leak protein resulting in phacolytic glaucoma.

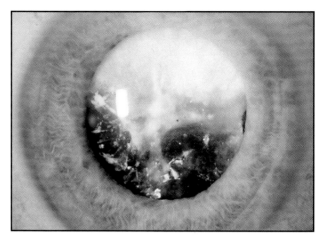

Figure 9-43b. Lens capsule and nucleus remain in lens that has undergone partial resorption of lens material, which may have produced secondary phacolytic glaucoma.

anterior chamber aspirates following needling procedures for soft cataracts.[450]

It also has been proposed that heavy molecular weight proteins from a leaking mature lens or fragments of cortical material may themselves block the trabecular meshwork.[451-453] In support of this contention, Epstein has noted that macrophages are not invariably found in phacolytic glaucoma.[453]

Cholesterol crystals and calcium oxalate crystals have been found in phacolytic glaucoma.[454,455]

SOAG Caused by Uveal Malignant Melanoma

In 1970, Yanoff reported that 20% of 96 eyes found to contain uveal malignant melanomas presented with glaucoma.[244] In previous classic studies, approximately 7% to 10% of enucleated eyes have been reported to contain melanomas that were unsuspected clinically.[456-460] Unsuspected melanomas are 10 times more prevalent in individuals presenting with glaucoma than in the control group of patients.[244] Recently unsuspected melanoma has decreased significantly in frequency. Nevertheless, such lesions must be positively excluded in any patient with a blind, painful eye having opaque media.

The mechanisms for angle-closure glaucoma secondary to uveal malignant melanomas have been discussed earlier in this chapter. One mechanism through which melanoma may produce SOAG glaucoma is melanomalytic glaucoma, which represents mechanical obstruction of the trabecular meshwork by

macrophages and debris from a necrotic uveal melanoma.[461-463] A similar process has been reported in association with necrotic iris melanocytomas.[464] Ring melanoma may infiltrate the anterior chamber angle structures thereby producing SOAG (Figure 9-44).[351,465]

Schwartz-Matsuo Syndrome

IOP usually is lowered in eyes with retinal detachment. Occasionally, however, an acute elevation in IOP may be found in association with retinal detachment. Such eyes characterize Schwartz-Matsuo syndrome.[466,467] Usually cellular material is present in the anterior chamber, and the material has been characterized as comprised of photoreceptor outer segments.

VARIABLE OUTFLOW

Normal (Low) Tension Glaucoma

By definition, normal tension glaucoma (NTG) is characterized by typical glaucomatous optic nerve head cupping and visual field loss at an IOP that is within the statistically normal range.[468-471] After simulating conditions such as optic nerve lesions, "burned out" POAG, wide diurnal swings in IOP, and systemic medication masking POAG have been excluded, approximately 30% of glaucoma patients can be classified as NTG.[2-4]

NTG patients have be divided into two groups by Levene.[470] The first group of patients have minimally

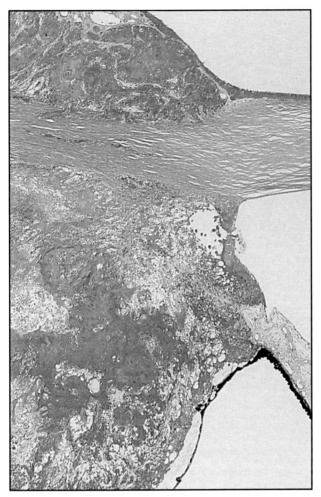

Figure 9-44. Photomicrograph of unusual instance of infiltration of angle structures and replacement of ciliary body by intraocular invasion of ocular surface squamous cell carcinoma. Ring melanoma may cause glaucoma through a similar mechanism.

elevated IOP with peak pressures near 24 mmHg. These patients really are a subset of more typical POAG and, not surprisingly, have been demonstrated to benefit most from pressure control. The second group have pressures at or below the "normal" range. Nevertheless, they exhibit characteristic optic nerve head cupping and visual field loss usually associated with POAG. The NTG patients more often exhibit early central visual field loss and decreased visual acuity compared to those with POAG. Moreover, NTG individuals have an increased prevalence of monocular cases, have cupping that is disproportionate in relation to the degree of field loss, have increased females sex prevalence, are associated with optic disc splinter hemorrhages, and are poorly responsive to IOP control.

Some authors would further subdivide the NTG population. For example, a more favorable prognosis is found in those patients with a previous history of hemodynamic crisis.[472] NTG also has been associated with multiple systemic and local hemodynamic factors such as orthostatic hypotension, carotid occlusive disease, blood viscosity, migraine, diabetes, and particularly the regulation of optic nerve head blood flow. [473-488] A common thread in all these studies is an association between NTG and a hemodynamic factor. Others have questioned a hemodynamic cause for NTG. [489] Recently, NTG has been demonstrated to be associated with calcification and ectasia of the carotid artery into the optic canal.[490]

NTG is discussed further in Chapter 6.

REFERENCES

1. Bathija R, Gupta N, Zangwill L, Weinreb RN. Changing definition of glaucoma. *J Glaucoma.* 1998;7:165-169.
2. Hollows FC, Graham PA. Intra-ocular pressure, glaucoma, and glaucoma suspects in a defined population. *Br J Ophthalmol.* 1966;50:570-586.
3. Bengtsson B. The prevalence of glaucoma. *Br J Ophthalmol.* 1981;65:46-49.
4. Klein BE, Klein R, Sponsel WE, et al. Prevalence of glaucoma. The Beaver Dam Eye Study. *Ophthalmology.* 1992;99:1499-1504.
5. Van Herick W, Shaffer RN, Schwartz A. Estimation of width of angle of anterior chamber. Incidence and significance of the narrow angle. *Am J Ophthalmol.* 1969;68:626-629.
6. Thomas R, George T, Braganza A, Muliyil J. The flashlight test and van Herick's test are poor predictors for occludable angles. *Aust N Z J Ophthalmol.* 1996;24:251-256.
7. Congdon NG, Quigley HA, Hung PT, Wang TH, Ho TC. Screening techniques for angle-closure glaucoma in rural Taiwan. *Acta Ophthalmol.* 1996;74:113-119.
8. Becker B, Keskey GG, Christensen RE. Hypersecretion glaucoma. *Arch Ophthalmol.* 1956;56:180-187.
9. deLuise VP, Anderson DR. Primary infantile glaucoma (congenital glaucoma). *Surv Ophthalmol.* 1983;28:1-19.
10. Lowe RF. A history of primary angle-closure glaucoma. *Surv Ophthalmol.* 1995;40:163-170.
11. Godel V, Stein R, Feiler-Ofry V. Angle-closure glaucoma. Postoperative acute glaucoma after phenylephrine eyedrops. *Am J Ophthalmol.* 1968;65:552-554.
12. Lowe RF. Plateau iris. *Aust J Ophthalmol.* 1981;9:71-73.
13. Wand M, Grant WM, Simmons RJ, Hutchinson BT. Plateau iris syndrome. *Trans Am Acad Ophthalmol Otolaryngol.* 1977;83:122-130.
14. Pavlin CJ, Ritch R, Foster FS. Ultrasound biomicroscopy in plateau iris syndrome. *Am J Ophthalmol.* 1992;113:390-395.
15. Wand M, Pavlin CJ, Foster FS. Plateau iris syndrome: ultrasound biomicroscopic and histologic study [letter]. *Ophthalmic Surg.* 1993;24:129-131.

16. Alper MG, Laubach JL. Primary angle-closure glaucoma in the American Negro. *Arch Ophthalmol.*1968;79:663-668.

17. Pavlin CJ, Harasiewicz K, Foster FS. An ultrasound biomicroscopic dark-room provocative test. *Ophthalmic Surg.* 1995;26:253-255.

18. Kondo T, Miyazawa D, Unigame K, Kurimoto Y. Ultrasound biomicroscopic findings in humans with shallow anterior chamber and increased intraocular pressure after the prone provocation test. *Am J Ophthalmol.* 1997;124:632-640.

19. Hong C, Park KH, Hyung SM, Song KY, Kim DM, Youn DH. Evaluation of pupillary block component in angle-closure glaucoma. *Jpn J Ophthalmol.* 1996;40:239-243.

20. Brini A, Flament J. Cataracta glaucomatosa acuta. *Exp Eye Res.* 1973;16:19-28.

21. Dayan M, Turner B, McGhee C. Acute angle-closure glaucoma masquerading as systemic illness. *BMJ.* 1996;313:413-415.

22. Lotery AJ, Frazer DG. Iatrogenic acute angle closure glaucoma masked by general anaesthesia and intensive care. *Ulster Med J.* 1995;64:178-180.

23. Siriwardena D, Arora AK, Fraser SG, McClelland HK, Claoue C. Misdiagnosis of acute angle closure glaucoma. *Age Ageing.* 1996;25:421-423.

24. Bertolini J, Pelucio M. The red eye. *Emer Med Clin North Am.* 1995;13:561-579.

25. Congdon N, Wang F, Tielsch JM. Issues in the epidemiology and population-based screening of primary angle-closure glaucoma. *Surv Ophthalmol.* 1992;36:411-23.

26. Arkell SM, Lightman DA, Sommer A, Taylor HR, Korshin OM, Tielsch JM. The prevalence of glaucoma among Eskimos of northwest Alaska. *Arch Ophthalmol.* 1987;105:482-485.

27. Van RG, Arkell SM, Charlton W, Doesburg W. Primary angle-closure glaucoma among Alaskan Eskimos. *Doc Ophthalmol.* 1988;70:265-276.

28. Seah SK, Foster PJ, Chew PT, et al. Incidence of acute primary angle-closure glaucoma in Singapore. An island-wide survey. *Arch Ophthalmol.* 1997;115:1436-1440.

29. Erie JC, Hodge DO, Gray DT. The incidence of primary angle-closure glaucoma in Olmsted County, Minnesota. *Arch Ophthalmol.* 1997;115:177-181.

30. Foster PJ, Baasanhu J, Alsbirk PH, Munkhbayar D, Uranchimeg D, Johnson GJ. Glaucoma in Mongolia. A population-based survey in Hovsgol province, northern Mongolia [see comments]. *Arch Ophthalmol.* 1996;114: 1235-1241.

31. Nguyen N, Mora JS, Gaffney MM, et al. A high prevalence of occludable angles in a Vietnamese population [see comments]. *Ophthalmology.* 1996;103:1426-1431.

32. Wolfs RC, Grobbee DE, Hofman A, de Jong PT. Risk of acute angle-closure glaucoma after diagnostic mydriasis in nonselected subjects: the Rotterdam Study. *Invest Ophthalmol Vis Sci.* 1997;38:2683-2687.

33. Patel KH, Javitt JC, Tielsch JM, et al. Incidence of acute angle-closure glaucoma after pharmacologic mydriasis [see comments]. *Am J Ophthalmol.* 1995;120:709-717.

34. Spaeth GL. Incidence of acute angle-closure glaucoma after pharmacologic mydriasis [letter; comment]. *Am J Ophthalmol.* 1996;122:283-284.

35. Goldstein JH. Incidence of acute angle-closure glaucoma after pharmacologic mydriasis [letter; comment]. *Am J Ophthalmol.* 1996;121:733-735.

36. Fivgas GD, Beck AD. Angle-closure glaucoma in a 10-year-old girl. *Am J Ophthalmol.* 1997;124:251-253.

37. Epstein NE, Goldbloom DS. Oral imipramine and acute angle-closure glaucoma [letter; comment]. *Arch Ophthalmol.* 1995;113:698.

38. Kramer M, Reines S. Oral imipramine and acute angle-closure glaucoma [letter; comment]. *Arch Ophthalmol.* 1995;113:698-699.

39. Geanon JD, Perkins TW. Bilateral acute angle-closure glaucoma associated with drug sensitivity to hydrochlorothiazide [letter]. *Arch Ophthalmol.* 1995;113:1231-1232.

40. Denis P, Charpentier D, Berros P, Touameur S. Bilateral acute angle-closure glaucoma after dexfenfluramine treatment. *Ophthalmologica.* 1995;209:223-224.

41. Kirwan JF, Subak-Sharpe I, Teimory M. Bilateral acute angle closure glaucoma after administration of paroxetine [letter]. *Br J Ophthalmol.* 1997;81:252.

42. Lewis CF, DeQuardo JR, DuBose C, Tandon R. Acute angle-closure glaucoma and paroxetine [letter]. *J Clin Psychiatry.* 1997;58:123-124.

43. Schlingemann RO, Smit AA, Lunel HF, Hijdra A. Amaurosis fugax on standing and angle-closure glaucoma with clomipramine [letter]. *Lancet.* 1996;347:465.

44. Mandak JS, Minerva P, Wilson TW, Smith EK. Angle closure glaucoma complicating systemic atropine use in the cardiac catheterization laboratory. *Cathet Cardiovasc Diagn.* 1996;39:262-264.

45. Mitchell JD, Schwartz AL. Acute angle-closure glaucoma associated with intranasal cocaine abuse. *Am J Ophthalmol.* 1996;122:425-426.

46. Lowe RF. Central corneal thickness. Ocular correlations in normal eyes and those with primary angle-closure glaucoma. *Br J Ophthalmol.* 1969;53:824-826.

47. Lowe RF. Corneal radius and ocular correlations. *Am J Ophthalmol.* 1969;67:864-868.

48. Lowe RF. Anterior lens curvature. Comparisons between normal eyes and those with primary angle-closure glaucoma. *Br J Ophthalmol.* 1972;56:409-413.

49. Lowe RF. Acute angle closure glaucoma and the crystalline lens. *Aust J Ophthalmol.* 1973;1:89-94.

50. Lowe RF, Clark BA. Radius of curvature of the anterior lens surface. Correlations in normal eyes and in eyes involved with primary angle-closure glaucoma. *Br J Ophthalmol.* 1973;57:471-474.

51. Lowe RF, Clark BA. Posterior corneal curvature. Correlations in normal eyes and in eyes involved with primary angle-closure glaucoma. *Br J Ophthalmol.* 1973;57: 464-470.

52. Panek WC, Christensen RE, Lee DA, Fazio DT, Fox LE, Scott TV. Biometric variables in patients with occludable anterior chamber angles. *Am J Ophthalmol.* 1990;110:185-188.

53. Markowitz SN, Morin JD. Angle-closure glaucoma: relation between lens thickness, anterior chamber depth and age. *Can J Ophthalmol.* 1984;19:300-302.

54. Markowitz SN, Morin JD. The ratio of lens thickness to axial length for biometric standardization in angle-closure glaucoma. *Am J Ophthalmol.* 1985;99:400-402.

55. Lin YW, Wang TH, Hung PT. Biometric study of acute primary angle-closure glaucoma. *J Formos Med Assoc.* 1997; 96:908-912.

56. Congdon NG, Youlin Q, Quigley H, et al. Biometry and primary angle-closure glaucoma among Chinese, white, and black populations. *Ophthalmology.* 1997;104:1489-1495.

57. Sawada A, Sakuma T, Yamamoto T, Kitazawa Y. Appositional angle closure in eyes with narrow angles: comparison between the fellow eyes of acute angle-closure glaucoma and normotensive cases. *J Glaucoma.* 1997;6:288-292.

58. Sakuma T, Sawada A, Yamamoto T, Kitazawa Y. Appositional angle closure in eyes with narrow angles: an ultrasound biomicroscopic study. *J Glaucoma.* 1997;6:165-169.

59. Talluto D, Feith M, Allee S. Simultaneous angle closure in twins. *J Glaucoma.* 1998;7:68-69.

60. Ritch R. Exfoliation syndrome and occludable angles. *Trans Am Ophthalmol Soc.* 1994;92:845-944.

61. Gross FJ, Tingey D, Epstein DL. Increased prevalence of occludable angles and angle-closure glaucoma in patients with pseudoexfoliation [see comments]. *Am J Ophthalmol.* 1994;117:333-336.

62. Brusini P, Tosoni C, Miani P. Increased prevalence of occludable angles and angle-closure glaucoma in patients with pseudoexfoliation [letter; comment] [see comments]. *Am J Ophthalmol.* 1994;118:540.

63. von der Lippe I, Kuchle M, Naumann GO. Pseudoexfoliation syndrome as a risk factor for acute ciliary block angle closure glaucoma. *Acta Ophthalmol.* 1993;71:277-279.

64. Wan WL, Minckler DS, Rao NA. Pupillary-block glaucoma associated with childhood cystinosis. *Am J Ophthalmol.* 1986;101:700-705.

65. Salmon JF, Murray AD. The association of iridoschisis and primary angle-closure glaucoma. *Eye.* 1992;6:267-272.

66. Pitts JF, Jay JL. The association of Fuchs's corneal endothelial dystrophy with axial hypermetropia, shallow anterior chamber, and angle closure glaucoma [see comments]. *Br J Ophthalmol.* 1990;74:601-604.

67. Loewenstein A, Geyer O, Hourvitz D, Lazar M. The association of Fuch's corneal endothelial dystrophy with angle closure glaucoma [letter; comment]. *Br J Ophthalmol.* 1991; 75:510.

68. Anonymous. Laser peripheral iridotomy for pupillary-block glaucoma. American Academy of Ophthalmology. *Ophthalmology.* 1994;101:1749-1758.

69. Fleck BW, Wright E, Fairley EA. A randomised prospective comparison of operative peripheral iridectomy and Nd:YAG laser iridotomy treatment of acute angle closure glaucoma: 3 year visual acuity and intraocular pressure control outcome. *Br J Ophthalmol.* 1997;81:884-888.

70. Schwenn O, Sell F, Pfeiffer N, Grehn F. Prophylactic Nd:YAG-laser iridotomy versus surgical iridectomy: a randomized, prospective study. *Ger J Ophthalmol.* 1995;4:374-379.

71. Lowe RF. Acute angle-closure glaucoma, the second eye. An analysis of 200 cases. *Br J Ophthalmol.* 1962;46:641-650.

72. Wishart PK, Batterbury M. Ocular hypertension: correlation of anterior chamber angle width and risk of progression to glaucoma. *Eye.* 1992;6:248-256.

73. Davidorf JM, Baker ND, Derick R. Treatment of the fellow eye in acute angle-closure glaucoma: a case report and survey of members of the American Glaucoma Society [see comments]. *J Glaucoma.* 1996;5:228-232.

74. Schwartz GF, Steinmann WC, Spaeth GL, Wilson RP. Surgical and medical management of patients with narrow anterior chamber angles: comparative results. *Ophthalmic Surg.* 1992;23:108-112.

75. Wilensky JT, Kaufman PL, Frohlichstein D, et al. Follow-up of angle-closure glaucoma suspects. *Am J Ophthalmol.* 1993;115:338-346.

76. Aminlari A, Sassani JW. Simultaneous bilateral malignant glaucoma following laser iridotomy. *Graefes Arch Clin Exp Ophthalmol.* 1993;231:12-14.

77. Wilensky JT, Ritch R, Kolker AE. Should patients with anatomically narrow angles have prophylactic iridectomy? *Surv Ophthalmol.* 1996;41:31-36.

78. Ritch R, Liebmann JM. Argon laser peripheral iridoplasty. *Ophthalmic Surg Lasers.* 1996;27:289-300.

79. Tielsch JM, Sommer A, Katz J, Royall RM, Quigley HA, Javitt J. Racial variations in the prevalence of primary open-angle glaucoma. The Baltimore Eye Survey [see comments]. *JAMA.* 1991;266:369-374.

80. Sacca SC, Rolando M, Marletta A, Macri A, Cerqueti P, Ciurlo G. Fluctuations of intraocular pressure during the day in open-angle glaucoma, normal-tension glaucoma and normal subjects. *Ophthalmologica.* 1998;212:115-119.

81. David R, Zangwill L, Briscoe D, Dagan M, Yagev R, Yassur Y. Diurnal intraocular pressure variations: an analysis of 690 diurnal curves. *Br J Ophthalmol.* 1992;76:280-283.

82. Zeimer RC, Wilensky JT, Gieser DK. Presence and rapid decline of early morning intraocular pressure peaks in glaucoma patients. *Ophthalmology.* 1990;97:547-550.

83. Wilensky JT, Gieser DK, Dietsche ML, Mori MT, Zeimer R. Individual variability in the diurnal intraocular pressure curve. *Ophthalmology.* 1993;100:940-944.

84. Georgopoulos G, Andreanos D, Liokis N, Papakonstantinou D, Vergados J, Theodossiadis G. Risk factors in ocular hypertension. *Eur J Ophthalmol.* 1997;7:357-363.

85. O'Brien C, Butt Z, Ludlam C, Detkova P. Activation of the coagulation cascade in untreated primary open-angle glaucoma. *Ophthalmology.* 1997;104:725-729.

86. Hamard P, Hamard H, Dufaux J. Blood flow rate in the microvasculature of the optic nerve head in primary open angle glaucoma. A new approach. *Surv Ophthalmol.* 1994;38:S87-S93.

87. Kaiser HJ, Flammer J, Graf T, Stumpfig D. Systemic blood pressure in glaucoma patients. *Graefes Arch Clin Exp Ophthalmol.* 1993;231:677-680.

88. Shin DH, Becker B, Kolker AE. Family history in primary open-angle glaucoma. *Arch Ophthalmol.* 1977;95:598-600.

89. Damji KF, Allingham RR. Molecular genetics is revolutionizing our understanding of ophthalmic disease. *Am J Ophthalmol.* 1997;124:530-543.

90. Teng CC, Paton RT, Katzin HM. Primary degeneration in the vicinity of the chamber angle. As an etiologic factor in wide-angle glaucoma. *Am J Ophthalmol.* 1955;40:619-631.

91. Teng CC, Katzin HM, Chi HH. Primary degeneration in the vicinity of the chamber angle. As an etiologic factor in wide-angle glaucoma: Part II. *Am J Ophthalmol.* 1957;43.

92. Ashton N. Doyne memorial lecture: The exit pathway of the aqueous. *Trans Ophthalmol Soc UK.* 1960;80:397-421.

93. Fine BS. Observations on the drainage angle in man and rhesus monkey: A concept of the pathogenesis of chronic simple glaucoma: A light and electron microscopic study. *Invest Ophthalmol Vis Sci.* 1964;3:609-646.

94. Tripathi RC. Aqueous outflow pathway in normal and glaucomatous eyes. *Br J Ophthalmol.* 1972;56:157-174.

95. Alvarado JA, Yun AJ, Murphy CG. Juxtacanalicular tissue in primary open angle glaucoma and in nonglaucomatous normals. *Arch Ophthalmol.* 1986;104:1517-1528.

96. Alvarado JA, Murphy CG. Outflow obstruction in pigmentary and primary open angle glaucoma. *Arch Ophthalmol.* 1992;110:1769-1778.

97. Rohen JW. Why is intraocular pressure elevated in chronic simple glaucoma? Anatomical considerations. *Ophthalmology.* 1983;90:758-765.

98. Tawara A, Varner HH, Hollyfield JG. Distribution and characterization of sulfated proteoglycans in the human trabecular tissue. *Invest Ophthalmol Vis Sci.* 1989;30:2215-2231.

99. Yun AJ, Murphy CG, Polansky JR, Newsome DA, Alvarado JA. Proteins secreted by human trabecular cells. Glucocorticoid and other effects. *Invest Ophthalmol Vis Sci.* 1989;30:2012-2022.

100. Freddo TF. The Glenn A. Fry Award Lecture 1992: aqueous humor proteins: a key for unlocking glaucoma? *Optom Vis Sci.* 1993;70:263-270.

101. Fine BS, Yanoff M, Stone RA. A clinicopathologic study of four cases of primary open-angle glaucoma compared to normal eyes. *Am J Ophthalmol.* 1981;91:88-105.

102. Grierson I. What is open angle glaucoma? Eye 1987;1:15-28.

103. Alvarado J, Murphy C, Juster R. Trabecular meshwork cellularity in primary open-angle glaucoma and nonglaucomatous normals. *Ophthalmology.* 1984;91:564-579.

104. Nelson LB, Maumenee IH. Ectopia lentis. *Surv Ophthalmol.* 1982;27:143-160.

105. Goldberg MF. Clinical manifestations of ectopia lentis et pupillae in 16 patients. *Trans Am Ophthalmol Soc.* 1988;86:158-177.

106. al-Salem M. Autosomal recessive ectopia lentis in two Arab family pedigrees. *Ophthalmic Paediatrics & Genetics.* 1990;11:123-127.

107. Colley A, Lloyd IC, Ridgway A, Donnai D. Ectopia lentis et pupillae: the genetic aspects and differential diagnosis. *J Med Genet.* 1991;28:791-794.

108. Edwards MJ, Challinor CJ, Colley PW, et al. Clinical and linkage study of a large family with simple ectopia lentis linked to FBN1. *Am J Med Genet.* 1994;53:65-71.

109. Bjerrum K, Kessing SV. Congenital ectopia lentis and secondary buphthalmos likely occurring as an autosomal recessive trait. *Acta Ophthalmologica.* 1991;69:630-634.

110. Meire FM. Hereditary ectopia lentis. A series of 10 cases of ectopia lentis et pupillae. *Bull Soc Belge Ophtalmol.* 1991;241:25-36.

111. Reichel E, Wiggs JL, Mukai S, DJ DA. Oxycephaly, bilateral ectopia lentis, and retinal detachment. *Ann Ophthalmol.* 1992;24:97-98.

112. Verloes A, Hermia JP, Galand A, Koulischer L, Dodinval P. Glaucoma-lens ectopia-microspherophakia-stiffness-shortness (GEMSS) syndrome: a dominant disease with manifestations of Weill-Marchesani syndromes. *Am J Med Genetics.* 1992;44:48-51.

113. Bawle E, Quigg MH. Ectopia lentis and aortic root dilatation in congenital contractural arachnodactyly. *Am J Med Genet.* 1992;42:19-21.

114. Noble KG, Bass S, Sherman J. Ectopia lentis, chorioretinal dystrophy and myopia. A new autosomal recessive syndrome. *Doc Ophthalmol.* 1993;83:97-102.

115. Lonnqvist L, Child A, Kainulainen K, Davidson R, Puhakka L, Peltonen L. A novel mutation of the fibrillin gene causing ectopia lentis. *Genomics* 1994;19:573-576.

116. Cruysberg JR, Pinckers A. Ectopia lentis et pupillae syndrome in three generations. *Br J Ophthalmol.* 1995;79:135-138.

117. Nelson LB, Spaeth GL, Nowinski TS, Margo CE, Jackson L. Aniridia. A review. *Surv Ophthalmol.* 1984;28:621-642.

118. Regenbogen L, Ilie S, Elian I. Homocystinuria—a surgical and anaesthetic risk. *Metabolic & Pediatric Ophthalmology.* 1980;4:209-211.

119. Favre JP, Becker F, Lorcerie B, Dumas R, David M. Vascular manifestations in homocystinuria. *Ann Vasc Surg.* 1992;6:294-297.

120. Lieberman ER, Gomperts ED, Shaw KN, Landing BH, Donnell GN. Homocystinuria: clinical and pathologic review, with emphasis on thrombotic features, including pulmonary artery thrombosis. *Perspectives in Pediatric Pathology.* 1993;17:125-147.

121. Mandel H, Brenner B, Berant M, et al. Coexistence of hereditary homocystinuria and factor V Leiden—effect on thrombosis. *N Engl J Med.* 1996;334:763-768.

122. Lowe S, Johnson DA, Tobias JD. Anesthetic implications of the child with homocystinuria [see comments]. *J Clin Anesth.* 1994;6:142-144.

123. Burke JP, M OK, Bowell R, Naughten ER. Ocular complications in homocystinuria—early and late treated. *Br J Ophthalmol.* 1989;73:427-431.

124. Luntz MH, Rosenblatt M. Malignant glaucoma. *Surv Ophthalmol.* 1987;32:73-93.

125. Levene RZ. Current concepts of malignant glaucoma. *Ophthalmic Surg.* 1986;17:515-18,20.

126. Shaffer RN, Hoskins HD, Jr. Ciliary block (malignant) glaucoma. *Ophthalmology.* 1978;85:215-221.

127. Mills DW, Willis NR. Malignant glaucoma - the long and short of it. *Can J Ophthalmol.* 1978;13:86-88.

128. Fanous S, Brouillette G. Ciliary block glaucoma: malignant glaucoma in the absence of a history of surgery and of miotic therapy. *Can J Ophthalmol.* 1983;18:302-303.

129. Manku MS. Spontaneous bilateral malignant glaucoma. *Aust N Z J Ophthalmol.* 1985;13:249-250.

130. Gonzalez F, Sanchez-Salorio M, Pacheco P. Simultaneous bilateral "malignant glaucoma" attack in a patient with no antecedent eye surgery or miotics. *Eur J Ophthalmol.* 1992;2:91-93.

131. Robinson A, Prialnic M, Deutsch D, Savir H. The onset of malignant glaucoma after prophylactic laser iridotomy. *Am J Ophthalmol.* 1990;110:95-96.

132. Cashwell LF, Martin TJ. Malignant glaucoma after laser iridotomy [see comments]. *Ophthalmology.* 1992;99:651-658.

133. Mastropasqua L, Ciancaglini M, Carpineto P, Lobefalo L, Gallenga PE. Aqueous misdirection syndrome: a complication of neodymium: YAG posterior capsulotomy. *J Cataract Refract Surg.* 1994;20:563-565.

134. DiSclafani M, Liebmann JM, Ritch R. Malignant glaucoma following argon laser release of scleral flap sutures after trabeculectomy. *Am J Ophthalmol.* 1989;108:597-598.

135. Macken P, Buys Y, Trope GE. Glaucoma laser suture lysis. *Br J Ophthalmol.* 1996;80:398-401.

136. Melamed S, Cahane M, Gutman I, Blumenthal M. Postoperative complications after Molteno implant surgery. *Am J Ophthalmol.* 1991;111:319-322.

137. Chin GN, Goodman NL. Aspergillus flavus keratitis. *Ann Ophthalmol.* 1978;10:415-418.

138. Lass JH, Thoft RA, Bellows AR, Slansky HH. Exogenous Nocardia asteroides endophthalmitis associated with malignant glaucoma. *Annals of Ophthalmology* 1981;13:317-321.

139. Kuriakose T, Thomas PA. Keratomycotic malignant glaucoma. *Indian Journal of Ophthalmology* 1991;39:118-121.

140. Chandler PA, Simmons RJ, Grant WM. Malignant glaucoma. Medical and surgical treatment. *Am J Ophthalmol.* 1968;66:495-502.

141. Weiss DI, Shaffer RN. Ciliary block (malignant) glaucoma. *Trans Am Acad Ophthalmol Otolaryngol.* 1972;76:450-461.

142. Tello C, Chi T, Shepps G, Liebmann J, Ritch R. Ultrasound biomicroscopy in pseudophakic malignant glaucoma [published erratum appears in Ophthalmology 1993 Dec;100(12):1747]. *Ophthalmology.* 1993;100:1330-1334.

143. Trope GE, Pavlin CJ, Bau A, Baumal CR, Foster FS. Malignant glaucoma. Clinical and ultrasound biomicroscopic features. *Ophthalmology.* 1994;101:1030-1035.

144. Park M, Unigame K, Kiryu J, Kondo T. Management of a patient with pseudophakic malignant glaucoma; role of ultrasound biomicroscopy [letter]. *Br J Ophthalmol.* 1996;80:676-677.

145. Epstein DL, Hashimoto JM, Anderson PJ, Grant WM. Experimental perfusions through the anterior and vitreous chambers with possible relationships to malignant glaucoma. *Am J Ophthalmol.* 1979;88:1078-1086.

146. Brown RH, Lynch MG, Tearse JE, Nunn RD. Neodymium-YAG vitreous surgery for phakic and pseudophakic malignant glaucoma. *Arch Ophthalmol.* 1986;104:1464-1466.

147. Liu Y, Yang W, Li S. Neodymium: YAG laser therapy in aphakic pupillary block glaucoma and aphakic malignant (ciliovitreal block) glaucoma. *Yen Ko Hsueh Pao* [Eye Science] 1990;6:11-16.

148. Melamed S, Ashkenazi I, Blumenthal M. Nd-YAG laser hyaloidotomy for malignant glaucoma following one-piece 7 mm intraocular lens implantation. *Br J Ophthalmol.* 1991;75:501-503.

149. Little BC. Treatment of aphakic malignant glaucoma using Nd:YAG laser posterior capsulotomy. *Br J Ophthalmol.* 1994;78:499-501.

150. Momoeda S, Hayashi H, Oshima K. Anterior pars plana vitrectomy for phakic malignant glaucoma. *Jpn J Ophthalmol.* 1983;27:73-79.

151. Lynch MG, Brown RH, Michels RG, Pollack IP, Stark WJ. Surgical vitrectomy for pseudophakic malignant glaucoma. *Am J Ophthalmol.* 1986;102:149-153.

152. Harbour JW, Rubsamen PE, Palmberg P. Pars plana vitrectomy in the management of phakic and pseudophakic malignant glaucoma. *Arch Ophthalmol.* 1996;114:1073-1078.

153. John T, Sassani JW, Eagle RCJ. The myofibroblastic component of rubeosis iridis. *Ophthalmology.* 1983;90:721-728.

154. Brown GC, Magargal LE, Schachat A, Shah H. Neovascular glaucoma. Etiologic considerations. *Ophthalmology.* 1984;91:315-320.

155. Tolentino MJ, Adamis AP. Angiogenic factors in the development of diabetic iris neovascularization and retinopathy. [Review] [121 refs]. *Int Ophthalmol Clin.* 1998;38:77-94.

156. Williamson TH. Central retinal vein occlusion: what's the story?. [Review] [145 refs]. *Br J Ophthalmol.* 1997;81:698-704.

157. O'Reilly MS. The preclinical evaluation of angiogenesis inhibitors. [Review] [87 refs]. *Invest New Drugs.* 1997;15:5-13.

158. Margo CE, Zimmerman LE. Retinoblastoma: the accuracy of clinical diagnosis in children treated by enucleation. *J Pediatr Ophthalmol Strabismus.* 1983;20:227-229.

159. Byrnes GA, Shields CL, Shields JA, De PP, Eagle RJ. Retinoblastoma presenting with spontaneous hyphema and dislocated lens. *J Pediatr Ophthalmol Strabismus.* 1993;30:334-336.

160. Tseng SS, Keys MP. Battered child syndrome simulating congenital glaucoma. *Arch Ophthalmol.* 1976;94:839-840.

161. Ghose S, Kishore K, Patil ND, Saxena R. Spontaneous hyphema in an infant with Christmas disease. *Can J Ophthalmol.* 1993;28:40-42.

162. Moazed K, Albert D, Smith TR. Rubeosis iridis in "pseudogliomas." *Surv Ophthalmol.* 1980;25:85-90.

163. Thieme R, Lukassek B, Keinert K. [Problems in juvenile xanthogranuloma of the anterior uvea (author's transl)]. *Klin Monatsbl Augenheilkd.* 1980;176:893-898.

164. Witmer R, Landolt E. [Juvenile nevoxanthogranuloma of the iris]. *Klin Monatsbl Augenheilkd.* 1980;176:658-660.

165. Canning CR, McCartney AC, Hungerford J. Medulloepithelioma (diktyoma). *Br J Ophthalmol.* 1988;72:764-767.

166. Gartner S, Henkind P. Neovascularization of the iris (rubeosis iridis). *Surv Ophthalmol.* 1978;22:291-312.

167. Campbell DG, Shields MB, Smith TR. The corneal endothelium and the spectrum of essential iris atrophy. *Am J Ophthalmol.* 1978;86:317-324.

168. Shields MB, Campbell DG, Simmons RJ. The essential iris atrophies. *Am J Ophthalmol.* 1978;85:749-759.

169. Eagle RJ, Font RL, Yanoff M, Fine BS. Proliferative endotheliopathy with iris abnormalities. The iridocorneal endothelial syndrome. *Arch Ophthalmol.* 1979;97:2104-2111.

170. Shields MB. Proliferative endotheliopathy with iris abnormalities. The iridocorneal endothelial syndrome. *Arch Ophthalmol.* 1979;97:2104-111.

171. Shields MB. Progressive essential iris atrophy, Chandler's syndrome, and the iris nevus (Cogan-Reese) syndrome: a spectrum of disease. *Surv Ophthalmol.* 1979;24:3-20.

172. Quigley HA, Forster RF. Histopathology of cornea and iris in Chandler's syndrome. *Arch Ophthalmol.* 1978;96:1878-1882.

173. Shields MB, McCracken JS, Klintworth GK, Campbell DG. Corneal edema in essential iris atrophy. *Ophthalmology.* 1979;86:1533-1550.

174. Eagle RJ, Font RL, Yanoff M, Fine BS. The iris naevus (Cogan-Reese) syndrome: light and electron microscopic observations. *Br J Ophthalmol.* 1980;64:446-452.

175. Bahn CF, Falls HF, Varley GA, Meyer RF, Edelhauser HF, Bourne WM. Classification of corneal endothelial disorders based on neural crest origin. *Ophthalmology.* 1984;91:558-563.

176. Alvarado JA, Murphy CG, Juster RP, Hetherington J. Pathogenesis of Chandler's syndrome, essential iris atrophy and the Cogan-Reese syndrome. II. Estimated age at disease onset. *Invest Ophthalmol Vis Sci.* 1986;27:873-882.

177. Alvarado JA, Murphy CG, Maglio M, Hetherington J. Pathogenesis of Chandler's syndrome, essential iris atrophy and the Cogan-Reese syndrome. I. Alterations of the corneal endothelium. *Invest Ophthalmol Vis Sci.* 1986;27:853-872.

178. Alvarado JA, Underwood JL, Green WR, et al. Detection of herpes simplex viral DNA in the iridocorneal endothelial syndrome. *Arch Ophthalmol.* 1994;112:1601-1609.

179. Alvarado JA, Underwood JL, Green WR, et al. Detection of herpes simplex viral DNA in the iridocorneal endothelial syndrome [see comments]. *Arch Ophthalmol.* 1994;112:1601-1609.

180. Denis P, Baudrimont M, Nordmann JP, Laroche L, Saraux H. Immunohistochemical and ultrastructural study of the cornea in Chandler's syndrome. Report of a case. *Ophthalmologica.* 1994;208:289-293.

181. Hirst LW, Green WR, Luckenbach M, de la Cruz Z, Stark WJ. Epithelial characteristics of the endothelium in Chandler's syndrome. *Invest Ophthalmol Vis Sci.* 1983;24:603-611.

182. Rodrigues MM, Phelps CD, Krachmer JH, Cibis GW, Weingeist TA. Glaucoma due to endothelialization of the anterior chamber angle. A comparison of posterior polymorphous dystrophy of the cornea and Chandler's syndrome. *Arch Ophthalmol.* 1980;98:688-696.

183. Rodrigues MM, Streeten BW, Spaeth GL. Chandler's syndrome as a variant of essential iris atrophy. A clinicopathologic study. *Arch Ophthalmol.* 1978;96:643-652.

184. Hetherington J, Jr. The spectrum of Chandler's syndrome. *Ophthalmology.* 1978;85:240-244.

185. Lichter PR. The spectrum of Chandler's syndrome: an often overlooked cause of unilateral glaucoma. *Ophthalmology.* 1978;85:245-251.

186. Wittebol-Post D, van Bijsterveld OP. Essential progressive iris atrophy. Report of two cases. *Ophthalmologica.* 1979;178:303-310.

187. Scheie HG, Yanoff M, Kellogg WT. Essential iris atrophy. Report of a case. *Arch Ophthalmol.* 1976;94:1315-1320.

188. Kaiser-Kupfer M, Kuwabara T, Kupfer C. Progressive bilateral essential iris atrophy. *Am J Ophthalmol.* 1977;83:340-346.

189. Kupfer C, Kaiser-Kupfer M, Kuwabara T. Progressive bilateral essential iris atrophy. *Trans Am Ophthalmol Soc.* 1977;74:341-356.

190. DeBroff BM, Thoft RA. Surgical results of penetrating keratoplasty in essential iris atrophy. *J Refract Corneal Surg.* 1994;10:428-432.

191. Kidd M, Hetherington J, Magee S. Surgical results in iridocorneal endothelial syndrome. *Arch Ophthalmol.* 1988;106:199-201.

192. Scheie HG, Yanoff M. Iris nevus (Cogan-Reese) syndrome. A cause of unilateral glaucoma. *Arch Ophthalmol.* 1975;93:963-970.

193. Khalil MK, Finlayson MH. Electron microscopy in iris nevus syndrome. *Can J Ophthalmol.* 1980;15:44-48.

194. Harris M, Tso AY, Kaba FW, Green WR, de la Cruz ZC. Corneal endothelial overgrowth of angle and iris. Evidence of myoblastic differentiation in three cases. *Ophthalmology.* 1984;91:1154-1160.

195. Colosi NJ, Yanoff M. Reactive corneal endothelialization. *Am J Ophthalmol.* 1977;83:219-24.

196. Terry TL, Chisholm JF, Schonberg AL. Studies on surface-epithelium invasion of the anterior segment of the eye. *Am J Ophthalmol.* 1939;22:1083-110.

197. Weiner MJ, Trentacoste J, Pon DM, Albert DM. Epithelial downgrowth: a 30-year clinicopathological review. *Br J Ophthalmol.* 1989;73:6-11.

198. Sugar A, Meyer RF, Hood CI. Epithelial downgrowth following penetrating keratoplasty in the aphake. *Arch Ophthalmol.* 1977;95:464-467.

199. Feder RS, Krachmer JH. The diagnosis of epithelial downgrowth after keratoplasty. *Am J Ophthalmol.* 1985;99:697-703.

200. Burris TE, Nordquist RE, Rowsey JJ. Model of epithelial downgrowth: III. Scanning and transmission electron microscopy of iris epithelialization. Cornea 1985;4:249-255.

201. Jensen P, Minckler DS, Chandler JW. Epithelial ingrowth. *Arch Ophthalmol.* 1977;95:837-842.

202. Iwamoto T, Srinivasan BD, DeVoe AG. Electron microscopy of epithelial downgrowth. *Ann Ophthalmol.* 1977;9:1095-1110.

203. Zavala EY, Binder PS. The pathologic findings of epithelial ingrowth. *Arch Ophthalmol.* 1980;98:2007-2014.

204. Sidrys LA, Demong T. Epithelial downgrowth after penetrating keratoplasty. *Can J Ophthalmol.* 1982;17:29-31.

205. Soong HK, Meyer RF, Wolter JR. Fistula excision and peripheral grafts in the treatment of persistent limbal wound leaks. *Ophthalmology.* 1988;95:31-6.

206. Schaeffer AR, Nalbandian RM, Brigham DW, ODonnell FEJ. Epithelial downgrowth following wound dehiscence after extracapsular cataract extraction and posterior chamber lens implantation: surgical management. *J Cataract Refract Surg.* 1989;15:437-441.

207. Smith RE, Parrett C. Specular microscopy of epithelial downgrowth. *Arch Ophthalmol.* 1978;96:1222-1224.

208. Holliday JN, Buller CR, Bourne WM. Specular microscopy and fluorophotometry in the diagnosis of epithelial downgrowth after a sutureless cataract operation [letter]. *Am J Ophthalmol.* 1993;116:238-240.

209. Hales RH, Spencer WH. Unsuccessful penetrating keratoplasties. Correlation of clinical and histologic findings. *Arch Ophthalmol.* 1963;70:805-810.

210. Kurz GH, D'Amico RA. Histopathology of corneal graft failures. *Am J Ophthalmol.* 1968;66:184-199.

211. Friedman AH, Henkind P. Corneal stromal overgrowth after cataract extraction. *Brit J Ophthalmol.* 1970;54:528-534.

212. Swan KC. Fibroblastic ingrowth following cataract surgery. *Arch Ophthalmol.* 1973;89:445-449.

213. Michels RG, Kenyon KR, Maumence AE. Retrocorneal fibrous membrane. *Invest Ophthalmol Vis Sci.* 1972;11:822-831.

214. Snip RC, Kenyon KR, Green WR. Retrocorneal fibrous membrane in the vitreous touch syndrome. *Am J Ophthalmol.* 1975;79:233-244.

215. Raitta C, Lehto I, Puska P, Vesti E, Harju M. A randomized, prospective study on the use of sodium hyaluronate (Healon) in trabeculectomy. *Ophthalmic Surg.* 1994;25:536-539.

216. Smith MF, Doyle JW, Sherwood MB. Comparison of the Baerveldt glaucoma implant with the double-plate Molteno drainage implant. *Arch Ophthalmol.* 1995;113:444-447.

217. Freedman J, Rubin B. Molteno implants as a treatment for refractory glaucoma in black patients [see comments]. *Arch Ophthalmol.* 1991;109:1417-1420.

218. Perkins TW, Cardakli UF, Eisele JR, Kaufman PL, Heatley GA. Adjunctive mitomycin C in Molteno implant surgery. *Ophthalmology.* 1995;102:91-97.

219. Chihara E, Nishida A, Kodo M, et al. Trabeculotomy ab externo: an alternative treatment in adult patients with primary open-angle glaucoma. [Review]. *Ophthalmic Surg.* 1993;24:735-739.

220. Susanna R, Jr., Nicolela MT, Takahashi WY. Mitomycin C as adjunctive therapy with glaucoma implant surgery. *Ophthalmic Surg.* 1994;25:458-462.

221. Tomlinson CP, Belcher CDd, Smith PD, Simmons RJ. Management of leaking filtration blebs. *Ann Ophthalmol.* 1987;19:405-408, 411.

222. Luntz MH, Berlin MS. Combined trabeculectomy and cataract extraction. Advantages of a modified technique and review of current literature. *Trans Ophthalmol Soc UK.* 1980;100:533-541.

223. Raitta C, Setala K. Trabeculectomy with the use of sodium hyaluronate. A prospective study. *Acta Ophthalmol.* 1986;64:407-413.

224. Blok MD, Greve EL, Dunnebier EA, Muradin F, Kijlstra A. Scleral flap sutures and the development of shallow or flat anterior chamber after trabeculectomy. *Ophthalmic Surg.* 1993;24:309-313.

225. Kolker AE, Kass MA, Rait JL. Trabeculectomy with releasable sutures. *Trans Am Ophthalmol Soc.* 1993;91:131-141; discussion 41-5.

226. Kolker AE, Kass MA, Rait JL. Trabeculectomy with releasable sutures. *Arch Ophthalmol.* 1994;112:62-66.

227. Wada Y, Nakatsu A, Kondo T. Long-term results of trabeculotomy ab externo. *Ophthalmic Surg.* 1994;25:317-320.

228. Weber PA, Henry MA, Kapetansky FM, Lohman LF. Argon laser treatment of the ciliary processes in aphakic glaucoma with flat anterior chamber. *Am J Ophthalmol.* 1984;97:82-85.

229. Epstein DL, Steinert RF, Puliafito CA. Neodymium-YAG laser therapy to the anterior hyaloid in aphakic malignant (ciliovitreal block) glaucoma. *Am J Ophthalmol.* 1984;98:137-143.

230. Tomey KF, Senft SH, Antonios SR, Shammas IV, Shihab ZM, Traverso CE. Aqueous misdirection and flat chamber after posterior chamber implants with and without trabeculectomy. *Arch Ophthalmol.* 1987;105:770-773.

231. Lockie P. Ciliary-block glaucoma treated by posterior capsulotomy. *Aust N Z J Ophthalmol.* 1987;15:207-209.

232. Burney EN, Quigley HA, Robin AL. Hypotony and choroidal detachment as late complications of trabeculectomy. *Am J Ophthalmol.* 1987;103:685-688.

233. Veldman E, Greve EL. Glaucoma filtering surgery, a retrospective study of 300 operations. *Doc Ophthalmol.* 1987;67:151-70.

234. Fourman S. Management of cornea-lens touch after filtering surgery for glaucoma [see comments]. *Ophthalmology.* 1990;97:424-8.

235. Chandler PA, Braconier HE. Spontaneous intra-epithelial cysts of the iris and ciliary body with glaucoma. *Am J Ophthalmol.* 1958;45:64-74.

236. Lichter PR, Shaffer RN. Interstitial keratitis and glaucoma. *Am J Ophthalmol.* 1969;68:241-248.

237. Farmer SG, Kalina RE. Epithelial implantation cyst of the iris. *Ophthalmology.* 1981;88:1286-1289.

238. Shields JA. Primary cysts of the iris. *Trans Am Ophthalmol Soc.* 1981;79:771-809.

239. Rummelt V, Naumann GO. Block excision of congenital and infantile nonpigmented epithelial iris cysts. Report on eight infants. *Ger J Ophthalmol.* 1992;1:361-366.

240. Finger PT, McCormick SA, Lombardo J, Tello C, Ritch R. Epithelial inclusion cyst of the iris. *Arch Ophthalmol.* 1995;113:777-80.

241. Shields JA, Sanborn GE, Augsburger JJ. The differential diagnosis of malignant melanoma of the iris. A clinical study of 200 patients. *Ophthalmology.* 1983;90:716-20.

242. Grant WM. Late glaucoma after interstitial keratitis. *Am J Ophthalmol.* 1975;79:87-91.

243. Anonymous. Secondary glaucoma due to inactive congenital syphilitic interstitial keratitis. (With 1 colour plate). *Ophthalmologica.* 1977;174:188-194.

244. Yanoff M. Glaucoma mechanisms in ocular malignant melanomas. *Am J Ophthalmol.* 1970;70:898-904.

245. Hittner HM, Rhodes LM, McPherson AR. Anterior segment abnormalities in cicatricial retinopathy of prematurity. *Ophthalmology.* 1979;86:803-816.

246. Hartnett ME, Gilbert MM, Richardson TM, Krug JH, Jr., Hirose T. Anterior segment evaluation of infants with retinopathy of prematurity. *Ophthalmology.* 1990;97:122-130.

247. Hartnett ME, Gilbert MM, Hirose T, Richardson TM, Katsumi O. Glaucoma as a cause of poor vision in severe retinopathy of prematurity. *Graefes Arch Clin Exp Ophthalmol.* 1993;231:433-438.

248. Haddad R, Font RL, Reeser F. Persistent hyperplastic primary vitreous. A clinicopathologic study of 62 cases and review of the literature. *Surv Ophthalmol.* 1978;23:123-134.

249. Pollard ZF. Results of treatment of persistent hyperplastic primary vitreous. *Ophthalmic Surg.* 1991;22:48-52.

250. Eiferman RA, Law M, Lane L. Iridoschisis and keratoconus [see comments]. *Cornea.* 1994;13:78-79.

251. Hersh PS. Iridoschisis following penetrating keratoplasty for keratoconus [letter; comment]. *Cornea.* 1994;13:545-546.

252. Foss AJ, Hykin PG, Benjamin L. Interstitial keratitis and iridoschisis in congenital syphilis. *J Clin Neuro-Ophthalmol.* 1992;12:167-170.

253. Salvador F, Linares F, Merita I, Amen M. Unilateral iridoschisis associated with syphilitic interstitial keratitis and glaucoma. *Ann Ophthalmol.* 1993;25:328-329.

254. Summers CG, Doughman DJ, Letson RD, Lufkin M. Juvenile iridoschisis and microphthalmos. *Am J Ophthalmol.* 1985;100:437-439.

255. Johnson MR, Bachynski BN. Juvenile iridoschisis and microphthalmos [letter]. *Am J Ophthalmol.* 1986;101:742-744.

256. Rodrigues MC, Spaeth GL, Krachmer JH, Laibson PR. Iridoschisis associated with glaucoma and bullous keratopathy. *Am J Ophthalmol.* 1983;95:73-81.

257. Campbell DG, Essigmann EM. Hemolytic ghost cell glaucoma. Further studies. *Arch Ophthalmol.* 1979;97:2141-2146.

258. Lambrou FH, Jr., Aiken DG, Woods WD, Campbell DG. The production and mechanism of ghost cell glaucoma in the cat and primate. *Invest Ophthalmol Vis Sci.* 1985;26:893-897.

259. Crouch ER, Jr., Frenkel M. Aminocaproic acid in the treatment of traumatic hyphema. *Am J Ophthalmol.* 1976;81:355-360.

260. McGetrick JJ, Jampol LM, Goldberg MF, Frenkel M, Fiscella RG. Aminocaproic acid decreases secondary hemorrhage after traumatic hyphema. *Arch Ophthalmol.* 1983; 101:1031-1033.

261. Cassel GH, Jeffers JB, Jaeger EA. Wills Eye Hospital Traumatic Hyphema Study. *Ophthalmic Surg.* 1985;16:441-443.

262. Palmer DJ, Goldberg MF, Frenkel M, Fiscella R, Anderson RJ. A comparison of two dose regimens of epsilon aminocaproic acid in the prevention and management of secondary traumatic hyphemas. *Ophthalmology.* 1986;93:102-108.

263. Lawrence T, Wilison D, Harvey J. The incidence of secondary hemorrhage after traumatic hyphema. *Ann Ophthalmol.* 1990;22:276-278.

264. Crouch ER, Jr., Williams PB. Secondary hemorrhage in traumatic hyphema [letter; comment]. *Am J Ophthalmol.* 1992;113:344-346.

265. Volpe NJ, Larrison WI, Hersh PS, Kim T, Shingleton BJ. Secondary hemorrhage in traumatic hyphema. *Am J Ophthalmol.* 1991;112:507-513.

266. Fong LP. Secondary hemorrhage in traumatic hyphema. Predictive factors for selective prophylaxis. *Ophthalmology.* 1994;101:1583-1588.

267. Kennedy RH, Brubaker RF. Traumatic hyphema in a defined population. *Am J Ophthalmol.* 1988;106:123-130.

268. Witteman GJ, Brubaker SJ, Johnson M, Marks RG. The incidence of rebleeding in traumatic hyphema. *Ann Ophthalmol.* 1985;17:525-6, 8-9.

269. Agapitos PJ, Noel LP, Clarke WN. Traumatic hyphema in children. *Ophthalmology.* 1987;94:1238-1241.

270. Wax MB, Ridley ME, Magargal LE. Reversal of retinal and optic disc ischemia in a patient with sickle cell trait and glaucoma secondary to traumatic hyphema. *Ophthalmology.* 1982;89:845-851.

271. Greenwald MJ, Crowley TM. Sickle cell hyphema with secondary glaucoma in a non-black patient. *Ophthalmic Surg.* 1985;16:170-171.

272. Kobayashi H, Honda Y. Intraocular hemorrhage in a patient with hemophilia. *Metabolic Ophthalmology.* 1984;8:27-30.

273. Friedman AH, Halpern BL, Friedberg DN, Wang FM, Podos SM. Transient open-angle glaucoma associated with sickle cell trait: report of 4 cases. *Br J Ophthalmol.* 1979;63:832-836.

274. Marcus DM, Albert DM. Recognizing child abuse. *Arch Ophthalmol.* 1992;110:766-767.

275. Zimmerman LE. Ocular lesions of juvenile xanthogranuloma. Nevoxanthoedothelioma. *Am J Ophthalmol.* 1965;60: 1011-1035.

276. Yoshizumi MO, Thomas JV, Smith TR. Glaucoma-inducing mechanisms in eyes with retinoblastoma. *Arch Ophthalmol.* 1978;96:105-110.

277. Mansour AM, Greenwald MJ, R OG. Diffuse infiltrating retinoblastoma. *J Pediatr Ophthalmol Strabismus.* 1989; 26:152-154.

278. Shields JA, Eagle RC, Shields CL, De Potter P. Congenital neoplasms of the nonpigmented ciliary epithelium (medulloepithelioma). *Ophthalmology.* 1996;103:1998-2006.

279. Caprioli J, Sears ML. The histopathology of black ball hyphema: a report of two cases. *Ophthalmic Surg.* 1984;15:491-495.

280. Beyer TL, Hirst LW. Corneal blood staining at low pressures. *Arch Ophthalmol.* 1985;103:654-655.

281. Messmer EP, Gottsch J, Font RL. Blood staining of the cornea: a histopathologic analysis of 16 cases. *Cornea.* 1984;3:205-12.

282. McDonnell PJ, Green WR, Stevens RE, Bargeron CB, Riquelme JL. Blood staining of the cornea. Light microscopic and ultrastructural features. *Ophthalmology.* 1985;92: 1668-74.

283. Gottsch GD, Messmer EP, McNair DS, Font RL. Corneal blood staining. An animal model. *Ophthalmology.* 1986;93:797-802.

284. McDonnell PJ, Gritz DC, McDonnell JM, Zarbin MA. Fluorescence of blood-stained cornea. *Cornea.* 1991;10:445-449.

285. Ritch R. Pathophysiology of glaucoma in uveitis. *Trans Ophthalmol Soc UK.* 1981;101:321-324.

286. Posner A, Schlossman A. Syndrome of unilateral recurrent attacks of glaucoma with cyclitic symptoms. *Arch Ophthalmol.* 1948;39:517-535.

287. Posner A, Schlossman A. Further observations on the syndrome of glaucomatocyclitic crises. *Trans Am Acad Ophthalmol Otolaryngol.* 1953;57:531-536.

288. Kass MA, Becker B, Kolker AE. Glaucomatocyclitic crisis and primary open-angle glaucoma. *Am J Ophthalmol.* 1973;75:668-673.

289. Raitta C, Vannas A. Glaucomatocyclitic crisis. *Arch Ophthalmol*. 1977;95:608-612.

290. Sokolic P. Observation of glaucomatocyclitic crisis associated with developmental glaucoma: contribution to the etiology. *Acta Ophthalmol*. 1966;44:607-612.

291. Sokolic P. Another case with recurrent glaucomatocyclitic crisis and anomalies in chamber angle, observed during and between hypertensive episodes. Contribution to etiology. *Acta Ophthalmol*. 1969;47:1129-1134.

292. Sokolic P. Developmental factor in the etiopathogenesis of glaucomatocyclitic crisis. *Ophthalmologica*. 1970;161:446-450.

293. Hart CT, Weatherill JR. Gonioscopy and tonography in glaucomatocyclitic crises. *Br J Ophthalmol*. 1968;52:682-687.

294. Yamamoto S, Pavan-Langston D, Tada R, et al. Possible role of herpes simplex virus in the origin of Posner-Schlossman syndrome. *Am J Ophthalmol*. 1995;119:796-798.

295. Setala K, Vannas A. Endothelial cells in the glaucomatocyclitic crisis. *Advances in Ophthalmology*. 1978;36:218-24.

296. Fuchs E. Ueber Komplikationen der Heterochromie. *Z. Augenheilk*. 1906;15:191-212.

297. OConnor GR. Doyne lecture. Heterochromic iridocyclitis. *Trans Ophthalmol Soc U K*. 1985;104:219-231.

298. Loewenfeld IE, Thompson HS. Fuchs's heterochromic cyclitis: A critical review of the literature. I. Clinical characteristics of the syndrome. *Surv Ophthalmol*. 1973;17:394-457.

299. Loewenfeld IE, Thompson HS. Fuchs's heterochromic cyclitis: A critical review of the literature. II. Etiology and mechanisms. *Surv Ophthalmol*. 1973;18:2-61.

300. Zamir E, Margalit E, Chowers I. Iris crystals in Fuchs' heterochromic iridocyclitis. *Arch Ophthalmol*. 1998;116:1394.

301. Noda S, Hayasaka S. Recurrent subconjunctival hemorrhages in patients with Fuchs' heterochromic iridocyclitis. *Ophthalmologica*. 1995;209:289-291.

302. Goble RR, Murray PI. Fuchs' heterochromic uveitis and sarcoidosis [see comments]. *Br J Ophthalmol*. 1995;79:1021-1023.

303. Fearnley IR, Rosenthal AR. Fuchs' heterochromic iridocyclitis revisited. *Acta Ophthalmol*. 1995;73:166-170.

304. La Hey E, de Vries J, Langerhorst CT, Baarsma GS, Kijlstra A. Treatment and prognosis of secondary glaucoma in Fuchs' heterochromic iridocyclitis. *Am J Ophthalmol*. 1993;116:327-340.

305. Berger BB, Tessler HH, Kottow MH. Anterior segment ischemia in Fuchs' heterochromic cyclitis. *Arch Ophthalmol*. 1980;98:499-501.

306. Norrsell K, Holmer AK, Jacobson H. Aqueous flare in patients with monocular iris atrophy and uveitis. A laser flare and iris angiography study. *Acta Ophthalmologica (Scand)*. 1998;76:405-412.

307. Bloch-Michel E, Lambin P, Debbia M, Tounsi Y, Trichet C, Offret H. Local production of IgG and IgG subclasses in the aqueous humor of patients with Fuchs heterochromic cyclitis, herpetic uveitis and toxoplasmic chorioretinitis. *Int Ophthalmol*. 1997;21:187-194.

308. Muhaya M, Calder V, Towler HM, Shaer B, McLauchlan M, Lightman S. Characterization of T cells and cytokines in the aqueous humour (AH) in patients with Fuchs' heterochromic cyclitis (FHC) and idiopathic anterior uveitis (IAU). *Clinical & Experimental Immunology*. 1998;111:123-128.

309. Perry HD, Yanoff M, Scheie HG. Rubeosis in Fuchs heterochromic iridocyclitis. *Arch Ophthalmol*. 1975;93:337-339.

310. Roussel TJ, Coster DJ. Fuchs's heterochromic cyclitis and posterior capsulotomy. *Br J Ophthalmol*. 1985;69:449-451.

311. Farrar SM, Shields MB, Miller KN, Stoup CM. Risk factors for the development and severity of glaucoma in the pigment dispersion syndrome. *Am J Ophthalmol*. 1989;108:223-229.

312. Farrar SM, Shields MB. Current concepts in pigmentary glaucoma. *Surv Ophthalmol*. 1993;37:233-252.

313. Becker B, Shin DH, Cooper DG, Kass MA. The pigment dispersion syndrome. *Am J Ophthalmol*. 1977;83:161-166.

314. Ritch R. A unification hypothesis of pigment dispersion syndrome. [Review] [118 refs]. *Trans Am Ophthalmol Soc*. 1996;94:381-405; discussion-9.

315. Roberts DK, Chaglasian MA, Meetz RE. Clinical signs of the pigment dispersion syndrome in blacks. *Optom Vis Sci*. 1997;74:993-1006.

316. Campbell DG. Pigmentary dispersion and glaucoma. A new theory. *Arch Ophthalmol*. 1979;97:1667-72.

317. Smith JP. Pigmentary open-angle glaucoma secondary to posterior chamber intraocular lens implantation and erosion of the iris pigment epithelium. *Journal-American Intra-Ocular Implant Society*. 1985;11:174-6.

318. Samples JR, Van Buskirk EM. Pigmentary glaucoma associated with posterior chamber intraocular lenses. *Am J Ophthalmol*. 1985;100:385-8.

319. Karickhoff JR. Pigmentary dispersion syndrome and pigmentary glaucoma: a new mechanism concept, a new treatment, and a new technique [see comments]. *Ophthalmic Surg*. 1992;23:269-77.

320. Karickhoff JR. Reverse pupillary block in pigmentary glaucoma: follow up and new developments [letter; comment]. *Ophthalmic Surg*. 1993;24:562-3.

321. Potash SD, Tello C, Liebmann J, Ritch R. Ultrasound biomicroscopy in pigment dispersion syndrome [see comments]. *Ophthalmology*. 1994;101:332-9.

322. Kaiser-Kupfer MI, Kupfer C, McCain L. Asymmetric pigment dispersion syndrome. *Trans Am Ophthalmol Soc*. 1983;81:310-24.

323. Pavlin CJ, Macken P, Trope GE, Harasiewicz K, Foster FS. Accommodation and iridotomy in the pigment dispersion syndrome. *Ophthalmic Surg Lasers*. 1996;27:113-20.

324. Liebmann JM, Tello C, Chew SJ, Cohen H, Ritch R. Prevention of blinking alters iris configuration in pigment dispersion syndrome and in normal eyes. *Ophthalmology*. 1995;102:446-55.

325. Pavlin CJ, Macken P, Trope G, Feldman F, Harasiewicz K, Foster FS. Ultrasound biomicroscopic features of pigmentary glaucoma. *Can J Ophthalmol*. 1994;29:187-92.

326. Pavlin CJ. Ultrasound biomicroscopy in pigment dispersion syndrome [letter; comment]. *Ophthalmology*. 1994;101:1475-1477.

327. Lagreze WD, Funk J. Iridotomy in the treatment of pigmentary glaucoma: documentation with high resolution ultrasound. *Ger J Ophthalmol*. 1995;4:162-166.

328. Sokol J, Stegman Z, Liebmann JM, Ritch R. Location of the iris insertion in pigment dispersion syndrome. *Ophthalmology*. 1996;103:289-293.

329. Semple HC, Ball SF. Pigmentary glaucoma in the black population. *Am J Ophthalmol.* 1990;109:518-522.

330. Migliazzo CV, Shaffer RN, Nykin R, Magee S. Long-term analysis of pigmentary dispersion syndrome and pigmentary glaucoma. *Ophthalmology.* 1986;93:1528-1536.

331. Smith DL, Kao SF, Rabbani R, Musch DC. The effects of exercise on intraocular pressure in pigmentary glaucoma patients. *Ophthalmic Surg.* 1989;20:561-567.

332. Haynes WL, Johnson AT, Alward WL. Effects of jogging exercise on patients with the pigmentary dispersion syndrome and pigmentary glaucoma. *Ophthalmology.* 1992;99:1096-1103.

333. Jensen PK, Nissen O, Kessing SV. Exercise and reversed pupillary block in pigmentary glaucoma. *Am J Ophthalmol.* 1995;120:110-112.

334. Ritch R, Chaiwat T, Harbin TS, Jr. Asymmetric pigmentary glaucoma resulting from cataract formation. *Am J Ophthalmol.* 1992;114:484-8.

335. Caplan MB, Brown RH, Love LL. Pseudophakic pigmentary glaucoma. *Am J Ophthalmol.* 1988;105:320-1.

336. Pignalosa B, Toni F, Liguori G. Pigmentary dispersion syndrome subsequent IOL implantation in P.C. *Doc Ophthalmol.* 1989;73:231-4.

337. Mastropasqua L, Lobefalo L, Gallenga PE. Iris chafing in pseudophakia. *Doc Ophthalmol.* 1994;87:139-44.

338. Gandolfi SA, Vecchi M. Effect of a YAG laser iridotomy on intraocular pressure in pigment dispersion syndrome. *Ophthalmology.* 1996;103:1693-5.

339. Carassa RG, Bettin P, Fiori M, Brancato R. Nd:YAG laser iridotomy in pigment dispersion syndrome: an ultrasound biomicroscopic study. *Br J Ophthalmol.* 1998;82:150-3.

340. Lagreze WD, Mathieu M, Funk J. The role of YAG-laser iridotomy in pigment dispersion syndrome. *Ger J Ophthalmol.* 1996;5:435-8.

341. Haynes WL, Alward WL, Tello C, Liebmann JM, Ritch R. Incomplete elimination of exercise-induced pigment dispersion by laser iridotomy in pigment dispersion syndrome. *Ophthalmic Surg & Lasers.* 1995;26:484-6.

342. Ritch R, Liebmann J, Robin A, et al. Argon laser trabeculoplasty in pigmentary glaucoma. *Ophthalmology.* 1993;100:909-913.

343. Scheie HG, Cameron JD. Pigment dispersion syndrome: a clinical study. *Br J Ophthalmol.* 1981;65:264-9.

344. Weseley P, Liebmann J, Walsh JB, Ritch R. Lattice degeneration of the retina and the pigment dispersion syndrome. *Am J Ophthalmol.* 1992;114:539-43.

345. Scuderi G, Papale A, Nucci C, Cerulli L. Retinal involvement in pigment dispersion syndrome. *Int Ophthalmol.* 1995;19:375-378.

346. Scuderi GL, Ricci F, Nucci C, Galasso MJ, Cerulli L. Electro-oculography in pigment dispersion syndrome. *Ophthalmic Res.* 1998;30:23-29.

347. Johnson DH. Does pigmentation affect the trabecular meshwork? *Arch Ophthalmol.* 1989;107:250-254.

348. Epstein DL, Freddo TF, Anderson PJ, Patterson MM, Bassett-Chu S. Experimental obstruction to aqueous outflow by pigment particles in living monkeys. *Invest Ophthalmol Vis Sci.* 1986;27:387-395.

349. Murphy CG, Johnson M, Alvarado JA. Juxtacanalicular tissue in pigmentary and primary open angle glaucoma. The hydrodynamic role of pigment and other constituents. *Arch Ophthalmol.* 1992;110:1779-1785.

350. Richter CU, Richardson TM, Grant WM. Pigmentary dispersion syndrome and pigmentary glaucoma. A prospective study of the natural history. *Arch Ophthalmol.* 1986;104:211-215.

351. Chaudhry IM, Moster MR, Augsburger JJ. Iris ring melanoma masquerading as pigmentary glaucoma. *Arch Ophthalmol.* 1997;115:1480-1481.

352. Naumann GO, Schlotzer-Schrehardt U, Kuchle M. Pseudoexfoliation syndrome for the comprehensive ophthalmologist. Intraocular and systemic manifestations. [Review] [52 refs]. *Ophthalmology.* 1998;105:951-968.

353. Theobald GD. Pseudo-exfoliation of the lens capsule. *Am J Ophthalmol.* 1954;37:1-12.

354. Prince AM, Streeten BW, Ritch R, Dark AJ, Sperling M. Preclinical diagnosis of pseudoexfoliation syndrome. *Arch Ophthalmol.* 1987;105:1076-82.

355. Ringvold A. Electron microscopy of the limbal conjunctiva in eyes with pseudo-exfoliation syndrome (PE syndrome). *Virchows Archiv-A: Pathology-Pathologische Anatomie.* 1972;355:275-283.

356. Streeten BW, Bookman L, Ritch R, Prince AM, Dark AJ. Pseudoexfoliative fibrillopathy in the conjunctiva. A relation to elastic fibers and elastosis. *Ophthalmology.* 1987;94:1439-1449.

357. Eagle RC, Jr., Font RL, Fine BS. The basement membrane exfoliation syndrome. *Arch Ophthalmol.* 1979;97:510-515.

358. Schlotzer-Schredhardt U, Kuchle M, Dorfler S, Naumann GO. Pseudoexfoliative material in the eyelid skin of pseudoexfoliation-suspect patients: a clinico-histopathological correlation. *Ger J Ophthalmol.* 1993;2:51-60.

359. Kuchle M, Schlotzer-Schrehardt U, Naumann GO. Occurrence of pseudoexfoliative material in parabulbar structures in pseudoexfoliation syndrome. *Acta Ophthalmol.* 1991;69:124-130.

360. Schlotzer-Schrehardt U, Kuchle M, Naumann GO. Electron-microscopic identification of pseudoexfoliation material in extrabulbar tissue. *Arch Ophthalmol.* 1991;109:565-570.

361. Streeten BW, Dark AJ, Wallace RN, Li ZY, Hoepner JA. Pseudoexfoliative fibrillopathy in the skin of patients with ocular pseudoexfoliation. *Am J Ophthalmol.* 1990;110:490-499.

362. Streeten BW, Li ZY, Wallace RN, Eagle RC, Jr., Keshgegian AA. Pseudoexfoliative fibrillopathy in visceral organs of a patient with pseudoexfoliation syndrome. *Arch Ophthalmol.* 1992;110:1757-1762.

363. Schlotzer-Schrehardt UM, Koca MR, Naumann GO, Volkholz H. Pseudoexfoliation syndrome. Ocular manifestation of a systemic disorder? *Arch Ophthalmol.* 1992;110:1752-1756.

364. Mitchell P, Wang JJ, Smith W. Association of pseudoexfoliation syndrome with increased vascular risk. *Am J Ophthalmol.* 1997;124:685-687.

365. Repo LP, Suhonen MT, Terasvirta ME, Koivisto KJ. Color Doppler imaging of the ophthalmic artery blood flow spectra of patients who have had a transient ischemic attack. Correlations with generalized iris transluminance and pseudoexfoliation syndrome [see comments]. *Ophthalmology.* 1995;102:1199-1205.

366. Rouhiainen H, Terasvirta M. Pigmentation of the anterior chamber angle in normal and pseudoexfoliative eyes. *Acta Ophthalmol.* 1990;68:700-702.

367. Sampaolesi R, Zarate J, Croxato O. The chamber angle in exfoliation syndrome. Clinical and pathological findings. *Acta Ophthalmol.* 1988;184(suppl):48-53.

368. Wishart PK, Spaeth GL, Poryzees EM. Anterior chamber angle in the exfoliation syndrome. *Br J Ophthalmol.* 1985;69:103-107.

369. Franks WA, Miller MH, Hitchings RA, Jeffrey MN. Secondary angle closure in association with pseudoexfoliation of the lens capsule. *Acta Ophthalmol.* 1990;68:350-352.

370. Baltatzis S, Georgopoulos G, Theodossiadis P. Fibrin reaction after extracapsular cataract extraction: a statistical evaluation. *Eur J Ophthalmol.* 1993;3:95-97.

371. Repo LP, Terasvirta ME, Tuovinen EJ. Generalized peripheral iris transluminance in the pseudoexfoliation syndrome. *Ophthalmology.* 1990;97:1027-1029.

372. Repo LP, Terasvirta ME, Koivisto KJ. Generalized transluminance of the iris and the frequency of the pseudoexfoliation syndrome in the eyes of transient ischemic attack patients. *Ophthalmology.* 1993;100:352-355.

373. Asano N, Schlotzer-Schrehardt U, Naumann GO. A histopathologic study of iris changes in pseudoexfoliation syndrome. *Ophthalmology.* 1995;102:1279-1290.

374. Sugar S. Pigmentary glaucoma and the glaucoma associated with the exfoliation-pseudoexfoliation syndrome: update. Robert N. Shaffer lecture. *Ophthalmology.* 1984;91:307-310.

375. Prince AM, Ritch R. Clinical signs of the pseudoexfoliation syndrome. *Ophthalmology.* 1986;93:803-807.

376. Repo LP, Naukkarinen A, Paljarvi L, Terasvirta ME. Pseudoexfoliation syndrome with poorly dilating pupil: a light and electron microscopic study of the sphincter area. *Graefes Arch Clin Exp Ophthalmol.* 1996;234:171-176.

377. Aasved H. Prevalence of fibrillopathia epitheliocapsularis (pseudoexfoliation) and capsular glaucoma. *Trans Ophthalmol Soc UK.* 1979;99:293-295.

378. Ye TC, Mao WS, Zhang J. Pseudoexfoliation syndrome in Chinese. *Jpn J Ophthalmol.* 1989;33:300-10.

379. Summanen P, Tonjum AM. Exfoliation syndrome among Saudis. *Acta Ophthalmol-Suppl.* 1988;184:107-111.

380. Shimizu K, Kimura Y, Aoki K. Prevalence of exfoliation syndrome in the Japanese. *Acta Ophthalmol-Suppl.* 1988;184:112-115.

381. Krause U, Alanko HI, Karna J, et al. Prevalence of exfoliation syndrome in Finland. *Acta Ophthalmol-Suppl.* 1988;184:120-122.

382. Colin J, Le Gall G, Le Jeune B, Cambrai MD. The prevalence of exfoliation syndrome in different areas of France. *Acta Ophthalmol-Suppl.* 1988;184:86-89.

383. Forsius H. Exfoliation syndrome in various ethnic populations. *Acta Ophthalmol-Suppl.* 1988;184:71-85.

384. Yalaz M, Othman I, Nas K, et al. The frequency of pseudoexfoliation syndrome in the eastern Mediterranean area of Turkey. Acta Ophthalmologica 1992;70:209-213.

385. Tarkkanen AHA. Exfoliation syndrome. *Trans Ophthalmol Soc U K.* 1986;105:233-236.

386. Friederich R. Eye disease in the Navajo indians. *Ann Ophthalmol.* 1982;14:38-40.

387. Jones W, White RE, Magnus DE. Increased occurrence of exfoliation in the male, Spanish American population of New Mexico. *J Am Optom Assoc.* 1992;63:643-648.

388. Hiller R, Sperduto RD, Krueger DE. Pseudoexfoliation, intraocular pressure, and senile lens changes in a population-based survey. *Arch Ophthalmol.* 1982;100:1080-1082.

389. Layden WE, Ritch R, King DG, Teekhasaenee C. Combined exfoliation and pigment dispersion syndrome. *Am J Ophthalmol.* 1990;109:530-4.

390. Psilas KG, Stefaniotou MJ, Aspiotis MB. Pseudoexfoliation syndrome and diabetes mellitus. *Acta Ophthalmol.* 1991;69:664-666.

391. Ringvold A, Blika S, Elsas T, et al. The middle-Norway eye-screening study. II. Prevalence of simple and capsular glaucoma. *Acta Ophthalmol.* 1991;69:273-280.

392. Kozart DM, Yanoff M. Intraocular pressure status in 100 consecutive patients with exfoliation syndrome. *Ophthalmology.* 1982;89:214-218.

393. Yanoff M, Klemetti A. Intraocular pressure in exfoliation syndrome. *Acta Ophthalmol-Suppl.* 1988;184:59-61.

394. Henry JC, Krupin T, Schmitt M, et al. Long-term follow-up of pseudoexfoliation and the development of elevated intraocular pressure. *Ophthalmology.* 1987;94:545-552.

395. Klemetti A. Intraocular pressure in exfoliation syndrome. *Acta Ophthalmol-Suppl.* 1988;184:54-58.

396. Crittendon JJ, Shields MB. Exfoliation syndrome in the southeastern United States. II. Characteristics of patient population and clinical course. *Acta Ophthalmol-Suppl.* 1988;184:103-106.

397. Konstas AG, Jay JL, Marshall GE, Lee WR. Prevalence, diagnostic features, and response to trabeculectomy in exfoliation glaucoma. *Ophthalmology.* 1993;100:619-627.

398. Konstas AG, Allan D. Pseudoexfoliation glaucoma in Greece. *Eye.* 1989;3:747-53.

399. Henke V, Naumann GO. [Incidence of the pseudo-exfoliation syndrome in enucleated eyes]. *Klin Monatsbl Augenheilkd.* 1987;190:173-175.

400. Netland PA, Ye H, Streeten BW, Hernandez MR. Elastosis of the lamina cribrosa in pseudoexfoliation syndrome with glaucoma. *Ophthalmology.* 1995;102:878-986.

401. Gottanka J, Flugel-Koch C, Martus P, Johnson DH, Lutjen-Drecoll E. Correlation of pseudoexfoliative material and optic nerve damage in pseudoexfoliation syndrome. *Invest Ophthalmol Vis Sci.* 1997;38:2435-2446.

402. Jonas JB, Papastathopoulos KI. Optic disk appearance in pseudoexfoliation syndrome. *Am J Ophthalmol.* 1997;123:174-180.

403. FitzSimon JS, Mulvihill A, Kennedy S, Finch A, Collum LM, Eustace P. Association of HLA type with pseudoexfoliation of the lens capsule [see comments]. *Br J Ophthalmol.* 1996;80:402-404.

404. Ringvold A, Blika S, Elsas T, et al. The middle-Norway eye-screening study. III. The prevalence of capsular glaucoma is influenced by blood-group antigens. *Acta Ophthalmol.* 1993;71:207-213.

405. Gradle HS, Sugar HS. Concerning the chamber angle. II. Exfoliation of the zonular lamella and glaucoma capsulare. *Am J Ophthalmol.* 1940;23:982-997.

406. Sampaolesi R, Argento C. Scanning electron microscopy of the trabecular meshwork in normal and glucomatous eyes. *Invest Ophthalmol Vis Sci.* 1977;16:302-314.

407. Gillies WE. Secondary glaucoma associated with pseudoexfoliation of the lens capsule. *Trans Ophthalmol Soc UK.* 1978;98:96-100.

408. Bartholomew RS. Effect of cataract extraction on the intraocular pressure in eyes with pseudoexfoliation of the lens. *Transactions of the Ophthalmological Societies of the United Kingdom.* 1979;99:312-3.

409. Morrison JC, Green WR. Light microscopy of the exfoliation syndrome. *Acta Ophthalmol-Suppl.* 1988;184:5-27.

410. Schlotzer-Schrehardt U, Naumann GO. Trabecular meshwork in pseudoexfoliation syndrome with and without open-angle glaucoma. A morphometric, ultrastructural study. *Invest Ophthalmol Vis Sci.* 1995;36:1750-1764.

411. Jerndal T, Lind A. New aspects on the heredity of open angle glaucoma. *Acta Ophthalmol.* 1979;57:826-831.

412. Tarkkanen A. Pseudoexfoliation of the lens capsule. *Acta Ophthalmol-Suppl.* 1962;71:1-98.

413. Takei Y, Mizuno K. Electron-microscopic study of pseudoexfoliation of the lens capsule. *Graefes Archiv Klin Exp Ophthalmol.* 1978;205:213-220.

414. Assia EI, Apple DJ, Morgan RC, Legler UF, Brown SJ. The relationship between the stretching capability of the anterior capsule and zonules. *Invest Ophthalmol Vis Sci.* 1991;32:2835-2839.

415. Pavlin CJ, Buys YM, Pathmanathan T. Imaging zonular abnormalities using ultrasound biomicroscopy. *Arch Ophthalmol.* 1998;116:854-857.

416. Goder GJ. Our experiences in planned extracapsular cataract extraction in the exfoliation syndrome. *Acta Ophthalmol-Suppl.* 1988;184:126-128.

417. Naumann GO. Exfoliation syndrome as a risk factor for vitreous loss in extracapsular cataract surgery (preliminary report). Erlanger-Augenblatter-Group. *Acta Ophthalmol-Suppl.* 1988;184:129-131.

418. Zetterstrom C, Olivestedt G, Lundvall A. Exfoliation syndrome and extracapsular cataract extraction with implantation of posterior chamber lens. *Acta Ophthalmol.* 1992; 70:85-90.

419. Moreno J, Duch S, Lajara J. Pseudoexfoliation syndrome: clinical factors related to capsular rupture in cataract surgery. *Acta Ophthalmol.* 1993;71:181-184.

420. Chitkara DK, Smerdon DL. Risk factors, complications, and results in extracapsular cataract extraction. *J Cataract Refract Surg.* 1997;23:570-574.

421. Drolsum L, Haaskjold E, Sandvig K. Phacoemulsification in eyes with pseudoexfoliation. *J Cataract Refract Surg.* 1998;24:787-792.

422. Scorolli L, Campos EC, Bassein L, Meduri RA. Pseudoexfoliation syndrome: a cohort study on intraoperative complications in cataract surgery. *Ophthalmologica.* 1998;212:278-280.

423. Kuchle M, Amberg A, Martus P, Nguyen NX, Naumann GO. Pseudoexfoliation syndrome and secondary cataract. *Br J Ophthalmol.* 1997;81:862-866.

424. Dark AJ, Streeten BW, Jones D. Accumulation of fibrillar protein in the aging human lens capsule, with special reference to the pathogenesis of pseudoexfoliative disease of the lens. *Arch Ophthalmol.* 1969;82:815-821.

425. Dark AJ, Streeten BW, Cornwall CC. Pseudoexfoliative disease of the lens: a study in electron microscopy and histochemistry. *Br J Ophthalmol.* 1977;61:462-72.

426. Streeten BW, Licari PA, Marucci AA, Dougherty RM. Immunohistochemical comparison of ocular zonules and the microfibrils of elastic tissue. *Invest Ophthalmol Vis Sci.* 1981;21:130-135.

427. Streeten BW, Gibson SA, Dark AJ. Pseudoexfoliative material contains an elastic microfibrillar-associated glycoprotein. *Trans Am Ophthalmol Soc.* 1986;84:304-320.

428. Li ZY, Streeten BW, Yohai N. Amyloid P protein in pseudoexfoliative fibrillopathy. *Curr Eye Res.* 1989;8:217-227.

429. Li ZY, Streeten BW, Wallace RN. Association of elastin with pseudoexfoliative material: an immunoelectron microscopic study. *Curr Eye Res.* 1988;7:1163-1172.

430. Seland JH. The ultrastructure of the deep layer of the lens capsule in fibrillopathia epitheliocapsularis (FEC), so-called senile exfoliation or pseudoexfoliation. A scanning electron microscopic study. *Acta Ophthalmol.* 1978;56:335-348.

431. Seland JH. Histopathology of the lens capsule in fibrillopathia epitheliocapsularis (FEC) or so-called senile exfoliation or pseudoexfoliation. An electron microscopic study. *Acta Ophthalmol.* 1979;57:477-499.

432. Seland JH. The ultrastructural changes in the exfoliation syndrome. *Acta Ophthalmol-Suppl.* 1988;184:28-34.

433. Ringvold A, Nicolaissen B, Jr. Culture of iris tissue from human eyes with and without pseudoexfoliation. *Acta Ophthalmol.* 1990;68:310-316.

434. Tetsumoto K, Schlotzer-Schrehardt U, Kuchle M, Dorfler S, Naumann GO. Precapsular layer of the anterior lens capsule in early pseudoexfoliation syndrome. *Graefes Arch Clin Exp Ophthalmol.* 1992;230:252-257.

435. Schlotzer-Schrehardt U, von der Mark K, Sakai LY, Naumann GO. Increased extracellular deposition of fibrillin-containing fibrils in pseudoexfoliation syndrome. *Invest Ophthalmol Vis Sci.* 1997;38:970-984.

436. Fitzsimmons TD, Fagerholm P, Wallin O. Hyaluronan in the exfoliation syndrome. *Acta Ophthalmol.* 1997;75:257-260.

437. Kuchle M, Vinores SA, Mahlow J, Green WR. Blood-aqueous barrier in pseudoexfoliation syndrome: evaluation by immunohistochemical staining of endogenous albumin. *Graefes Arch Clin Exp Ophthalmol.* 1996;234:12-18.

438. Kuchle M, Nguyen NX, Hannappel E, Naumann GO. The blood-aqueous barrier in eyes with pseudoexfoliation syndrome. *Ophthalmic Res.* 1995;27 Suppl 1:136-142.

439. Dotsenko V, Neshkova E, Namazova I, Vavilova L, Yarovaya G. Hageman factor and kallikrein in pathogenesis of senile cataracts and the pseudoexfoliation syndrome. *Immunopharmacology.* 1996;32:141-145.

440. Moreno-Montanes J, Lajara Blesa J. IgG, albumin and total IgG index in the aqueous humour of eyes with pseudoexfoliation syndrome. *Acta Ophthalmol.* 1995;73:249-251.

441. Streeten BW, Dark AJ, Barnes CW. Pseudoexfoliative material and oxytalan fibers. *Exp Eye Res.* 1984;38:523-531.

442. Garner A, Alexander RA. Pseudoexfoliative disease: histochemical evidence of an affinity with zonular fibres. *Br J Ophthalmol.* 1984;68:574-80.

443. Hietanen J, Tarkkanen A. Glycoconjugates in exfoliation syndrome. A lectin histochemical study of the ciliary body and lens. *Acta Ophthalmol.* 1989;67:288-294.

444. Ermilov VV. [Amyloidosis of the eye combined with other senile pathology]. *Arkh Patol.* 1993;55:43-45.

445. Schlotzer-Schrehardt U, Dorfler S, Naumann GO. Immunohistochemical localization of basement membrane components in pseudoexfoliation material of the lens capsule. *Curr Eye Res.* 1992;11:343-355.

446. Kubota T, Khalil A, Tawara A, Zhang X, Inomata H. Double staining of proteoglycans and the HNK-1 carbohydrate epitope in pseudoexfoliation material. *Curr Eye Res.* 1998;17:60-64.

447. Kubota T, Schlotzer-Schrehardt U, Inomata H, Naumann GO. Immunoelectron microscopic localization of the HNK-1 carbohydrate epitope in the anterior segment of pseudoexfoliation and normal eyes. *Curr Eye Res.* 1997;16:231-238.

448. Hiscott P, Schlotzer-Schrehardt U, Naumann GO. Unexpected expression of thrombospondin 1 by corneal and iris fibroblasts in the pseudoexfoliation syndrome. *Hum Pathol.* 1996;27:1255-1258.

449. Flocks M, Littwin CS, Zimmerman LE. Phacolytic glaucoma. *Arch Ophthalmol.* 1955;54:37-45.

450. Yanoff M, Scheie HG. Cytology of human lens aspirate. Its relationship to phacolytic glaucoma and phacoanaphylactic endophthalmitis. *Arch Ophthalmol.* 1968;80:166-170.

451. Epstein DL, Jedziniak JA, Grant WM. Identification of heavy-molecular-weight soluble protein in aqueous humor in human phacolytic glaucoma. *Invest Ophthalmol Vis Sci.* 1978;17:398-402.

452. Epstein DL, Jedziniak JA, Grant WM. Obstruction of aqueous outflow by lens particles and by heavy-molecular-weight soluble lens proteins. *Invest Ophthalmol Vis Sci.* 1978;17:272-277.

453. Epstein DL. Diagnosis and management of lens-induced glaucoma. *Ophthalmology.* 1982;89:227-230.

454. Brooks AM, Grant G, Gillies WE. Comparison of specular microscopy and examination of aspirate in phacolytic glaucoma. *Ophthalmology.* 1990;97:85-89.

455. Bartholomew RS, Rebello PF. Calcium oxalate crystals in the aqueous. *Am J Ophthalmol.* 1979;88:1026-1028.

456. Kirk HQ, Petty RW. Malignant melanoma of the choroid. A correlation of clinical and histological findings. *Arch Ophthalmol.* 1956;56:843-860.

457. Makley TA, Teed RW. Unsuspected intraocular malignant melanomas. *Arch Ophthalmol.* 1958;60:475-478.

458. Litricin O. Unsuspected uveal melanomas. *Am J Ophthalmol.* 1973;76:734-738.

459. Robertson DM, Campbell RJ. Errors in the diagnosis of malignant melanoma of the choroid. *Am J Ophthalmol.* 1979;87:269-275.

460. Davidorf FH, Letson AD, Weiss ET, Levine E. Incidence of misdiagnosed and unsuspected choroidal melanomas. A 50-year experience. *Arch Ophthalmol.* 1983;101:410-412.

461. Yanoff M, Scheie HG. Melanomalytic glaucoma. Report of a case. *Arch Ophthalmol.* 1970;84:471-473.

462. Van Buskirk EM, Leure-duPree AE. Pathophysiology and electron microscopy of melanomalytic glaucoma. *Am J Ophthalmol.* 1978;85:160-166.

463. McMenamin PG, Lee WR. Ultrastructural pathology of melanomalytic glaucoma. *Br J Ophthalmol.* 1986;70:895-906.

464. Fineman MS, Eagle RC, Shields JA, Shields CL, De Potter P. Melanocytomalytic glaucoma in eyes with necrotic iris melanocytoma. *Ophthalmology.* 1998;105:492-496.

465. Manschot WA. Ring melanoma. *Arch Ophthalmol.* 1964;71:625-632.

466. Callender D, Jay JL, Barrie T. Schwartz-Matsuo syndrome: atypical presentation as acute open angle glaucoma [letter]. *Br J Ophthalmol.* 1997;81:609-610.

467. Matsuo T. Photoreceptor outer segments in aqueous humor: key to understanding a new syndrome. *Surv Ophthalmol.* 1994;39:211-233.

468. Sugar HS. Low tension glaucoma: a practical approach. *Ann Ophthalmol.* 1979;11:1155-1171.

469. Levene RZ. Low tension glaucoma. Part II. Clinical characteristics and pathogenesis [editorial]. *Ann Ophthalmol.* 1980;12:1383.

470. Levene RZ. Low tension glaucoma: a critical review and new material. *Surv Ophthalmol.* 1980;24:621-664.

471. Grosskreutz C, Netland PA. Low-tension glaucoma. *Int Ophthalmol Clin.* 1994;34:173-185.

472. Drance SM. Some factors in the production of low tension glaucoma. *Br J Ophthalmol.* 1972;56:229-242.

473. Pillunat LE, Stodtmeister R, Wilmanns I. Pressure compliance of the optic nerve head in low tension glaucoma. *Br J Ophthalmol.* 1987;71:181-187.

474. Stroman GA, Stewart WC, Golnik KC, Cure JK, Olinger RE. Magnetic resonance imaging in patients with low-tension glaucoma. *Arch Ophthalmol.* 1995;113:168-172.

475. Carter CJ, Brooks DE, Doyle DL, Drance SM. Investigations into a vascular etiology for low-tension glaucoma [see comments]. *Ophthalmology.* 1990;97:49-55.

476. Butt Z, McKillop G, C OB, Allan P, Aspinall P. Measurement of ocular blood flow velocity using colour Doppler imaging in low tension glaucoma. *Eye.* 1995;9:29-33.

477. Quaranta L, Manni G, Donato F, Bucci MG. The effect of increased intraocular pressure on pulsatile ocular blood flow in low tension glaucoma. *Surv Ophthalmol.* 1994;38:S177-181; discussion S82.

478. Klaver JH, Greve EL, Goslinga H, Geijssen HC, Heuvelmans JH. Blood and plasma viscosity measurements in patients with glaucoma. *Br J Ophthalmol.* 1985;69:765-770.

479. Bito LZ. Impact of intraocular pressure on venous outflow from the globe: a hypothesis regarding IOP-dependent vascular damage in normal-tension and hypertensive glaucoma. *J Glaucoma*. 1996;5:127-134.

480. Rankin SJ, Walman BE, Buckley AR, Drance SM. Color Doppler imaging and spectral analysis of the optic nerve vasculature in glaucoma [see comments]. *Am J Ophthalmol*. 1995;119:685-693.

481. Kaiser HJ, Flammer J, Wenk M, Luscher T. Endothelin-1 plasma levels in normal-tension glaucoma: abnormal response to postural changes. *Graefes Arch Clin Exp Ophthalmol*. 1995;233:484-488.

482. Yamazaki Y, Hayamizu F. Comparison of flow velocity of ophthalmic artery between primary open angle glaucoma and normal tension glaucoma. *Br J Ophthalmol*. 1995;79:732-734.

483. Sugiyama T, Moriya S, Oku H, Azuma I. Association of endothelin-1 with normal tension glaucoma: clinical and fundamental studies. *Surv Ophthalmol*. 1995;39:S49-S56.

484. Lietz A, Kaiser HJ, Stumpfig D, Flammer J. Influence of posture on the visual field in glaucoma patients and controls. *Ophthalmologica*. 1995;209:129-131.

485. Harris A, Sergott RC, Spaeth GL, Katz JL, Shoemaker JA, Martin BJ. Color Doppler analysis of ocular vessel blood velocity in normal-tension glaucoma. *Am J Ophthalmol*. 1994;118:642-649.

486. Kaiser HJ, Flammer J, Burckhardt D. Silent myocardial ischemia in glaucoma patients. *Ophthalmologica*. 1993;207:6-7.

487. Rojanapongpun P, Drance SM, Morrison BJ. Ophthalmic artery flow velocity in glaucomatous and normal subjects. *Br J Ophthalmol*. 1993;77:25-29.

488. Cartwright MJ, Grajewski AL, Friedberg ML, Anderson DR, Richards DW. Immune-related disease and normal-tension glaucoma. A case-control study. *Arch Ophthalmol*. 1992;110:500-502.

489. Muller M, Kessler C, Wessel K, Mehdorn E, Kompf D. Low-tension glaucoma: a comparative study with retinal ischemic syndromes and anterior ischemic optic neuropathy. *Ophthalmic Surg*. 1993;24:835-838.

490. Gutman I, Melamed S, Ashkenazi I, Blumenthal M. Optic nerve compression by carotid arteries in low-tension glaucoma. *Graefes Arch Clin Exp Ophthalmol*. 1993;231:711-717.

Chapter Ten

CONGENITAL AND PEDIATRIC GLAUCOMA

Ali Aminlari, MD, FACS

Primary congenital glaucoma is the most common type of glaucoma in children, however, it occurs much less frequently than the primary glaucomas that are seen in adults (Figure 10-1). It has been estimated that every ophthalmologist will have the chance to see only one case every 5 years, and an ophthalmic resident has the opportunity to see only two or three cases of congenital glaucoma during his or her training. Approximately 60% to 70% of congenital glaucoma cases are bilateral.

Primary congenital glaucoma usually is diagnosed at birth or shortly thereafter. Most cases are diagnosed in the first year of life; however, it may become apparent at anytime throughout childhood or early adult life. Photophobia, blepharospasm, and epiphora are the most common presenting symptoms of congenital glaucoma (Figures 10-2 and 10-3).

During the first 3 years of life, the collagen fibers of the eye are softer and more elastic than in older individuals. Thus, elevation of intraocular pressure (IOP) in children younger than 3 years of age (infan-

tile glaucoma) causes rapid enlargement of the globe. The globe enlargement occurs primarily at the corneo-scleral junction. As the cornea and limbus enlarge, the endothelium of the cornea and Descemet's membrane are stretched. This stretching can result in a linear rupture of the Descemet's membrane (Haab's striae). The Descemet's membrane rupture may occur acutely, causing an influx of aqueous into the stoma and epithelium, resulting in sudden corneal edema. The corneal edema produces photophobia, blepharospasm, and tearing. The child becomes very irritable and may hide his or her face from bright lights.

Continuous enlargement of the eye leads to progressive myopia and scleral thinning. In very advanced cases, these changes result in a bluish appearance of the sclera and severe stretching of the corneo-scleral junction to the extent that the limbus cannot be identified (Figure 10-4). The iris also is stretched and appears very thin. The iris root and trabecular meshwork become degenerated and Schlemm's canal collapses. The ciliary body, choroid,

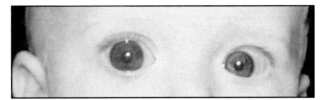

Figure 10-1. Unilateral primary congenital glaucoma.

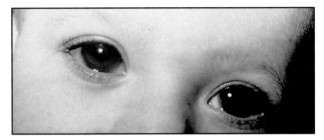

Figure 10-3. Epiphora with congenital glaucoma.

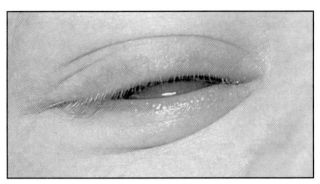

Figure 10-2. Photophobia and blepharospasm in congenital glaucoma.

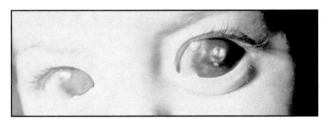

Figure 10-4. Very advanced primary congenital glaucoma.

and the retina are atrophic. Zonular fibers may break resulting in dislocation of the lens. The optic disc eventually becomes totally cupped. In such advanced cases, the prognosis is very poor, and any intraocular procedure may lead to phthisis bulbi.

Late onset glaucoma, after age 3 years, is termed *juvenile glaucoma* (Figures 10-5 and 10-6). These patients develop glaucoma from the same anomalies as neonates and infants with primary congenital glaucoma. Their glaucoma presents at a later date either as a primary process or as a recurrence after seemingly successful surgery. They usually present like chronic glaucoma in adults. This group often is overlooked because the possibility of juvenile glaucoma is not considered.

In juvenile glaucoma, the posterior sclera may still have some elasticity permitting it to expand secondary to high IOP. Progressive myopia results from such expansion, however, the cornea does not enlarge. Therefore, progressive myopia, although is not a pathognomonic sign, should prompt consideration of congenital glaucoma in this age group.

CLASSIFICATION OF GLAUCOMA IN CHILDREN

Glaucoma in infants and children are classified into three groups.
1. **Primary congenital or infantile glaucoma.** This refers to a type of glaucoma resulting from an isolated maldevelopment of the trabecular meshwork region not associated with other developmental ocular or systemic anomalies, nor any ocular diseases that can cause an increase in IOP. It is the most common type of glaucoma in infancy, occurring in approximately one per 10,000 live births.[1]
2. **Secondary glaucoma.** This refers to glaucoma resulting from ocular pathology (eg, inflammation or tumors). This form of glaucoma is usually said to be less common than primary type; however, Barsoum-Homsy and Chevrette studied 63 cases (95 eyes) of glaucoma in children and found that secondary glaucoma to be the most common type of glaucoma in children.[2]
3. **Developmental glaucoma.** This term refers to a type of congenital glaucoma associated with developmental anomalies of the eye and other parts of the body, which present at birth (Figure 10-7).

Hoskins has classified congenital glaucoma on the basis of clinically identifiable anatomic defects of the eye.[3] These congenital anatomical defects may involve trabecular meshwork, cornea, iris, or a combinations of these structures.

The Shaffer-Weis classification divides the developmental glaucomas into primary, secondary, and acquired glaucoma.[4]

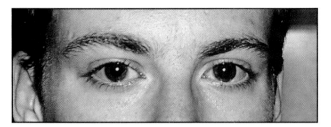

Figure 10-5. Juvenile glaucoma.

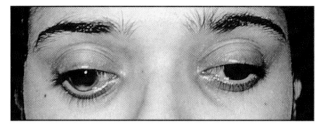

Figure 10-6. Juvenile glaucoma.

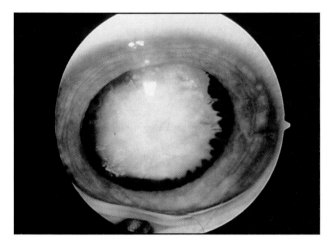

Figure 10-7. PHPV with congenital glaucoma.

HEREDITARY

Approximately 90% of primary congenital glaucoma cases are sporadic in occurrence. In 10% of patients where a hereditary pattern is evident, it is believed to be autosomal recessive.[5]

HISTOPATHOLOGY AND EMBRYOLOGY

A basic understanding of embryology of the anterior segment of the eye is helpful in relation to pathogenesis of childhood glaucoma.

Tissue derived from the neural crest has been demonstrated to contribute extensively to the embryologic development of the head and neck, particularly ocular tissues. In the head and neck, tissue derived from neural crest functions embryologically in a manner similar to mesoderm in other bodily regions. The reader is referred to extensive reviews, which discuss the role of neural crest tissue in cephalic embryology and in the classification of the glaucomas.[6-9] Only a brief overview will be presented in this chapter. It is derived from these and other sources.[10-15]

The anterior chamber angle is formed by three primordial embryonic tissues:

1. **Surface ectoderm.** This gives rise to the crystalline lens and corneal epithelium. The lens develops as an invagination during the third week of gestation and separates from the surface ectoderm by the sixth week.
2. **Neural ectoderm.** This forms the optic cup. The margins of the optic cup give rise to the iris epithelium.
3. **Neural crest.** The structure of the anterior chamber arises from neural crest-derived tissue. The undifferentiated mesenchymal tissue, between surface ectoderm and the lens, forms the following structures during seventh and eighth weeks of gestation:
   - Corneal endothelium—this later secretes Descemet's membrane
   - Corneal stoma
   - Iris stroma

The anterior surface of the iris meets the corneal endothelium at 5 months of gestation to form the peripheral aspect of the anterior chamber angle.[16] Adjacent and posterior to this area cells form the trabecular meshwork, the ciliary body overlaps the trabecular meshwork.

The trabecular meshwork gradually is exposed to the anterior chamber as the iridocorneal angle deepens and moves posteriorly.

The mechanism of the tissue changes that lead to the formation of the anterior chamber angle is not well known. There are several theories including atrophy of tissue and cell death in the angle.[17] Another theory proposes that the angle is formed by a process of cleavage between the cells that form the trabecular meshwork and the cells that form the root of the iris and ciliary body.[18] Anderson believes that the trabecular meshwork becomes exposed to the anterior chamber by posterior sliding of the iris and ciliary body.[16] Continued posterior sliding of the uveal tissue occurs during the first 6 to 12 months of life. This forms the angle recess which is not normally present at birth.

The iris and ciliary body in primary congenital glaucoma are similar to the one of seventh or eighth month of gestation rather than the one which is at full-term development.[16] The iris insertion and anterior ciliary body overlap the posterior portion of the trabecular meshwork. Histopathologic examination of the angle structure in primary congenital glaucoma demonstrates thickening of trabecular beams, thickened cords of uveal meshwork, and compression of trabecular meshwork with a resultant decrease of trabecular spaces.[19] These changes may be the cause of obstruction to the outflow of aqueous fluid and, therefore, result in elevation of IOP.

Thickening of juxtacanalicular tissue and production of an amorphous material in the subendothelial area of the inner wall of Schlemm's canal also have been found in histopathologic examination of infants' eyes with congenital glaucoma.[19,20]

Anterior insertion of longitudinal and circular fibers of ciliary muscle into trabecular meshwork rather than into scleral spur is suggested by Maumenee to be typical histopathologic finding in primary congenital glaucoma.[21]

Barkan's membrane is a postulated semitransparent membrane that extends over trabecular meshwork is suggested to be the cause of elevated IOP in childhood glaucoma.[22] The existence of such a membrane has not been verified.[23]

Ocular embryology will be discussed further relative to some specific congenital glaucoma syndromes.

DIAGNOSIS OF CONGENITAL GLAUCOMA

The clinical presentation of primary congenital glaucoma leads, in the majority of cases, to the diagnosis of this disease. A complete office examination or an examination under anesthesia is necessary in evaluating children suspected to have glaucoma.

An office examination can be performed on children as young as 3 years of age using chloral hydrate sedation, if needed. A short office examination frequently can be performed on children younger than 6 months of age. Pacifying the child with a bottle is helpful in checking IOP. Various tonometers (eg, Schiötz, Perkins applanation, or hand-held electronic tonometers [Tono-Pen, Mentor O&O, Inc, Norwell, Mass]) can be used.

For a complete ophthalmological examination, general anesthesia is usually required in infantile glaucoma. Mask anesthesia is adequate and safe for a short follow-up examination, but endotracheal intubation is necessary if surgery is required, or examination is expected to be prolonged.

TONOMETRY

Except for ketamine, which may increase IOP, general anesthetics usually lower the pressure. It is recommended that the pressure be checked in early stage of anesthesia to reduce errors.

Different types of tonometers can be used for IOP check. The Schiötz tonometer occasionally is used, however, it is not as accurate as the Perkins hand-held applanation tonometer. The Tono-Pen is very convenient and easy to use. In my experience, Tono-Pen reading may be 2 to 3 mmHg lower than an applanation measurement.

The normal IOP in infants under anesthesia is usually in the low teens (in mmHg). A pressure of 20 mmHg or more should be considered abnormal.

Elevated IOP alone is not sufficient to confirm a diagnosis of congenital glaucoma. Other signs of this disease (eg, corneal haze, increased corneal diameter, and increased optic disc cupping) are as important as elevated pressure.

CORNEAL DIAMETER

Accurate measurement of corneal size is important in the diagnosis and follow-up examination of children with glaucoma. Using calipers for this purpose, the corneal diameter measurement should be taken from limbus to a similar point 180 degrees away at the opposite limbus. The 95% ranges of normal corneal diameters are: 9.4 to 11.0 mm at age 1 month, 10.5 to 11.7 mm at age 6 months, and 10.8 to 12.0 mm at age 12 months.[24] Morin and colleagues found a corneal diameter of 11 mm or less in only 24% of primary congenital glaucoma patients at age less than 3 months, and only in 9% of those over 3 months.[25] In congenital glaucoma sometimes the diameter of cornea enlarges to as much as 17 mm. Changes in corneal diameter less than 0.5 mm in follow-up examination should be interpreted cautiously.

GONIOSCOPY

A 14-mm Koeppe lens provides a clear view of the angle of the eye, and a hand-held microscope with a Barkan light or any type of illuminator are necessary for gonioscopy during anesthesia. If the cornea is cloudy, removing the corneal epithelium clears the view. During gonioscopy, the site of iris insertion should be evaluated carefully. In congenital glaucoma, the iris usually is inserted anterior to scleral spur, and the angle recess is poorly formed.

FUNDUSCOPY

Dilated fundus examination and disc evaluation are essential in diagnosing congenital glaucoma. Cupping of the optic disc occurs much faster than in adults. Optic disc cupping larger than 30% of disc diameter, especially if asymmetric between two eyes, is strong evidence that the disc is under pressure and may be glaucomatous.

The normal infant optic disc is as pink as in the normal adult. In the past, it had been thought that the optic disc in the newborn was paler than in adults; however, Khodadoust,[26] and Shaffer and Hetherington[27] have demonstrated the ease with which blood could be shunted from the infant's optic disc by a small increase in IOP. Even the pressure of a lid speculum or the pressure generated by separating the lids may cause shunting of blood and a pale appearing disc.

Changes in the optic disc occur readily with changes in IOP in infants.[28] Richardson and Shaffer[28] in 1966, and Khodadoust in 1968[26] documented the early response of the infant disc to elevated IOP. These findings demonstrate the greater vulnerability of the infant optic disc to increased IOP compared to the adult disc.

How rapidly does this cupping occur in infant eyes? When congenital glaucoma is diagnosed at birth, it is not uncommon to find a large degree of optic disc cupping. This finding proves that disc damage can start during intrauterine development. If IOP is not controlled, increased cupping can be demonstrated in 4 to 6 weeks. This early rapid change in disc contour probably is related to mechanical distortion in the disc supporting elements, and in its initial stages may not represent neuronal loss. Thus, posterior bowing of the lamina cribrosa is a late occurrence in adult glaucoma but it occurs early in infants.

Glaucomatous cupping in infants, unlike in adults, is usually reversible following normalization of IOP.

This was first reported in 1965 by Chandler and Grant.[29] Marked decreases in cupping commonly are seen at 4 to 6 weeks after normalization of pressure. The younger the child, the faster this reversibility. This phenomenon is so constant that it can be used as the main criterion for control of glaucoma in infants rather than using the height of IOP. I have observed a marked decrease in cup disc ratio in some of our patients in just 2 weeks following a successful goniotomy. Such a rapid change in optic disc cupping is probably related to mechanical changes cited earlier. Improvement in the amount of cupping may be limited by many factors including the extent of nerve fiber loss.

DIFFERENTIAL DIAGNOSIS

Children under age 3 with epiphora and photophobia should be suspected as having congenital glaucoma. Nasolacrimal duct obstruction also must be considered, however, it is rarely accompanied with photophobia.

Conjunctivitis, corneal abrasion, some types of corneal dystrophies (eg, Meesman's and Reis-Buckler's) also may present with irritation and tearing. A careful history and examination will reveal the correct diagnosis.

High myopia can present with a large eye, but without other signs and symptoms of congenital glaucoma. Similarly, megalocornea, a condition with very large corneal diameter, may mimic the corneal enlargement of congenital glaucoma (Figure 10-8). Eyes with (congenital) megalocornea have very deep anterior chambers and the corneal diameter may be as large as 16 mm; however, the IOP is normal and no Descemet's rupture or corneal edema should be present. Photophobia or tearing are not present with this condition.

Megalocornea is a sex-linked disorder and occurs mainly in males. The IOP of these patients should be monitored closely, as they may develop glaucoma. I have followed a 4-year-old boy with megalocornea who developed glaucoma at the age of 10.

Traumatic rupture of Descemet's membrane is another condition to be differentiated from congenital glaucoma. Forceps delivery is a common cause of unilateral Descemet's rupture, mostly in the left eye, which is due to the high incidence of left anterior occiput presentation at birth. These types of Descemet's ruptures are commonly vertical but they may run in various directions. Corneal edema may be present with photophobia, lacrimation, and ble-

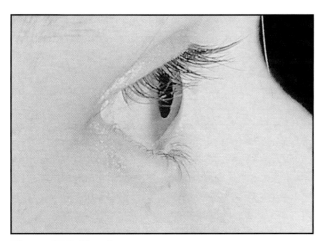

Figure 10-8. Megalocornea.

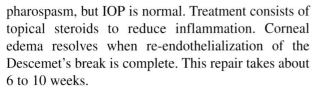

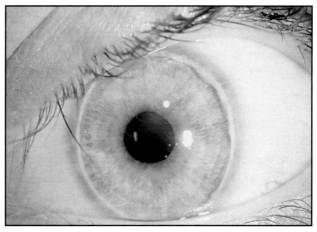

Figure 10-9. Posterior embryotoxon.

pharospasm, but IOP is normal. Treatment consists of topical steroids to reduce inflammation. Corneal edema resolves when re-endothelialization of the Descemet's break is complete. This repair takes about 6 to 10 weeks.

Congenital hereditary endothelial dystrophy (CHED) and posterior polymorphous corneal dystrophy (PPED) can have cloudy cornea at birth or later in life. The differentiation from congenital glaucoma is crucial. Normal IOP and corneal diameter, which do not increase in time, and mainly stromal rather than epithelial edema speak in favor of dystrophy rather than glaucoma. Corneal cloudiness is due to corneal edema and thickening of stroma. These may sometimes be accompanied by photophobia and tearing. Occasionally these patients may have been misdiagnosed and subjected to unnecessary glaucoma surgery. I have observed this misdiagnosis on one occasion.

Other congenital anomalies such as sclerocornea, cystinosis, and mucopolysaccharidosis, which may be accompanied by a cloudy cornea, should be differentiated from congenital glaucoma.

Anomalies of the optic nerve head are sometimes difficult to distinguish from glaucomatous cupping. Tilted disc, coloboma of the nerve head, pits, hypoplasia, and highly myopic discs are among this category.

Corneal edema due to keratitis in newborns (eg, rubella keratitis) should be differentiated from congenital glaucoma.

DEVELOPMENTAL GLAUCOMA

Several developmental anomalies of the eye have been described, which have traditionally been believed to represent dysgenesis of mesoderm of the anterior ocular segment but are probably secondary to abnormalities in development of neural crest derived tissue. These conditions may involve the cornea, iris, lens, or irido-corneal angle. Glaucoma may be present with any of these conditions including Axenfeld's, Rieger's, and Peter's anomalies.

Posterior embryotoxon or prominent Schwalbe's line is present in about 15% of the general population [30] (Figure 10-9). Axenfeld reported a condition in which strands of peripheral iris traversed the angle of the eye and attached to the prominent Schwalbe's line [31] (Figure 10-10). In Rieger's anomaly there also is stromal hypoplasia of the iris in addition to Axenfeld changes.[32] There may be some iris hole formation, ectropion uveae, and corectopia. If Rieger's anomaly is part of a systemic manifestation of this disorder, then it is called Rieger's syndrome. These systemic findings include facial and dental anomalies, including broad and flat nasal bridge, telecanthus (wide interorbital distance), hypertelorism (wide intercanthal distance), maxillary hypoplasia, and a protruding lower lip.[33]

About 50% of patients with Axenfeld's or Rieger's anomaly develop glaucoma. The incidence is slightly higher in Rieger's. Diagnosis is generally made between age 5 and 30 years.[34]

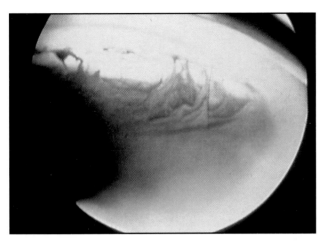
Figure 10-10. Strands of iris to Schwalbe's Line.

In 1897, Von Hippel reported a case of buphthalmos with bilateral central corneal opacities and adhesion of these opacities to the iris.[35] Peters described similar cases in 1906, which became generally known as Peters' anomaly.[36] Most of these cases are hereditary with autosomal recessive inheritance. They are generally bilateral and present at birth. Corneal endothelium and Descemet's membrane are missing in the center of the cornea with thinning and opacification of overlying stroma. Cataract may be present. Approximately 50% of patients with this anomaly have glaucoma. Goniotomy or trabeculotomy are not as effective as in primary congenital glaucoma, and trabeculectomy may offer the best chance of success. Corneal graft frequently is necessary.

Table 10-1 lists other developmental anomaly that may be accompanied by congenital.

Sturge-Weber syndrome is characterized by a hemangioma of the skin along the trigeminal distribution and ipsilateral lepto-meningeal angioma. The latter may cause a seizure disorder. Involvement is usually unilateral but bilateral lesions may occur. Cortical calcification is a characteristic radiographic sign (railroad tracks). Fifty percent of these patients develop glaucoma, which is more common when the hemangioma involves the upper eyelid (Figures 10-11 and 10-12). Glaucoma may occasionally be present on the side opposite the upper lid involvement (Figure 10-13).

The cause of glaucoma in Sturge-Weber syndrome is believed to be increased episcleral venous pressure. A congenital anomaly of the anterior chamber angle similar to primary congenital glaucoma also has been described.[37]

Table 10-1
Developmental Anomaly with Congenital Glaucoma

1. Phakomatoses
    a. Sturge-Weber syndrome or encephalotrigeminal angiomatosis
    b. Von Recklinghausen's neurofibromatosis
    c. Von Hippel Lindau disease
2. Aniridia
3. Lowe's syndrome
4. Stickler syndrome
5. Hallermann-Streiff syndrome
6. Rubenstein's broad-thumb syndrome
7. Hurler's and Ehlers Danlos syndrome

The management of glaucoma in Sturge-Weber syndrome is primarily surgical when it presents early in life; however, medical treatment should be tried when it occurs in later life.

Combined trabeculotomy-trabeculectomy may offer the best hope of surgical success.

Aniridia is a bilateral condition, which may be associated with multiple ocular defects including corneal opacity, cataract, and foveal hypoplasia. It is inherited as autosomal dominant. The name *aniridia* is misnomer, because the iris is only partially absent. A rudimentary stump always is present. Wilms tumor of kidney or other genito-urinary anomalies may be present.

Glaucoma occurs in 50% to 75% of patients with aniridia, but usually does not appear before late childhood or early adolescence. Medical therapy may control the pressure for a short period of time, however, the majority of patients finally require surgery to control the pressure. Trabeculotomy or goniotomy may not be helpful, and filtration procedures often fail. Cyclocryotherapy is effective in some cases.

TREATMENT OF CONGENITAL GLAUCOMA

The management of primary congenital glaucoma is essentially surgical.[38] Goniotomy and trabeculoto-

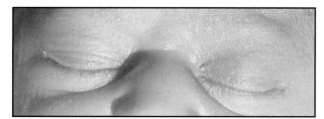

Figure 10-11. Unilateral Sturge-Weber with congenital glaucoma.

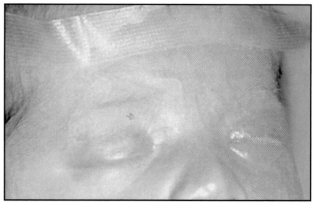

Figure 10-12. Bilateral Sturge-Weber with bilateral congenital glaucoma.

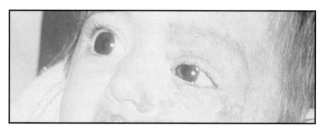

Figure 10-13. Unilateral Sturge-Weber with contralateral congenital glaucoma.

my have been the most successful procedures for congenital glaucoma.[39,40] Goniopuncture was proposed by Scheie and is believed to increase success rate.[41] These procedures are more successful in infants under 1 year of age.

Medical treatment is used primarily in the preoperative management of these patients. Beta blockers (eg, timolol or betaxolol) may be administered one drop twice daily for a short time period. Nevertheless, one must be aware of the comparatively large medication dose of one drop of such medications applied to an infant. Thus, such patients must be watched carefully for the development of side effects, which may be life threatening. Pilocarpine, in low concentration, and carbonic anhydrase inhibitors (eg, acetazolamide, 5 to 10 mg/kilo body weight), as the suspension, can be given. Dorzolamide, a topical carbonic anhydrase inhibitor, may not be as effective as the oral suspension. The newer glaucoma drops, brimonidine and latanoprost have not yet been approved to be used in children.

Surgical procedures such as goniotomy and trabeculotomy are effective when performed skillfully (Figures 10-14 and 10-15). One or two goniotomies can cure 94% of children with congenital glaucoma presenting within the first 2 years of life.[42] Congenital glaucoma presenting within the first month of life or after age 2 years has a poorer surgical outcome.

Others and myself prefer trabeculotomy to goniotomy. Nevertheless, others indicate no preference between the two procedures.[40,43,44]

Serious complications in trabeculotomy or goniotomy are rare. Difficulty locating Schlemm's canal, transient hyphema, cyclodialysis or iridodialysis, and cataract or lens dislocation rarely occur. Hyphema can be prevented by injecting air into the anterior chamber if bleeding occurs intraoperatively. Residual hyphema is usually cleared within 24 hours; however, hyphema may at times be large and persistent.

Should two or three goniotomies or trabeculotomies fail, trabeculectomy is the next best treatment. Antimetabolites can be used in low doses. Glaucoma setons can be inserted if trabeculectomy fails. Cyclodestructive procedures have a very low success rate.[45]

FOLLOW-UP EVALUATION

Topical steroids and antibiotics should be used for 4 to 6 weeks. The patient should be examined 2 to 4 weeks after the initial procedure, sooner if indicated. Decreased photophobia and tearing is a good indication that the treatment has been successful, at least partially. If there is no increase in corneal diameter or optic disc cupping, or if there is a decrease in corneal cloudiness and in IOP, reexamination is performed 3 to 4 months later, then every 6 months for 1 year and yearly thereafter. During the follow-up period a cycloplegic refraction should not be forgotten and any evidence of amblyopia, if present, should be managed aggressively. Amblyopia can be due to anisometropia, significant astigmatism, or corneal cloudiness.

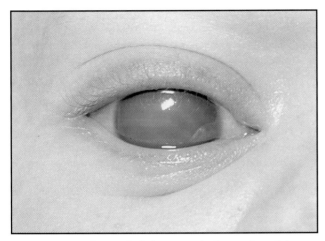

Figure 10-14. Congenital glaucoma before trabeculotomy.

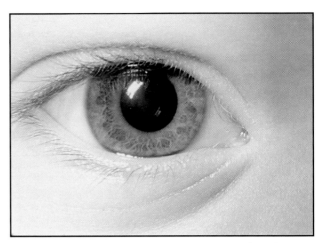

Figure 10-15. Congenital glaucoma 14 months after trabeculotomy.

The long-term prognosis for patients with primary congenital glaucoma is excellent when successfully treated.

SUMMARY

If congenital glaucoma is recognized early and appropriate treatment is instituted, prognosis is excellent. There is a poor prognosis if glaucoma presents within the first month or after 2 years of age. Treatment is primarily surgical; however, medical therapy is indicated immediately following the diagnosis in the preoperative period if surgery is to be delayed. It is also indicated in difficult patients who do not respond well to the surgical treatment. Patients with congenital glaucoma require long-life follow-up. An IOP rise can occur anytime and must be detected early and treated appropriately.

REFERENCES

1. Walton DS. Primary congenital open angle glaucoma: a study of the anterior segment abnormalities. *Trans Am Ophthalmol Soc.* 1979;77:746-768.
2. Barsoum-Homsy M, Chevrette L. Incidence and prognosis of childhood glaucoma. A study of 63 cases. *Ophthalmology.* 1986;93:1323-1327.
3. Hoskins HD Jr, Shaffer RN, Hetherington J. Anatomical classification of the developmental glaucomas. *Arch Ophthalmol.* 1984;102:1331-1336.
4. Shaffer RN, Weiss DI. *Congenital and Pediatric Glaucomas.* St Louis, Mo: CV Mosby; 1970.
5. Shaffer RN. Genetics and congenutal glaucoma. *Am J Ophthalmol.* 1965;60:981-994.
6. Kupfer C, Kaiser-Kupfer MI. New hypothesis of developmental anomalies of the anterior chamber associated with glaucoma. *Trans Ophthalmol Soc UK.* 1978;98:213-215.
7. Kupfer C, Kaiser-Kupfer MI. Observations on the development of the anterior chamber angle with reference to the pathogenesis of congenital glaucomas. *Am J Ophthalmol.* 1979;88:424-426.
8. Tripathi B, Tripathi R, ed. Embryology of the anterior segment of the human eye. In: Ritch R, Shields MB, Krupin T, eds. *The Glaucomas.* St Louis, Mo: CV Mosby; 1989.
9. Ozanics V, Jakobiec FA, ed. Prenatal development of the eye and its adnexa. In: Tasman W, ed. *Duane's Foundations of Clinical Ophthalmology.* Vol 1. Philadelphia, Pa: JB Lippincott Co; 1994:
10. Johnston MC, Noden DM, Hazelton RD, Coulombre JL, Coulombre AJ. Origins of avian ocular and periocular tissues. *Exp Eye Res.* 1979;29:27-43.
11. Beauchamp GR, Knepper PA. Role of the neural crest in anterior segment development and disease. *J Pediatr Ophthalmol Strabismus.* 1984;21:209-214.
12. Cook CS. Experimental models of anterior segment dysgenesis. *Ophthalmic Paediatr Genet.* 1989;10:33-46.
13. Tripathi BJ, Tripathi RC. Neural crest origin of human trabecular meshwork and its implications for the pathogenesis of glaucoma [see comments]. *Am J Ophthalmol.* 1989;107:583-590.
14. Doran RM. Anterior segment malformations: aetiology and genetic implications [editorial]. *Br J Ophthalmol.* 1991;75:579.
15. Williams DL. A comparative approach to anterior segment dysgenesis. *Eye.* 1993;7:607-616.
16. Anderson DR. The development of the trabecular meshwork and its abnormality in primary infantile glaucoma. *Trans Am Ophthalmol Soc.* 1981;79:458-485.
17. Allen L, Burian HM, Braley AE. A new concept of the development of the anterior chamber angle. *Arch Ophthalmol.* 1955;53:783.

18. Burian HM, Braley AE, Allen L. Viability of the ring of Schwalbe and the trabecular zone. *Arch Ophthalmol.* 1955;53:767-782.

19. Maul E, Strozzi L, Munoz C, Reyes C. The outflow pathway in congenital glaucoma. *Am J Ophthalmol.* 1980;89:667-673.

20. Tawara A, Inomata H. Developmental immaturity of the trabecular meshwork in congenital glaucoma. *Am J Ophthalmol.* 1981;92:508-525.

21. Maumenee AE. The pathogenesis of congenital glaucoma. *Am J Ophthalmol.* 1959;47:827.

22. Barkan O. Pathogenesis of congenital glaucoma. *Am J Ophthalmol.* 1955;40:1-11.

23. Worst JG. Congenital glaucoma. Remarks on the aspect of chamber angle, ontogenetic and pathogenetic background, and mode of action of goniotomy. *Invest Ophthalmol.* 1968;7:127-134.

24. Kiskis AA, Markowitz SN, Morin JD. Corneal diameter and axial length in congenital glaucoma. *Can J Ophthalmol.* 1985;20:93-97.

25. Morin JD, Merin S, Sheppard RW. Primary congenital glaucoma—a survey. *Can J Ophthalmol.* 1974;9:17-28.

26. Khodadoust AA, Ziai M, Biggs SL. Optic disc in normal newborns. *Am J Ophthalmol.* 1968;66:502-504.

27. Shaffer RN, Hetherington J, Jr. The glaucomatous disc in infants. A suggested hypothesis for disc cupping. *Trans Am Acad Ophthalmol Otolaryngol.* 1969;73:923-935.

28. Richardson KT, Shaffer RN. Optic-nerve cupping in congenital glaucoma. *Am J Ophthalmol.* 1966;62:507-509.

29. Chandler PA, Grant WM. *Lectures on Glaucoma.* Philadelphia, Pa: Lea & Febiger; 1986.

30. Burian HM, Braley AE, Allen L. External and gonioscopic visibility of the ring of Schwalbe and trabecular zone. An interpretation of posterior corneal embryotoxon and the so called congenital hyaline membrane on the posterior corneal surface. *Trans Am Ophthalmol Soc.* 1955;51:389-410.

31. Axenfeld T. Embryotoxon corneae posterius. *Klin Monatsbl Augenh.* 1920;65:381-382.

32. Rieger H. Verlagerung und Shlitzform der pupille mit hypoplasie des irisverderblattes. *Z Augenheilkd.* 1934;84:98.

33. Shields MB. Axenfeld-Rieger syndrome: a theory of mechanism and distinctions from the iridocorneal endothelial syndrome. *Trans Am Ophthalmol Soc.* 1983;81:736-784.

34. Waring GO, Rodrigues MM, Laibson PR. Anterior chamber cleavage syndrome. A stepladder classification. *Surv Ophthalmol.* 1975;20:3-27.

35. Von Hippel E. Uber hydrophthalmos congenitus nebst Bemerkungen uber die ver farbung der cornea duich blutfarbstoff, Pathologisch-anatomische untersuchungen. *Graefe Arch Klin Exp Ophthalmol.* 1897;4:539.

36. Peters A. Ueber angeborene defektbildung der descemetschen memberane. *Klin Monatsbl Augenheilk.* 1906;44:27.

37. Weiss DI. Congenital mesodermal anomalies and glaucoma. *Invest Ophthalmol and Vis Sci.* 1968;7:123-126.

38. Scheie HG. The management of infantile glaucoma. *Arch Ophthalmol.* 1959;62:35-54.

39. Barkan O. Operation for congenital glaucoma. *Am J Ophthalmol.* 1950;25:552.

40. McPherson SD, Jr., Berry DP. Goniotomy vs external trabeculotomy for developmental glaucoma. *Am J Ophthalmol.* 1983;95:427-431.

41. Scheie HG. Goniopuncture: A new filtering operation for glaucoma. *Arch Ophthalmol.* 1950;44:761-782.

42. Shaffer RN. Prognosis of goniotomy in primary infantile glaucoma (trabeculodysgenesis). *Trans Am Ophthalmol Soc.* 1982;80:321-325.

43. Anderson DR. Trabeculotomy compared to goniotomy for glaucoma in children. *Ophthalmology.* 1983;90:805-806.

44. Luntz MH, Livingston DG. Trabeculotomy ab externo and trabeculectomy in congenital and adult-onset glaucoma. *Am J Ophthalmol.* 1977;83:174-179.

45. Aminlari A. Cyclocryotherapy in congenital glaucoma. *Glaucoma.* 1981;3:331.

Chapter Eleven

GLAUCOMA PHARMACOLOGY

Jody R. Piltz, MD
Annapurna Singh, MD

INTRODUCTION

Most patients diagnosed with glaucoma in the United States first are started on topical medications. The decision-making process involved in initiating and selecting the appropriate therapy for an individual patient is complex. There are currently more than 20 different glaucoma drugs available from six broad classes. It is important to have a complete understanding of the mechanism of action of each drug, their interactions, and the potential complications of therapy. Understanding the available therapies enables physicians to make intelligent choices for their patients and choose a therapeutic plan that provides the greatest benefit and least risk.

In this chapter, we use a pharmacological basis for classifying these drugs (Table 11-1). We also discuss the rationale for treatment of glaucoma and outline basic principles involved in selecting appropriate medical therapy (Table 11-2). Brand names and companies are provided if generic formulations are not available.

AUTONOMIC OVERVIEW

The autonomic nervous system, which consists of the sympathetic and parasympathetic sub-systems, is responsible for regulating IOP. Acetylcholine is the neurotransmitter of the entire parasympathetic system. Cholinergic receptors are nicotinic (autonomic ganglia and striated muscle) or muscurinic (secretory glands and smooth muscle of multiple organ systems). Norepinephrine, the main transmitter of the sympathetic nervous system, is produced in the sympathetic nerve terminals. After release, its action is terminated by re-uptake and degradation by the enzyme catechol-O-methyl transferase. Adrenergic receptors are divided into alpha and beta type receptors. Alpha-1 receptors (α-1) are post-synaptic and mediate vasoconstriction, while α-2 receptors are pre-synaptic and inhibit the release of norepinephrine from the sympathetic nerve terminals. Beta-1 receptors (β-1) are more prevalent in cardiac tissue, while β-2 receptors are found in the lungs, glands, and eye.[1]

Table 11-1

Glaucoma Medications

Medication Class	Generic Name	Brand Name	Manufacturer	Strengths (%)	Sizes (mL)	Top Color
Parasympathomimetics						
Cholinergic Agents	Pilocarpine HCl	Multiple	Multiple	0.25 to 10	15, 30	Green
		Pilopine HS gel	Alcon (Ft. Worth, Tex)	4	4 gm	Green
	Pilocarpine nitrate	Pilagan	Allergan (Irvine, Calif)	1, 2, 4	15	Green
	Pilocarpine	Ocusert Pilo	Alza (Palo Alto, Calif)	20, 40	Box of 8	Inserts
Cholinesterase	Echothiophate	Phospholine	Storz (St. Louis, Mo)	0.03, 0.06, 0.125,	5	Dropper Bottle
	Iodide	Iodide		0.25		
Inhibitors	Demecarium	Humorsol	Merck (West Point, Pa)	0.125, 0.25	5	Dropper Bottle
Mixed	Carbachol	Isopto Carbachol	Alcon	0.75, 1.5, 2.25, 3	10, 30	Green
Adrenergic Agonists						
Non-Selective	Epinephrine HCl	Epifrin	Allergan	0.5, 1, 2	5, 10, 15	White
		Glaucon	Alcon	1, 2	10	White
	Epinephrine Borate	Epinal	Alcon	0.5, 1	7.5	White
	Dipivefrin HCl	Propine	Allergan	0.1	5, 10, 15	Purple
		Generics Available				
Selective	Aproclonidine	Iopidine	Alcon	0.5	5, 10	White
α Agonist				1.0	Dropperettes	
	Brimonidine	Alphagan	Allergan	0.2	5, 10, 15	Purple
β-Adrenergic Antagonists						
β-1 Selective	Betaxolol HCl	Betoptic S	Alcon	0.25 suspension	2.5, 5, 10, 15	Blue
		Betoptic	Alcon	0.5 solution	2.5, 5, 10, 15	Blue
Non-Selective	Timolol Maleate	Timoptic	Merck	0.25, 0.5	2.5, 5, 10, 15	Blue
		Generics Available			Ocudose	
		Timoptic-XE	Merck	0.25, 0.5	2.5, 5	Blue, Yellow
	Timolol	Betimol	Ciba (Duluth, Ga)	0.25, 0.5	2.5, 5, 10, 15	White
	Hemihydrate					
	Levobunolol HCl	Betagan	Allergan	0.25, 0.5	2, 5, 10, 15	Blue, Yellow
		Generics Available				
	Carteolol	Ocupress	Ciba	1.0	5, 10, 15	White
	Metipranolol	Optipranolol	Bausch & Lomb (Tampa, Fla)	0.3	2, 5, 10	White
Prostaglandins						
	Latanoprost	Xalatan	Pharmacia (Kalamazoo, Mich)	0.005	2.5	White
CAIs						
Oral	Acetazolamide	Diamox	Storz	125, 250 mg	Tablets	
		Tablets available generically		500 mg	Time release capsules	
	Methazolamide	Multiple	Multiple	25, 50 mg	Tablets	
Topical	Dorzolamide	Trusopt	Merck	2	5, 10	Orange
	Brinzolamide	Azopt	Alcon	1	5, 10, 15	Orange
Combination β-Blocker/CAI						
	Timolol Maleate & Dorzolamide	Cosopt	Merck	0.5 / 2	5, 10	Yellow

CHOLINERGIC DRUGS (MIOTICS, PARASYMPATHOMIMETICS)

Cholinergic drugs have been in use for more than 100 years. Although quite effective in lowering IOP, their use has decreased in recent years as new agents with fewer ocular side effects have been introduced. Cholinergic drugs often are called miotics because they stimulate pupillary constriction.

Mechanism of Action

Parasympathometic agents can be direct acting acetylcholine agonists (eg, pilocarpine), or they can act indirectly by inhibiting acetylcholinesterase (eg, echothiophate), thereby preventing the breakdown of endogenous acetylcholine and increasing the availability of acetylcholine at the receptor sites.[2] Pilocarpine stimulates only muscurinic receptors, while echothiophate stimulates both nicotinic and muscurinic receptors.[3] Cholinergic agents are bound to melanin, so higher concentrations are needed in patients with more darkly pigmented irides.

Most cholinergics lower IOP by 20 to 30% and are additive to most other agents. Cholinergic stimulation causes contraction of the fibers of the longitudinal ciliary muscle, which exerts traction on the scleral spur. This contraction enhances outflow through the trabecular meshwork, which normally accounts for 80% of aqueous outflow. Cholinergics decrease uveoscleral outflow, which accounts for 20% of aqueous egress from the eye.[4] Recent evidence suggests that pilocarpine also may act directly on the trabecular meshwork cells.[5]

Preparation and Administration

Pilocarpine drops are the most commonly prescribed cholinergic agonists. They are available as a nitrate or hydrochloride salt in concentrations ranging from 0.25% to 10%. Increasing the concentration increases the magnitude of IOP reduction,[6] however, with punctal occlusion, the maximal effect may be achieved with 2% pilocarpine in blue-eyed patients and 4% pilocarpine in brown-eyed patients.[7] Although dosing is generally four times daily, punctal occlusion may increase the duration of action, particularly at the higher concentrations. Peak action is achieved 2 hours after administration.

Pilocarpine is also available as Ocuserts (Alza) and in a gel formation (Pilopine gel 4%, Alcon) which are useful in decreasing the frequency of administration and minimizing ocular side effects. Ocuserts are a membrane-controlled delivery system with zero order kinetics (constant release rate) and need to be inserted only once a week.[8] They are available as P20 (20 µg/hour, equivalent to a 1% to 2% solution) and P40 (40 µg/hour, roughly equivalent to a 4% solution). Their use minimizes the miosis and accommodative spasm of Pilocarpine, but many patients find it difficult to insert and keep them in their eyes. Pilocarpine 4% gel is applied once daily at bedtime,[9] but may not provide IOP lowering for the full 24 hours.

Echothiophate iodide (phospholine iodide, Storz Ophthalmics) is the most commonly prescribed indirect acting cholinergic agent. It is available as 0.03%, 0.06%, 0.125%, and 0.25% solutions. It is administered two times daily. Because of the potential for cataract and iris cyst formation, it is used predominantly in aphakic and pseudophakic eyes. Systemic build up of acetylcholine may occur leading to possible systemic side effects.

Carbachol has both direct and indirect acting activity. Although it is 100 times more effective than acetylcholine and 200 times more effective than pilocarpine, it has poor corneal penetration.[3] It has similar efficacy to pilocarpine and is administered three times daily.

Adverse Effects

Superficial ocular hyperemia, epithelial toxicity, miosis with darkening of vision, spasm of accommodation with a myopic shift in refraction, and headache/brow ache are common ocular side effects. Although not serious, they are the most frequent cause of discontinuation of cholinergic agents. Visual side effects are more pronounced in people with cataracts, and cataract surgery can sometimes be delayed by discontinuing the cholinergic. Ocular side effects can be minimized by starting with a very low dose (0.5% to 1% in whites, 1% to 2% in African Americans), and increasing the strength only if needed.

Paradoxical increase in IOP associated with anterior chamber shallowing and increase in pupillary block also can occur. Retinal detachments develop rarely, particularly in people with pre-existing retinal breaks. Systemic side effects such as diarrhea, bradycardia, diaphoresis, salivation, and nausea rarely

Table 11-2

Side Effects of Glaucoma Medications

Medication Class	Mechanism of Action	Efficacy	Ocular Side Effects	Systemic Side Effects	Relative Contraindications
Parasympathomimetics	Increased outflow through the trabecular meshwork	++(+)	Miosis, dim vision accommodative spasm, induced myopia, posterior synechiae, cataracts*, iris cysts*, pseudo-pemphigoid*, retinal detachments	Headache, brow ache	Uveitis, neovascular glaucoma, retinal breaks, succinylcholine-induced general anesthesia*
Non-Selective Adrenergic Agonists	Increased outflow	+(+)	Hyperemia, blepharoconjunctivitis, adrenochrome deposition, mydriasis, pseudopemphigoid, cystoid macular edema, stains soft contacts lenses	Headache, anxiety, palpitations, elevated blood pressure incidence (fewer side effects with Dipivefrin)	Aphakia; pseudophakia, narrow angles, patients using reserpine, MAO inhibitors or tricyclic antidepressants, labile hypertension, cardiac arrhythmias thyrotoxicosis
α Adrenergic Agonists	Decreased aqueous production Increased uveoscleral outflow‡	++(+) ++	Toxic dermatitis, blepharoconjunctivitis, lid retraction†, conjunctival blanching†, hypotension and apnea in babies and children‡	Dry mouth, lethargy‡	Babies and young children‡; patients using MAO inhibitors or sedatives, significant cardiac, renal, hepatic, or cerebro-vascular disease, Raynaud's disease, thromboangiitis obliterans
β Adrenergic Antagonists	Decreased aqueous production	+++ ++betaxalol	Corneal anesthesia, blepharoconjunctivitis, delayed choroidal detachments	Bronchoconstriction, bradycardia, exacerbates heart block and congestive heart failure, fatigue, malaise, depression, dizziness, impotency, memory loss (fewer side effects with betaxolol)	Asthma, chronic obstructive pulmonary disease, bradycardia, second or third degree heart block, congestive heart failure, brittle diabetes, thyrotoxicosis, myasthemia gravis. Use with caution in patients taking reserpine, guanethidine, quinidine. (Contraindications of greater concern with non-selective β-blockers.)

Table 11-2 (continued)

Side Effects of Glaucoma Medications

Medication Class	Mechanism of Action	Efficacy	Ocular Side Effects	Systemic Side Effects	Relative Contraindications
Prostaglandins	Increases uveoscleral outflow	++++	Iris color change (hazel and mixed green/brown irides), conjunctival hyperemia, uveitis, cystoid macular edema, hypertrichosis	Myalgias	
CAIs	Decreases aqueous production				
Oral		+++	Transient myopia, delayed choroidal detachments	Metallic taste to food, malaise, depression, weight loss, anorexia, chronic diarrhea, kidney stones, Stevens-Johnson syndrome, aplastic anemia, metabolic acidosis, hypokalemia, acidosis with chronic aspirin use	Sulfa allergy, kidney stones, diabetic ketoacidosis, chronic respiratory acidosis, hypo-kalemia, patients using thiazide diuretics or phenytoin sodium, sickle cell anemia, hepatic disease
Topical		++(+)	Burning on instillation (dorzolamide)	Metallic taste, theoretical potential for same side effects as oral CAIs but no definitive evidence to date	Significant sulfa allergy

*Indirect acting parasympathetic agents (cholinesterase inhibitors)
† Aproclonidine
‡ Brimonidine

occur with routine dosing, but may develop after repeated dosing to treat an attack of angle-closure glaucoma.

Echothiophate iodide can induce formation of iris cysts, cataracts, pemphigoid-like syndrome, and punctal stenosis.[10] Systemic side effects such as nausea, diarrhea, abdominal cramps, anxiety, and confusion can occur secondary to cholinesterase depletion, but are rare at typical therapeutic doses.[11] Impaired ability to inactive succinyl choline secondary to irreversible cholinesterase inhibitors can lead to prolonged apnea if succinyl choline is used for induction during general anesthesia due.[12] Accidental ingestion of a single bottle of an anticholinesterase can be lethal in children.[13]

Contraindications

Cholinergic drugs are contraindicated in patients with synechial angle closure or neovascular glaucoma. They should be avoided if there are peripheral retinal breaks or in eyes at high risk for retinal detachment. They can exacerbate uveitis and worsen vision profoundly in patients with cataracts, particularly posterior subcapsular cataracts.

ADRENERGIC DRUGS

Adrenergic agonists are the second oldest class of glaucoma medications, introduced in the early part of the 20th century and used routinely since the 1950s. The older, non-selective agonists with alpha and beta effects (epinephrine and dipivefrin) are used less frequently since the newer selective alpha agonists were introduced in the 1990s.

Non-Selective Adrenergic Agonists

Mechanism of Action

Non-selective adrenergic agonists lower IOP by increasing outflow facility through the trabecular meshwork and by increasing uveoscleral outflow.[14,15] The effects are mediated predominantly by stimulation of the α-2 adrenergic receptor.[3] These agents are poorly additive to beta-blockers.

Preparation and Administration

Epinephrine is available as hydrochloride (0.25% to 2%), borate (0.5% to 2%), and bitartarate (1% to 2%). The hydrochloride 1%, borate 1%, and bitartarate 2% have equal potency. In addition, epinephrine is available as a pro drug, dipivalyl epinephrine (dipivefrin 0.1%). The two pivalic acid groups attached to epinephrine increase the corneal penetration 17 times. Dipivefrin (Propine, Allergan) is hydrolyzed in the cornea to epinephrine. It is administered twice daily.[16]

Adverse Effects

When first administered, epinephrine and dipivefrin cause conjunctival vasoconstriction, but this often is followed by conjunctival hyperemia within a few hours. Hypersensitivity, follicular conjunctival reaction, and mydriasis are common.[17] Adrenochrome deposits can occur with prolonged use.[18] Cystoid macular edema may develop in aphakic or pseudophakic eyes.[19] Systemic absorption is rare, but can lead to adrenergic over activity in the form of anxiety, palpitation, hypertension, and cardiac arrhythmia.

Contraindications

Epinephrine and dipivefrin should be avoided in aphakic and pseudophakic eyes due to its potential to cause cystoid macular edema. The cystoid macular edema usually is reversible upon cessation of the drug. These medications can discolor soft contact lenses. They should be avoided in patients taking MAO inhibitors or reserpine.

Selective Alpha Agonists

Mechanism of Action

Apraclonidine (Iopidine, Alcon), the first approved alpha agonist, initially was developed to reduce iris bleeding during Nd:YAG laser iridectomy, but it was found simultaneously to reduce IOP.[20] Apraclonidine increases outflow facility and decreases episcleral venous pressure.[21] Brimonidine (Alphagan, Allergan), a newer alpha-2 agonist, available since 1996, is 23 times more selective for the alpha-2 receptor than apraclonidine.[22] Blockade of the alpha-2 receptor causes increased release of norepinephrine from the nerve terminal. Brimonidine reduces IOP by a dual mechanism of decreasing aqueous production and increasing uveoscleral outflow.[23] Preliminary evidence in experimental models suggests that it also may act as a neuroprotective agent.[22,24]

Preparation and Administration

Apraclonidine was first used in the 1% concentration to prevent IOP spikes after anterior segment laser surgery or in other acute situations. It then was developed in a 0.5% solution for short-term adjunctive therapy. The 1% and 0.5% solutions lower IOP by comparable amounts.

Brimonidine was FDA approved in 1996. It is available in a 0.2% solution. IOP reduction of apraclonidine and brimonidine are comparable to that of timolol. The recommended dosage is three times daily, but similar efficacy can be achieved with twice daily dosage, particularly when combined with other classes of drops. Brimonidine is additive to beta-blockers and most other classes of drops.

Adverse Effects

Long-term administration of apraclonidine is hampered by tachyphylaxis and allergy. About one third of patients develop ocular allergy with conjunctival follicular reaction and toxic dermatitis.[25] Patients may experience eyelid retraction, conjunctival blanching, and dry mouth. Ocular allergy is less common with brimonidine than with apraclonidine. Brimonidine also causes less tachyphylaxis, mydriasis, and eyelid retraction.

Both medications are well tolerated systemically in adults, although drowsiness has been reported in 15% of subjects taking brimonidine.[26] Dry mouth is also frequently reported. Severe hypotension has been reported with brimonidine use in infants and young children.

Contraindications

Care should be taken when using these agents in subjects with hypotension or severe vascular disease. They should not be used in patients taking MAO inhibitors. Brimonidine should not be used in infants and young children.

ADRENERGIC ANTAGONISTS (BETA-BLOCKERS)

Beta adrenergic blockers are the most commonly prescribed medical therapy for glaucoma. First introduced in the 1970s,[27] they rapidly became the gold standard against which all other treatments are compared.

Mechanism of Action

Beta-blockers bind to beta adrenergic receptors and block sympathetic transmission. They lower IOP by reducing aqueous production 30% to 50%.[28] Blockade of other receptors such as serotonin subtypes also may contribute to the response.[5]

Most beta-blockers are non-selective β-1/β-2 antagonists. Carteolol (Ocupress, Ciba) is a non-selective β-1/β-2 antagonist with intrinsic sympathomimetic activity (ISA). ISA provides partial agonist activity and may help to diminish side effects. Betaxolol (Betoptic, Alcon) is a β-1 selective antagonist.

Preparation and Administration

Currently, there are numerous types of beta-blockers available. Timolol maleate 0.25%, 0.5%, and the long-acting, gel-forming Timoptic XE (Merck) formulation 0.25%, 0.5%, timolol hemihydrate (Betimol, Ciba) 0.25%, levobunolol 0.25%, 0.5%, metipranolol (Optipranolol, Bausch & Lomb) 0.3%, betaxolol 0.5%, betaxolol 0.25% suspension (Betoptic-S, Alcon), and carteolol 1%.

Although timolol 0.5% is the most commonly prescribed beta-blocker, most people have the maximal response using timolol 0.25%. Patients with dark irides may require the 0.5% strength. Most beta-blockers are prescribed twice daily; however, levobunolol and Timoptic XE have been shown to be effective with once daily dosing. In the XE formulation of timolol, the drop is transformed into a gel after it is instilled; this increases the contact time with the cornea permitting once daily dosing, and partially decreasing systemic absorption. It is preferable to administer once daily beta-blockers in the morning because beta-blockers are not active aqueous suppressants during sleep,[29] and because they have the potential to exacerbate nocturnal hypotension (systemic blood pressure dips during sleep), which may be a risk factor for glaucomatous optic nerve damage.

Betaxolol is available as a 0.5% solution (Betoptic) or a 0.25% suspension (Betoptic-S). Both formulations have similar efficacy and there is less burning with instillation of Betoptic-S. The efficacy of timolol and levobunolol are comparable,[30] but the β-1 selective betaxolol has slightly less IOP lowering effect.[31] Recent research has been addressing possible calcium channel blocking and neuroprotective effects of betaxolol. Non-selective beta-blockers lower IOP 25% to 30%. They are additive to most other classes of drops except the non-selective adrenergic agonists (epinephrine and dipivefrin). The selective β-1 blocker, betaxolol, may be more additive to epinephrine and dipivefrin than the other non-selective antagonists.

Adverse Effects

When first introduced, topical beta-blockers were thought to have minimal side effects. Ocular side effects were much less pronounced than with the previously available adrenergic agonists and cholinergic compounds. Significant and even fatal systemic side effects, however, soon became apparent.

The most common systemic side effects include depression, malaise, and fatigue.[32] Elderly patients are particularly susceptible to confusion and dizziness, and topical beta-blocker use has been associated with an increased incidence of falls in the elderly. Other serious side effects include bronchospasm in patients with reactive pulmonary disease, bradycardia and worsening of heart block, and congestive heart failure. Beta-blockers can mask the signs of hypoglycemia in diabetics, diminish exercise tolerance, exacerbate myasthenia gravis, and cause impotence and alopecia. They can decrease high density lipoprotein levels in serum lipid levels, but the impact on potential cardiac disease is unclear given the overall favorable effect of beta-blockers on heart disease. Carteolol has been shown to have less effect on plasma lipids than timolol, probably secondary to ISA. Beta-blockers may cause apnea in infancy. Even though betaxolol is a β-1, cardioselective beta-blocker, the risk of systemic side effects, including cardiac side effects, is lower than with non-selective beta-blockers. Ocular side effects of beta-blockers include corneal anesthesia and punctate keratitis. Allergy develops occasionally even after years of therapy. Changing to a different beta-blocker or to non-preserved timolol may be helpful.[33]

Contraindications

Non-selective beta-blockers should not be used in patients with asthma, chronic obstructive pulmonary disease, congestive heart failure, bradycardia, second- and third-degree heart block, and in diabetics prone to hypoglycemia. Care must be taken when prescribing beta-blockers to anyone with a history of depression, impotence, myasthenia gravis, and in neonates.

PROSTAGLANDIN ANALOGUES

Latanoprost (0.005%) is the first of the class of IOP reducing drugs known as prostaglandin analogues. Latanoprost (Xalatan, Pharmacia) was FDA approved in 1996 for adjunctive therapy in eyes in which IOP either was not controlled on current medications, or in which there was intolerance to other agents.

Mechanism of Action

Latanoprost reduces IOP by increasing uveoscleral outflow.[34] It is a pro-drug derivative of $PGF_{2\alpha}$. It causes relaxation of the ciliary muscle, enlarging the spaces between the muscle fibers. It also may have direct effects on the extraocular matrix of the ciliary muscle thereby increasing permeability.[5] It is slightly more effective than timolol in lowering IOP. When used alone, latanoprost reduces IOP by more than 30%.[35-39] Tachyphylaxis was not noted.[37] Adding Xalatan to a topical beta-blocker further reduced IOP by 13% to 28%.[40,41] Latanoprost is additive to most other classes of IOP lowering medications. Although it was initially thought to be poorly additive to miotics, recent studies have demonstrated additive effects, even with the stronger miotic agents.[42]

Preparation and Administration

Latanoprost 0.005% is administered once daily; it works around the clock with a peak response 12 hours after dosing. It may be more effective when administered at night.[35] Latanoprost maintains its efficacy for 6 weeks at room temperature; for long-term storage, latanoprost needs to be refrigerated.

Another $PGF_{2\alpha}$ prostaglandin derivative, unoprostone, is in use outside the United States, and is currently undergoing clinical trials in the United States.

Adverse Effects

The systemic safety profile for latanoprost is very good, owing to its short plasma half life (17 minutes). No systemic side effects on heart rate, blood pressure, and pulmonary function have been detected to date. The most common ocular side effect is increased iris pigmentation, particularly in eyes with mixed color, hazel, green, and light brown irides.[35] Histopathologic studies have demonstrated increased melanin content of the melanosomes rather than cellular proliferation of melanocytes.[43] It is important to discuss the potential for the iris color change with patients prior to starting latanoprost because the change is irreversible.

There is some evidence that latanoprost may cause or exacerbate cystoid macular edema or uveitis in susceptible individuals.[44,45] Other ocular side effects include conjunctival hyperemia, stinging sensation, foreign body sensation, blurred vision, and hypertrichosis of lashes and the surrounding skin. A flu-like syndrome, myalgias, and headache have been associated with latanoprost.

Contraindications

At present, there are no absolute contraindications to latanoprost use. One might consider avoiding it in patients who have recently had intraocular surgery or have had episodes of recurrent uveitis. It is worthwhile to consider using agents other than latanoprost as first line therapy in younger people because the long-term effects of the intracellular melanogenesis is not known.

CARBONIC ANHYDRASE INHIBITORS (CAIs)

Systemic CAIs were first introduced to treat glaucoma by Becker in 1954.[46] Although highly effective in lowering IOP, they cause extensive systemic side effects, which often limit chronic use. After more than 10 years of research, the first topical CAI was approved in 1995. These topical agents exhibit far fewer side effects and have lead to wider use of CAIs in the treatment of glaucoma.

Mechanism of Action

Carbonic anhydrase is involved in aqueous production by catalyzing the reversible reaction:

$$CO_2 + H_2O \rightleftharpoons H_2CO_3$$

The H_2CO_3 (carbonic acid) quickly dissociates to HCO_3^- and H^+ in the ciliary epithelium. Newly formed HCO_3^- enters the posterior chamber (with poorly understood sodium entry) creating a net flow of fluid into the posterior chamber. CAIs block the reversible reaction thereby preventing the formation of bicarbonate in the aqueous and, hence, reducing aqueous fluid production.[47]

The carbonic anhydrase enzyme is widely distributed in the body. In addition to the ciliary body, it is also found in the cornea, lens, and retina in the eye, and in the red blood cells, pancreas, stomach, and renal tubules. More than 99% of the enzyme has to be inhibited before effects on IOP can be observed.[47]

Preparation and Administrations

Acetazolamide and methazolamide are the most commonly prescribed CAIs. Acetazolamide usually is administered either as 250 mg tablets four times daily or as 500 mg sustained release Diamox Sequels twice daily. The Diamox Sequels (Storz) may be better tolerated than the tablets when the full 1000 mg/day dose is administered. In many people, the drug is highly efficacious at doses as low as 62.5 or 125 mg four times daily. The lowest dose possible should be used because the side effects are dose related. Methazolamide is less potent but better tolerated than acetazolamide because it causes less systemic acidosis. It usually is prescribed as 25 or 50 mg tablets twice daily.

Dorzolamide 2% solution (Trusopt, Merck), the first topical CAI, was introduced in 1994; brinzolamide 1% suspension (Azopt, Alcon) received FDA approval in 1998. When used as monotherapy, the topical CAIs are administered three times daily, but twice daily dosing is usually adequate when they are added to other medications. Dorzolamide decreases IOP by 18% to 22% at peak doses.[48] Dorzolamide has a similar IOP lowering effect as betaxolol, and is slightly less effective than timolol at trough; it has been shown to maintain its effect with long-term use.[49] The efficacy of brinzolamide appears to be similar to that of dorzolamide.

Dorzolamide provides an additional 13% to 21% lowering of IOP when added to timolol,[50] and an 8% decrease when added to latanoprost.[51] In most cases, a topical CAI can replace an oral CAI without any loss of IOP control.[44]

Adverse Effects

Oral Agents

The oral CAIs are very potent ocular hypotensive agents, but their use is limited by their propensity to cause systemic side effects. The most common side effect is an overall malaise complex associated with anorexia, weight loss, fatigue, and depression. Patients often have marked gastrointestinal symptoms including nausea and diarrhea, and notice a metallic taste to food. Unnecessary evaluations for occult malignancy have been performed when it was not appreciated that symptoms were a side effect to medication. Paresthesias, notably of the fingertips and around the mouth, are very common.

Acetazolamide causes a significant metabolic acidosis, which precludes its use in patients with hepatic and renal disease. It may precipitate or worsen red blood cell sickling in patients with sickle cell disease. Patients with severe pulmonary disease, who may have an underlying respiratory acidosis, should also avoid acetazolamide. Renal lithiasis formation is increased more than 10-fold.[52] Hypokalemia may develop in patients taking thiazide diuretics or steroids; this side effect may lead to severe untoward effects in association with many medications including digitalis and quinidine. Bone marrow depression may develop. Fatalities have been reported as a result of aplastic anemia, Stevens-Johnson syndrome, and other blood dyscrasias. Aplastic anemia usually develops between 2 to 3 months after starting the CAI, although cases have occurred anytime within the first 6 months. Complaints include fever, bruisability, epistaxis, purpura, sore throat, or jaundice. The development of aplastic anemia is not dose dependent.[53] Although routine blood screening is not currently a standard of care, it is important to warn patients of the signs and symptoms of aplastic anemia, and urge them to seek immediate care if any symptoms develop.[3] The oral CAIs have minimal ocular side effects. They can cause transient myopia. Delayed hypotony with choroidal detachments after filtration surgery can occur.

Topical Agents

Topical CAIs are well tolerated systemically. They have not been studied in patients with severe renal or hepatic disease and therefore should be avoided in these individuals. They are absorbed systemically, however systemic levels are insufficient to cause extra-ocular inhibition of carbonic anhydrase. Their potential to cause life-threatening side effects is unknown; no fatalities have been reported to date.

Ocular side effects occur most commonly; they include burning, stinging, superficial punctate keratitis, and discomfort. Bitter taste and contact dermatitis also can occur. Brinzolamide is claimed to cause less stinging than dorzolamide due to its more physiologic pH,[54] but may cause transient blurring of vision because it is a suspension, rather than a solution.

Contraindications

Since the true cross reactivity with other sulfa-based drugs is not known, both oral and topical CAIs should not be used in patients with a history of serious sulfa allergy. Systemic CAIs also should not be used by people with severe chronic obstructive pulmonary disease, diabetic ketoacidosis, renal lithiasis, renal insufficiency, or hepatic disease. Caution must be taken when prescribing oral CAIs in patients taking thiazide diuretics and steroids.

TIMOLOL-DORZOLAMIDE FIXED COMBINATION DROP

Timolol-dorzolamide fixed combination drop (Cosopt, Merck) is the newest addition to our glaucoma armamentarium and the first combination drop using the newer agents to be FDA approved. It was approved in 1998 for use in patients who do not respond adequately to beta-blockers alone. Combination drops help simplify medication regimens and improve compliance. Physicians must be diligent not to abuse their use, and reserve combination drops for instances when monotherapy is inadequate.

Cosopt lowers IOP more than either component alone.[55] It has comparable efficacy to concomitant administration of timolol twice daily and dorzolamide three times daily. The side effects are similar to those seen with the two components. The formulation is similar to that of dorzolamide (acidic pH), and it is, therefore, associated with the same ocular side effects as dorzolamide.

WHEN TO START THERAPY

The initiation of therapy for glaucoma is a very serious step. When started, therapy is usually continued for the remainder of the patient's life. Patients may be burdened by untoward side effects, costs, and inconvenience. The patient and physician together must decide if the benefits of therapy outweigh the risks and inconvenience.

For most people with definite glaucoma, the scales tip readily toward treatment. Recent evidence from the Collaborative Normal Tension Glaucoma Study Group provides prospective evidence that IOP reduction reduces the incidence of progression in glaucoma patients with baseline IOP <24 mmHg.[56] Because the risk of future glaucoma damage depends on the amount of damage already present and the current rate of progression,[57,58] IOP lowering treatment usually is initiated in subjects with definite glaucomatous damage.

The goal of treatment, however, is not to lower IOP to a certain level or to prevent progressive visual field changes. The goal of glaucoma therapy is to prevent or minimize a decline in a patient's perceived visual function and/or quality of life during his or her lifetime. Most patients are unaware of moderate field defects identified on formal visual field testing. The patient's risk factors for progression must be assessed in relation to a patient's life expectancy. Observation rather than treatment may be considered in an elderly patient with early disease who is unlikely to develop symptomatic field defects within his or her lifetime. The decision to treat also must take into account the patient's systemic health and medication use, risk of side effects, and psychosocial issues such as his or her understanding and feelings about the disease and its treatment, level of compliance, level of independence, and financial impact of the treatment.

Additional considerations are required when considering therapy in a glaucoma suspect. An open discussion between doctor and patient about the risks and benefits of treatment is especially important. Ocular hypertension affects 3 to 6 million people in the United States and the prevalence of ocular hypertension increases with age. It affects 1.2% of people in their 30s and 10% of people in their 70s.[59,60] Because only a minority of subjects with ocular hypertension develop glaucoma, all ocular hypertensive subjects do not need treatment. The conversion rate from ocular hypertension to glaucoma is 0.5% to 1% per year in the older studies,[61-64] but 3% to 4% per year in newer studies where more sophisticated diagnostic evaluations have been performed.[65-67]

In the past, many studies have been done to evaluate the efficacy of prophylactic treatment for ocular hypertension. Interestingly, only half of the studies favor medical therapy. Despite this fact, 1.5 million glaucoma suspects in the United States are treated costing approximately $300,000,000 yearly.[68] Fortunately, the National Eye Institute is currently sponsoring the Ocular Hypertension Treatment Study (OHTS), a multi-center clinical trial to evaluate if medical therapy prevents or delays the onset of glaucomatous damage. Until the results of OHTS are available, therapy should be reserved for patients with significant risk factors for glaucoma.

RISK FACTOR ASSESSMENT
IOP

Susceptibility of the optic nerve to damage from IOP varies between individuals. Interestingly, only 50% of patients with glaucoma have a screening IOP more than 21 mmHg and one out of six patients never have IOP measured more than 21 mmHg on repeat testing.[69,70] A majority of glaucoma patients have IOP of 25 mmHg or less. In patients with asymmetric disease, the risk of progressive glaucoma damage is greater in the eye with higher IOP, even when the IOP remains within the normal range.[71] There is no IOP level below which glaucoma damage never develops.

Age

The prevalence of glaucoma increases with age from 0.2% in 50- to 54-year-olds to 2% in 70- to 74-year-olds.[72] This prevalence may relate to a greater susceptibility for damage from IOP with age or to more prolonged exposure to higher IOP.

Race

The Baltimore and Barbados eye studies have shown that race is an important risk factor for POAG. The Baltimore eye survey noted that the prevalence of POAG is 4.3 times greater in African Americans and other races, and that African Americans are four to eight times more likely to go blind from glaucoma than white Americans. In African Americans, the prevalence of glaucoma was 1.2% in 40- to 59-year-olds and 11.3% in subjects 80 years of age or greater.[60]

The Barbados eye study also found a high prevalence of POAG in the black population of Barbados; 7% of black adults vs 0.8% of white adults were affected.[73] It is not known why POAG is more common and why it tends to occur at a younger age in blacks.

Family History

Family history also is an important risk factor for POAG. The Baltimore eye survey found a 3.7-fold increase in POAG in individuals who had a sibling with POAG and a 2.2-fold increased risk in people with an affected parent.[74]

Other possible risk factors include myopia, systemic hypertension, systemic hypotension, diabetes mellitus, and vasospastic disease such as migraine headaches, Prinzmetal angina, and Raynaud's disease.

MEDICATIONS, LASERS, AND BEYOND

In the United States, most patients are started on medications as initial therapy for glaucoma. The National Eye Institute-sponsored Glaucoma Laser Trial showed that argon laser trabeculoplasty may be a good first line therapy for glaucoma.[75] Evidence from the Moorfields Primary Treatment Study[76,77] and the Glasgow Glaucoma Trial[78] favor surgical trabeculectomy as initial therapy for glaucoma. The role of trabeculectomy as the first treatment for glaucoma is currently under investigation in the United States in the National Eye Institute-sponsored Collaborative Initial Glaucoma Treatment Study (CIGTS).

HOW TO INITIATE THERAPY
Establish a Baseline

It is important to have more than a single measure of IOP prior to starting therapy. The IOP in most subjects without glaucoma varies by less than 4 mmHg during a 24-hour period while subjects with glaucoma can have changes greater than 10 mmHg. Vary the time of day when the IOP is checked.

Know Your Patient

Be familiar with all aspects of the patient's ocular and medical history and perform a complete eye exam.

Try to know as much as possible about pertinent social aspects of your patient's life—home situation, career, and lifestyle. Learn about particular concerns your patients may have regarding their glaucoma and its treatment (eg, Is cost an issue? Is the patient unable to instill drops? Is once daily dosing important?).

Try to Do No Harm

Tailor your therapy to each individual patient, taking into account his or her ocular, medical, and psychosocial history. Know the ocular and medical contraindications to every medication. Be aware of serious drug interactions.

Educate Your Patient

The more your patient knows about glaucoma and the treatment options, the better you are able to help orchestrate his or her care. Most patients with glaucoma feel fine and have no visual symptoms. You need to help your patients understand why they need to take medication every day for the rest of their lives even if such medications are costly, inconvenient, uncomfortable, or have modest side effects. Teach your patient about potential side effects of each medication.

Set a Target IOP

Take into account the extent of glaucomatous damage and the baseline IOP. Choose a lower target with more extensive glaucomatous damage. A 20% to 30% reduction of IOP is a typical goal in most cases. Modify your goal based on subsequent progression or stability of the optic nerves and visual field.

Use a One-Eyed Drug Trial Whenever Feasible

Start therapy in one eye and recheck the IOP in 1 to 6 weeks, depending on the medication. This technique helps to distinguish therapeutic effect from diurnal variation. Take into account, however, that many drugs, particularly the topical beta-blockers, exhibit some crossover effect and lower the IOP in the contralateral untreated eye. This contralateral effect (crossover effect) tends to mask the true therapeutic effect.

Use the Least Amount of Medication Needed to Achieve the Target Pressure

If the one-eyed drug trial lowered the IOP sufficiently, prescribe the medication in both eyes (if the disease is bilateral). If there is minimal pressure lowering, discontinue the trial medication and institute a new one-eyed trial using a medication of a different class. If the IOP was lowered modestly but the goal was not achieved, a new medication is either substituted for or added to the trial medication. Continue medications only if they are effective; stop any medications that do not lower IOP.

Keep It Simple

Good compliance is crucial for the success of glaucoma therapy. The simpler the regimen, the more likely the patient is to be compliant. Keep the frequency of administration to a minimum. Re-evaluate compliance at each visit.

Question Your Patient

At each visit, question your patient about side effects and any other issues regarding their treatment. Remember, this is a lifelong disease and patients should not have to go through life with medication side effects that significantly impact on their quality of life. Some side effects may not develop immediately. Be sure your patients are aware of the potential side effects of their treatment so they can help you stay informed. Address any new compliance issues.

Teach Your Patients How to Instill Drops

Encourage them not to use more than one drop of each medicine if possible. Teach nasolacrimal duct occlusion with eyelid closure to decrease systemic absorption and to increase the therapeutic effect. Encourage patients to wait at least 10 minutes between drops if possible.

Write It Down

Compliance will be enhanced if patients are given written instructions about their medications. A schedule of when to take drops can be very effective for many patients. Written information about how to instill eye drops, nasolacrimal duct obstruction, side effects of medications, etc can be very helpful when the patient returns home and becomes confused about his or her instructions.

WHERE TO BEGIN?

There is no dogmatic answer to this question. Beta-blockers remain the most commonly prescribed first-line treatment. Their long-term use has a well-documented safety profile. Beta-blockers are additive to most other classes of medications, except for the nonselective adrenergic agonists (epinephrine and Propine). In most patients, the 0.25% solution of timolol maleate or levobunolol provides as much IOP lowering as the 0.5% solutions with fewer side effects. Once daily dosing helps improve patient compliance and decreases systemic absorption. The XE formulation of Timoptic increases the contact time in the eye permitting once daily dosing, and it seems to decrease systemic absorption. Timoptic XE 0.25% once in the morning is, therefore, an excellent first-line choice. Levobunolol 0.5%, also has been shown to provide effective 24-hour effect with once daily dosing and is a useful alternative. The β-1 selective beta-blocker, betaxolol, is also useful as first line therapy because it has fewer pulmonary side effects than the non-selective beta-blockers. Betaxolol lowers IOP slightly less effectively than the non-selective beta-blockers but some studies have shown improved long-term visual field performance in relation to non-selective beta-blockers.[79,80] Betaxolol is administered twice daily.

Latanoprost, timolol-dorzolamide fixed combination drop, and apraclonidine are not FDA approved for first-line use. Although it may be tempting to use these highly effective agents as initial therapy, it may be preferable from a medicolegal perspective to not use them. Another reason to avoid the combination timolol-dorzolamide drop for first-line treatment is that it prevents determining which components are effective or even allergenic. The topical CAIs and brimonidine are useful treatments but they require two or three times daily dosing and may be slightly less effective than non-selective beta-blockers. The choice for initial treatment will continue to evolve as we gain greater experience and a better understanding of the long-term safety profile of the newer agents.

The first medication prescribed lowers IOP more than secondary adjunctive therapy. If another medication is needed in addition to a beta-blocker, useful second-line treatments include topical CAIs, brimonidine, and latanoprost. The topical CAIs can be given as combination therapy with timolol allowing the patient to use a single bottle of drops twice daily. Adding latanoprost to the non-selective beta-blocker still permits the patient to administer only two drops daily. Brimonidine has good additivity to the beta-blockers but requires a regimen with a minimum of three drops per day. Cholinergics and systemic CAIs usually are reserved for those patients who do not respond to the beta-blockers plus newer agents; non-selective adrenergic agonists rarely are used now.

CONCLUSION

How and when to initiate glaucoma therapy cannot be simplified into a straightforward algorithm. A myriad of objective and subjective factors must be taken into account. The physician must be aware of each medication, its mechanism of action, potential side effects, and contraindications. The IOP cannot be treated in isolation. The unique complexities of each patient's physiology and psychosocial functioning needs to be understood. People change over time; thus, each patient's therapy for this lifelong disease must be routinely re-evaluated. The approach to glaucoma therapy will continue to evolve as we learn more about the disease and our current treatments and as new therapies become available.

REFERENCES

1. Shields MB. *Textbook of Glaucoma* (pp. 374-386). Baltimore, Md: Williams and Wilkins; 1998.
2. Leopold IH. The use and side effects of cholinergic agents in the management of intraocular pressure. In: Drance SM, Newfeld AH, eds. *Glaucoma: Applied Pharmacology and Medical Treatment* (pp. 357-393). Orlando, Fla: Grunn and Stratton; 1984.
3. Sherwood MB, Spaeth GL. *Complications of Glaucoma Therapy.* Thorofare, NJ: SLACK Incorporated; 1990.
4. Kaufman PL. Mechanisms of actions of the cholinergic drugs in the eye. In: Drance SM, Newfeld AH, eds. *Glaucoma: Applied Pharmacology and Medical Treatment* (pp. 395-427). Orlando, Fla: Grunn and Stratton; 1984.
5. Gabelt BT, Kaufman PL. A rational approach to adding glaucoma medications. *Review of Ophthalmology.* 1998;44-57.
6. Drance SM, Nash PA. The dose response of human intraocular pressure to pilocarpine. *Can J Ophthalmol.* 1971;6:9-13.
7. Zimmerman TJ, Sharir M, Nardin GF, Fuqua M. Therapeutic index of Pilocarpine, Carbachol, and Timolol with nasolacrimal occlusion. *Am J Ophthalmol.* 1992;114:1-7.
8. Worthen DM, Zimmerman TJ, Wind CA. An evaluation of the pilocarpine ocuserts. *Invest Ophthalmol Vis Sci.* 1974;13:296-299.
9. March WF, Stewart RM, Mandell AI, Bruce LA. Duration of effect of pilocarpine gel. *Arch Ophthalmol.* 1982;100:1270.
10. Morton WR, Drance SM, Fairlough M. The effect of echothiophate iodide on the lens. *Am J Ophthalmol.* 1969;63:1003-1020.
11. Ellis PP. Systemic effects of locally applied anticholinesterase agents. *Invest Ophthalmol Vis Sci.* 1966;5:146-151.
12. Leopold IH, Krishna N, Lehman RA. The effects of anticholinesterase agents on the blood cholinesterase levels of normal and glaucoma subjects. *Trans Am Ophthalmol Soc.* 1959;57:63.
13. Havener WH. *Ocular Pharmacology* (p. 357). St Louis, Mo: CV Mosby Co; 1983.
14. Sears ML, Neufeld AH. Adrenergic modulation of the outflow of aqueous humor. *Invest Ophthalmol Vis Sci.* 1975;14:83.
15. Neufeld AH. The mechanisms of action of adrenergic drugs in the eye. In: Drance SM, Newfeld AH, eds. *Glaucoma: Applied Pharmacology and Medical Treatment* (pp. 277-301). Orlando, Fla: Grunn and Stratton; 1984.
16. Mandell AI, Stentz F, Kitabchi AE. Dipivalyl epinephrine: a new prodrug in the treatment for glaucoma. *Ophthalmology.* 1978;85:268-275.
17. Aronson SB, Wyamamoto EA. Ocular hypersensitivity to epinephrine. *Invest Ophthalmol Vis Sci.* 1966;5:75-80.
18. Cashwell LF, Shields MB, Reed JW. Adrenochrome pigmentation. *Arch Ophthalmol.* 1977;95:514-515.
19. Kolker AE, Becker B. Epinephrine maculopathy. *Arch Ophthalmol.* 1968;79:552-562.
20. Robin AL, Pollack IP. Uses of ALO 2145 in anterior segment glaucoma laser surgery. In: Shields MB, Pollack IP, Kolker AE, eds. *Perspectives in Glaucoma. Transactions of the First Scientific Meeting of the American Glaucoma Society.* Thorofare, NJ: SLACK Incorporated; 1988.
21. Toris CB, Lafoya ME, Camras CB, Yablonski ME. Effects of aproclonidine on aqueous humor dynamics in human eyes. *Ophthalmology.* 1995;102:456-461.
22. Burke J, Schwartz M. Preclinical evaluation of brimonidine. *Surv Ophthalmol.* 1996;41(suppl 1):S9-S18.
23. Toris CB, Gleason Ml, Camras CB, Yablonski ME. Effects of brimonidine on aqueous humor dynamics in human eyes. *Arch Ophthalmol.* 1995;113:1514-1517.
24. Mitchell CK, Nguyen PT, Feldman RM. Neuroprotection of retinal ganglion cells. *Invest Ophthalmol Vis Sci.* 1998; 39:S261.
25. Butler P, et al. Clinical experience with the long term use of 1% aproclonidine. Incidence of allergic reactions. *Arch Ophthalmol.* 1995;113:293-296.
26. Schuman JS. Clinical experience with brimonidine 0.2% and timolol 0.5% in glaucoma and ocular hypertension. *Surv Ophthalmol.* 1996;41(suppl 1):S27-S37.
27. Ulrych M, Franciosa J, Conway J. Comparison of a new beta adrenergic blocker (MK-950) and propranolol in man. *Clin Pharmacol Ther.* 1972;13:232-238.

28. Zimmerman TJ. Timolol maleate—a new glaucoma medication? *Invest Ophthalmol Vis Sci.* 1977;16:687-688.
29. Reiss GR, Lee DA, Topper JE, Brubaker RF. Aqueous humor flow during sleep. *Invest Ophthalmol Vis Sci.* 1984;25:776-778.
30. Duzman E, Ober M, Scharrer A, Leopold IH. A clinical evaluation of the effects of topically applied levobunolol and timolol on increased intraocular pressure. *Am J Ophthalmol.* 1982;94:318-327.
31. Stewart RH, Kimbrough RL, Ward RL. Betaxolol versus timolol. A six month double blind comparison. *Arch Ophthalmol.* 1986;104:46-48.
32. Fraunfelder FT, Meyer SM. Systemic adverse reactions to glaucoma medications [review]. *Int Ophthalmol Clin.* 1989;29:143-146.
33. Novak GD. Ophthalmic beta-blockers since timolol. *Surv Ophthalmol.* 1987;31: 307-327.
34. Ziai N, Dolan JW, Kacere RD, Brubaker RF. The effects on aqueous dynamics of PhXA41 a new prostaglandin F2 alpha analogue after topical application in normal and ocular hypertensive human eyes. *Arch Ophthalmol.* 1993;111:351-358.
35. Alm A, Stjernschaantz J, et al. Effects on intraocular pressure and side effects of 0.005% latanoprost applied once daily, evening or morning. A comparison with timolol. *Ophthalmology.* 1995;102:1743-1752.
36. Camras CB, et al. Comparison of latanoprost and timolol in patients with ocular hypertension and glaucoma. A six month masked multi center trial in the United States. *Ophthalmology.* 1996;103:138-147.
37. Camras CB, et al. Latanoprost treatment for glaucoma: effects of treating for one year and of switching from timolol. *Am J Ophthalmol.* 1998;126:390-399.
38. Watson P, et al. A six-month, randomized, double-masked study comparing latanoprost with timolol in open-angle glaucoma and ocular hypertension. *Ophthalmology.* 1996;103: 126-137.
39. Watson PG, et al. Latanoprost: two years experience of its use in the United Kingdom. *Ophthalmology.* 1998;105:82-87.
40. Rulo AH, Greve EL, Hoyng PF. Additive effect of latanoprost, a prostaglandin PGF2 alpha and timolol in patients with elevated IOP. *Br J Ophthalmol.* 1994;78:899-902.
41. Alm A, Wiodengard I, Kjellgren D, et al. Latanoprost administered once daily caused a maintained reduction of intraocular pressure in glaucoma patients treated concomitantly with timolol. *Br J Ophthalmol.* 1995;79:12-16.
42. Linden C, Alm A. Latanoprost and physostigmine have mostly additive ocular hypotensive effects in human eyes. *Arch Ophthalmol.* 1997;115:857-861.
43. Selen G, Stjernschantz J, Resul B. Prostaglandin induced pigmentation in primates. *Surv Ophthalmol.* 1997;41(suppl 2):S125-S128.
44. Fechtner R, et al. Anterior uveitis associated with latanoprost. *Am J Ophthalmol.* 1998;126:37-41.
45. Warwar RE, et al. Cystoid macular edema and anterior uveitis associated with latanoprost use. *Ophthalmology.* 1998;105:263-268.
46. Becker B. Decrease in intraocular pressure in man by a carbonic anhydrase inhibitor, Diamox. *Am J Ophthalmol.* 1954;37:13-15.
47. Maren TH. Carbonic anhydrase: chemistry physiology and inhibition. *Physiol Rev.* 1967;47:595-766.
48. Lippa EA, Carlson LE, Ehinger B, et al. Dose-response and duration of action of dorzolamide, a topical carbonic anhydrase inhibitor. *Arch Ophthalmol.* 1992;100:495.
49. Strahlman ER, Tipping R, Vogel R. A double-masked, randomized 1-year study comparing dorzolamide (Trusopt), timolol, and betaxolol. *Arch Ophthalmol.* 1995;113:1009-1016.
50. Parfitt AM. Acetazolamide and sodium bicarbonate-induced nephrocalcinosis and nephrolithiasis: relationship to citrate and calcium excretion. *Arch Intern Med.* 1969;124:736.
51. Vanlandingham B, Brubaker R. Combined effect of dorzolamide and latanoprost on the rate of aqueous humor flow. *Am J Ophthalmol.* 1998;126:191-196.
52. Kass MA, Kolker AE, Gordon M, et al. Acetazolamide and urolithiasis. *Ophthalmology.* 1981;88:261-265.
53. Fraunfelder FT, Meyer SM, Bagby GC, Jr., Dreis MW. Hematologic reactions to carbonic anhydrase inhibitors. *Am J Ophthalmol.* 1985;100:79.
54. Silver LH, et al. Clinical efficacy and safety of brinzolamide (Azopt), a new topical carbonic anhydrase inhibitor for primary open angle glaucoma and ocular hypertension. *Am J Ophthalmol.* 1998;126:400-408.
55. Boyle JE, et al. A randomized trial comparing the dorzolamide-timolol combination given twice daily to monotherapy with dorzolamide and timolol. *Ophthalmology.* 1998;105:1945-1951.
56. Collaborative Normal-Tension Glaucoma Study Group. Comparison of glaucomatous progression between untreated patients with normal tension glaucoma and patients with therapeutically reduced intraocular pressures. *Am J Ophthalmol.* 1998;126:487-497.
57. Anderson DR. Glaucoma: the damage caused by pressure. XLVI Edward Jackson Memorial Lecture. *Am J Ophthalmol.* 1989;108:485-495.
58. Grant VM, Burke JF Jr. Why do some people go blind from glaucoma? *Ophthalmology.* 1982;89:991-998.
59. Armaly MF. On the distribution of applanation pressure. I. Statistical features and the effect of age, sex, and family history of glaucoma. *Arch Ophthalmol.* 1965;83:11-18.
60. Tielsch JM, Sommer A, Katz J, et al. Racial variations in the prevalence of primary open-angle glaucoma. The Baltimore Eye Survey. *JAMA.* 1991;266:369-374.
61. Walker WM. Ocular hypertension: follow-up of 109 case from 1963 to 1974. *Eye.* 1974;94:525-534.
62. Kitazawa Y, Horie T, Aoki S, et al. Untreated ocular hypertension: a long-term prospective study. *Arch Ophthalmol.* 1977;95:1180-1184.
63. Sorenson PN, Nielson NV, Norkov K. Ocular hypertension: a 15-year follow-up. *Acta Ophthalmol.* 1978;56:363-372.
64. Lundberg L, Wettrell K, Linner E. Ocular hypertension: a prospective twenty-year follow-up study. *Acta Ophthalmol.* 1987;65:705-708.
65. Schulzer M, Drance SM, Douglas GR. A comparison of treated and untreated glaucoma suspects. *Ophthalmology.* 1991;98:301-307.

66. Epstein DL, Krug JH, Hertzmark E, et al. A long-term clinical trial of timolol therapy versus no treatment in the management of glaucoma suspects. *Ophthalmology.* 1989;96: 1460-1467.

67. Kass MA, Gordon MO, Hoff, MR, et al. Topical timolol administration reduces the incidence of glaucomatous damage in ocular hypertensive individuals. *Arch Ophthalmol.* 1989;107:1590-1598.

68. Kass MA. The Ocular Hypertension Treatment Study. *J Glaucoma.* 1994;3:97-100.

69. Sommer A, Tielsch JM, Katz J, et al. Relationship between intraocular pressure and primary open angle glaucoma among white and black Americans. The Baltimore Eye Survey. *Arch Ophthalmol.* 1991;109:1090-1095.

70. Kahn HA, Milton RC. Alternative definitions of open-angle glaucoma. *Arch Ophthalmol.* 1980;98:2172-2177.

71. Cartwright MJ, Anderson DR. Correlation of asymmetric damage with asymmetric intraocular pressure in normal-tension glaucoma (low tension glaucoma). *Arch Ophthalmol.* 1988;106:898-900.

72. Viggosson G, Bjornsson G, Ingvasson JG. The prevalence of open-angle glaucoma in Iceland. *Acta Ophthalmol.* 1986;64: 138-141.

73. Leske MC, Connell AM, Schachat AP, et al. The Barbados Eye Study. Prevalence of open angle glaucoma. *Arch Ophthalmol.* 1994;112:821-829.

74. Tielsch JM, Katz J, Sommer A. Family history and risk of primary open angle glaucoma. The Baltimore Eye Survey. *Arch Ophthalmol.* 1994;112:69-73.

75. Glaucoma Laser Trial Research Group. The Glaucoma Laser Trial (GLT) and Glaucoma Laser Trial Follow-up Study: 7. Results. *Am J Ophthalmol.* 1995;120:718-731.

76. Migdal C, Hitchings R. Control of chronic simple glaucoma with primary medical, surgical and laser treatment. *Trans Ophthalmol Soc UK.* 1986;105:653-656.

77. Migdal C, Gregory W, Hitchings R. Long term functional outcome after early surgery compared with laser and medicine in open angle glaucoma. *Ophthalmology.* 1994;101:1651-1657.

78. Jay JL, Allan D. The benefit of early trabeculectomy versus conventional management in primary open angle glaucoma relative to the severity of the disease. *Eye.* 1989;3:528-535.

79. Messmer C, Flammer J, Stümpfig D. Influence of betaxolol and timolol on the visual fields of patients with glaucoma. *Am J Ophthalmol.* 1991;112:678-681.

80. Collignon-Brach J. Long-term effect of ophthalmic (-adreno-ceptor antagonists on intraocular pressure and retinal sensitivity in primary open-angle glaucoma. *Curr Eye Res.* 1992; 11:1-3 .

Chapter Twelve

NONINCISIONAL GLAUCOMA SURGERY

Richard A. Hill, MD

INTRODUCTION

In glaucoma therapy, lasers are used primarily in either a photocoagulation mode or a photodisruptive mode. Photocoagulation depends on the tissue's ability to absorb the incident laser wave length. For this reason, blue irises respond very poorly to argon lasers because the major chromophore for this laser is melanin. Thermal effects to adjacent tissue may be minimized by using shorter laser exposure times. In procedures where the goal is to remove tissue, such as iridotomy, a shorter pulse width with higher continuous wave power is more effective (0.1 seconds; 600 mW). This technique limits thermal conduction and increases transfer of energy to target tissues. If a significant, deep thermal effect is desired in performing a procedure (such as iridoplasty), a longer pulse length (0.5 seconds) is desirable.

Incident laser light may be reflected, absorbed, transmitted, scattered, or go on to produce plasma formation (Figure 12-1). Plasma formation, causing subsequent photodisruption, is produced primarily with Q-switched neodymium:YAG (or Nd:YAG) lasers. These ultra short pulse lasers produce a focal energy density sufficient to remove electrons from the outer orbital shells, which results in a localized production of plasma. The resulting shock wave and blast from this plasma production exceeds the local tissue structural integrity limits and results in tissue disruption. Although these two mechanisms are widely separate from each other, they are complimentary to one another and sometimes useful in the care of the glaucoma patient. Examples of this would be a patient on chronic anticoagulant therapy requiring iridotomy or the need to perform an iridoplasty after iridotomy.

LASER PERIPHERAL IRIDOTOMY

Laser peripheral iridotomy is used to treat pupillary block glaucoma (primary angle closure glaucoma) and the reverse pupillary block resulting from large, floppy irises (pigment dispersion glaucoma). The basic principles involve the effective spatial con-

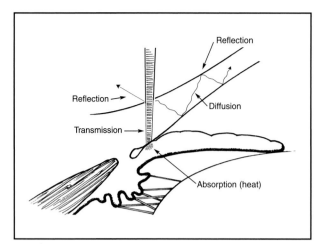

Figure 12-1. Many possible laser-tissue interactions can occur. The interactions may vary with pulse length, laser wavelength, or type of tissue.

finement of laser energy leading to either disruption (Q-switched Nd:YAG) or photocoagulation/ablation (Ar, Ar-Dye, Kr, or frequency-doubled Nd:YAG). In the case of the Nd:YAG laser, careful focus by the clinician will place the resultant plasma created by the application of the laser energy in an appropriate location. In the case of continuous wave and quasi-continuous wave lasers (frequency-doubled Nd:YAG lasers), chromophores (molecules that absorb laser energy at certain wavelengths) are utilized to retain laser energy in an appropriate area, heating tissue and causing photoablation/photocoagulation. For pigment dispersion glaucoma, some clinicians prefer the argon laser because it releases less pigment during iridotomy formation.

Patient Selection

Patients are selected based on clinical findings at gonioscopy. Optically occluded filtering angles, which open with pressure (compression gonioscopy), anatomically narrow angles (Shaffer grades 1 and 2), and q-shaped irises (pigment dispersion glaucoma) are indicators for a laser peripheral iridotomy. In pupillary block glaucoma, equalization of pressures in the posterior and anterior chambers allows for a posterior repositioning of the peripheral iris with subsequent deepening of the filtering angle. In pigment dispersion glaucoma, a large floppy iris leads to reverse pupillary block and equalization of pressures allows a more planer orientation of the iris and relief of irido-

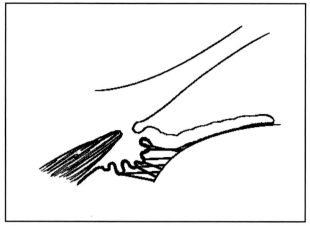

Figure 12-2a. Relief of reverse pupillary block by laser iridotomy can have a dramatic effect on iris position. A patient with pigment dispersion glaucoma and reverse pupillary block has this iris position before laser iridotomy.

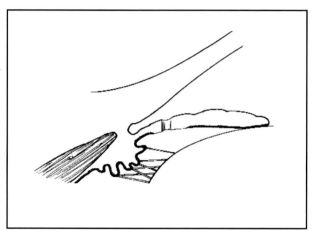

Figure 12-2b. After laser iridotomy, there is relief of iridozonular touch.

zonular touch (Figures 12-2a and 12-2b). Because the conversion from pigment dispersion syndrome to pigment dispersion glaucoma varies between 10% and 50%, most glaucoma specialists restrict laser iridotomy in pigment dispersion to young patients in whom the IOP has risen from their baseline or early pigment dispersion glaucoma patients. Presurgical patients are poor candidates because the effects of iridotomy may take years to show benefit (Figure 12-3).

Preoperative Preparation

Preoperative preparation ensures a successful and safe laser iridotomy. Preoperatively, both pilocarpine 1% (to firm the surface of the iris and allow more

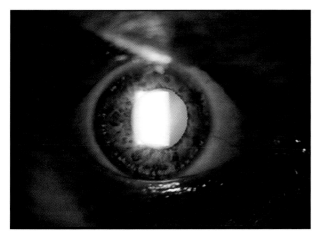

Figure 12-3. Nd:YAG laser iridotomy in a patient with pigment dispersion glaucoma. IOPs have normalized without medications 1 year post treatment.

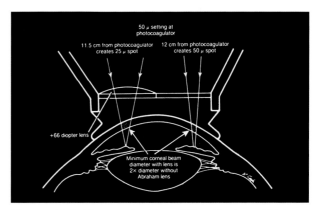

Figure 12-4. The construction of the Abraham iridotomy lens creates a rapidly converging laser beam. This minimizes both corneal and potential retinal irradiation while maximizing irido-irradiation. Courtesy of Ocular Instruments, Bellevue, Wash.

peripheral iridotomy placement) and apraclonidine 0.5% or 1.0 % or brimonidine 2% (as prophylaxis against postoperative pressure spikes) are given twice to the patient. If the patient is currently using an alpha agonist, then another medication from a pharmaceutical class that the patient is not currently using should be substituted for prophylaxis (prostaglandin/beta-blocker). In addition, extra vigilance is required in pigment dispersion and pseudoexfoliation patients because postoperative pressure spikes occur more commonly in this group of patients.

Contact Lenses

A contact lens such as the Abraham or Wise lens with coated optics should be used for laser iridotomy creation. The contact lens acts as a lid speculum, provides magnified viewing of the operative area, and the optical coating reduces laser reflections. The construction of these lenses with a high plus power operative area creates a rapidly converging laser beam. This allows for a lower corneal irradiance (power/area) while creating a much higher irradiance at the focal plane of the iris (Figure 12-4). These contact lenses are placed on the eye under topical anesthesia with the aid of an artificial tear solution such as Celluvisc (Allergan, Irvine, Calif).

Surgical Technique

The placement site of an iridotomy should vary slightly with choice of laser. In using the Nd:YAG

laser any superior or inferior region that is covered by the patient's eyelid is a reasonable site for a laser iridotomy. However, because the upper eyelid covers more of the iris, most clinicians prefer to place this superiorly in order to avoid a second pupil effect. When using the argon and other continuous wave or quasi-continuous wave lasers, the superior and nasal quadrant is selected because of the lower risk of macular radiation. Laser settings for the Nd:YAG laser are typically in the 2.0 to 3.0 mJ range with one to two pulses per burst. If bleeding occurs, simple pressure with the contact lens can usually stop it by transiently elevating IOP. In the case of bleeding recalcitrant to contact lens pressure (Figure 12-5), a continuous wave laser can be used at low power (350 to 500 mW), with a large spot size (500 µm) and longer duration burn (0.2 to 0.5 seconds) to stop the bleeding.

Settings for the argon and other continuous wave or quasi-continuous wave lasers are an exposure time of 0.1 seconds, spot size of 50 µm, and continuous wave energies in the 600 to 800 mW range to start with. These settings should be adjusted based on the observed laser-tissue interactions. In creating Nd:YAG iridotomies, at least one radial iris strand should be cut. If the Nd:YAG laser simply forces apart iris strands, this type of iridotomy will close rapidly with posterior pigment proliferation. In the performance of an argon iridotomy, continuous wave or quasi-continuous wave lasering it is not necessary to perform ancillary laser spots to tighten the area of laser ablation. Laser spots are placed on top of one another until full thickness iridotomy results. If a clinician has access to both lasers, a patient who is on anticoagulants can be pretreated heavily with an argon laser to coagulate vessels, and then the iridotomy can be completed either with an argon laser or with low-dose Nd:YAG laser pulses. This combination technique also may be used in thick, spongy brown irises to provide a more esthetic laser iridotomy when excessive tissue shredding is encountered.

Postoperative Care

Postoperatively, patients should have their IOP checked at approximately 1 hour's time. The patient should also be given a prescription for a topical corticosteroid used four times a day for 1 week. If the patient does not have an IOP spike after surgery, then the patient may be seen at 1 week after the procedure. If Zeiss gonioscopy can be performed at the 1-hour pressure check and the angle is found to be open to Shaffer grade 3 or better, then pilocarpine need not be used postoperatively. If the angle is Shaffer grade 2 or less, then pilocarpine may need to be used continuously by this patient or peripheral iridoplasty may be required if the patient is pilocarpine-intolerant. The patient should also be seen at 1 week and 1 month postoperatively for Zeiss gonioscopy to evaluate the angle and to ensure continuing patency of the laser iridotomy. It should be noted that pilocarpine inhibits exercise-induced pigment release and secondary pressure elevation, whereas iridotomy does not fully reduce this in pigment dispersion glaucoma.

PERIPHERAL IRIDOPLASTY

Patient Selection

Peripheral iridoplasty is useful in situations of acute angle-closure glaucoma where a laser peripheral iridotomy cannot be performed, and in cases of plateau iris in which the filtering angle is occludable on pilocarpine therapy or occludable after iridotomy, and the patient cannot tolerate pilocarpine therapy.

Preoperative Preparation

The patient is given pilocarpine preoperatively to maintain miosis during the procedure and to facilitate access to the peripheral iris. Apraclonidine should also be administered to minimize postoperative IOP spikes.

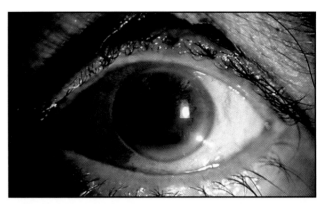

Figure 12-5. This patient presented in angle-closure while on aspirin therapy. Iridotomy with a Nd:YAG laser resulted in hyphema formation. Low irradiance (power/area), large spot size treatment with a continuous wave laser was not used.

Contact Lenses

For most applications of iridoplasty, an Abraham or Wise contact lens is sufficient. These lenses reduce corneal irradiation, increase iris irradiation, act as a lid speculum, and provide magnified viewing of the operative area. The lenses are placed on the eye under topical anesthesia with the aid of an artificial tear solution such as Celluvisc.

Surgical Technique

To perform iridoplasty, a continuous wave laser (such as argon or krypton) or a quasi-continuous wave laser (such as a frequency-doubled Nd:YAG laser) is utilized. Long exposures (0.5 seconds) and low power (250 to 350 mW) are typically used with a 500- to 1000-μm spot size. Spots are placed as far peripheral as the Abraham or Wise lens will allow with part of the aiming beam overlapping the peripheral limbus. The intent is to achieve a deep contraction burn (Figure 12-6). If release of pigment occurs, the laser power, not exposure duration should be turned down. Approximately eight to nine spots per quadrant are placed. Iris blood vessels that are visible as well as the 3 and 9 o'clock positions should be avoided.

Postoperative Care

Postoperatively, patients who have undergone iridoplasty should be placed on a topical corticosteroid four times a day for at least 1 week. Gonioscopy should be performed and quadrants retreated as needed. If retreatment is necessary, laser spots should be placed

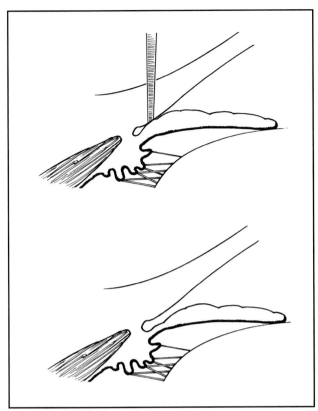

Figure 12-6. Iridoplasty for plateau iris. Long exposures (0.5s) with low continuous wave energy (325 mw) have a favorable mechanical effect on peripheral iris contour. Note the change in iris contour secondary to tissue contraction and the stromal thinning.

on the old laser burn to minimize the chances for iris ischemia. On occasion, a one-mirrored lens may be used for retreatment to access more peripheral iris.

LASER TRABECULOPLASTY

Laser trabeculoplasty is one of the most commonly performed glaucoma procedures. It predictably creates a 20% drop in IOP for approximately 80% of patients. Certain glaucomas, such as pigment dispersion and pseudoexfoliation glaucoma, may have somewhat better response to this technique. A poor effect is seen in younger patients and in patients with pseudophakia. In general, diode lasers are equally efficacious when compared to argon lasers. Diode lasers, however, may produce more discomfort when used for trabeculoplasty, perhaps secondary to a deeper penetration of laser light and stimulation of nerve fibers.

Patient Selection

In general clinical practice, most patients are offered laser trabeculoplasty after an attempt to use one or two topical medications. Laser trabeculoplasty is utilized earlier if the patient has allergy/intolerance to medical therapy or has medical contraindications (eg, early dementia, depression, noncompliance, or cardiopulmonary problems).

Preoperative Preparation

The patient undergoing laser trabeculoplasty should be pretreated with apraclonidine or brimonidine drops to minimize the incidence of postoperative laser-induced IOP spikes.

Contact Lenses

A variety of lenses are available for the performance of argon laser trabeculoplasty. The Ritch lens (Figure 12-7) provides variable angles of viewing, which facilitates treatment of the entire angle. It also creates a somewhat smaller spot size. Alternatively, a one-mirrored lens with coated optics may be used to perform this procedure. The one-mirrored lens can be tilted and its smaller size has an advantage in patients with overhanging brows or narrow fissures.

Surgical Technique

After pretreatment and use of a topical anesthetic, the contact lens is placed on the eye. The laser is set to a 50-μm spot size with an exposure time of 0.1 seconds; continuous wave or quasi-continuous wave power is set around 700 mW. Typically 50 to 60 spots are placed over 180 to 270 degrees. The spots are placed at the anterior pigmented border of the trabecular meshwork. This is the junction of the filtering and nonfiltering trabecular meshwork. This area is located just posterior to the terminus of the parallel piped (Schwalbe's line) produced by a thin slit beam (Figure 12-8). Spots placed posterior to this will result in pain and pectinate peripheral anterior synechiae with possible iatrogenic angle closure. The initial power selected is a function of the amount of pigment present in the trabecular meshwork. More pigmented angles will require lower continuous wave power, whereas less pigmented angles will

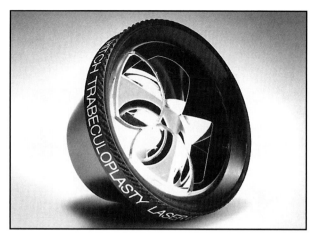

Figure 12-7. The Ritch lens is constructed to provide two different viewing angles for the superior and inferior angles, 64 and 59 degrees respectively. To reduce a 50 μm spot laser to 35 μm, a plano-convex button is placed over each mirror which also provides 1.4X magnification. Courtesy of Ocular Instruments, Bellevue, Wash.

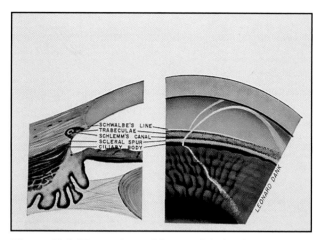

Figure 12-8. The teminus of the parallel piped produced by a thin slit beam marks the location of Schwalbe's line. This is one of the most reliable landmarks for gonioscopy. Adapted from Gorin G, Posner A. *Slit-Lamp Gonioscopy.* Baltimore, Md: Williams and Wilkins; 1961.

require more continuous wave power. The desired tissue effect is a blanch or formation of a small bubble (Figure 12-9). If the physician is treating the eye with a diode laser, the observed tissue effects are quite different. Diode lasers penetrate much more deeply secondary to longer wavelength and decreased absorption by melanin. There may be little superficial effect visible when using this laser.

Postoperative Care

If the patient was not on an alpha agonist preoperatively or does not have pigment dispersion or pseudoexfoliation glaucoma, the chances of a postoperative IOP spike are small. If the patient does not have an IOP spike, a return in 1 week should be scheduled to ensure discontinuation of topical cortical steroids started four times a day after this procedure. Patients should be seen again approximately 4 to 6 weeks postoperatively to determine the efficacy of this treatment.

SELECTIVE LASER TRABECULOPLASTY

A new type of trabeculoplasty has been described and developed by Dr. Mark Latina. This technique uses a Q-switched frequency doubled Nd:YAG laser (Coherent Selectra 7000). Fifty 400-μm spots are placed over 180 degrees. The described pulse durations of 10 ns to 1μs are under the thermal relaxation time for collagen-based tissues. This fact is important as no

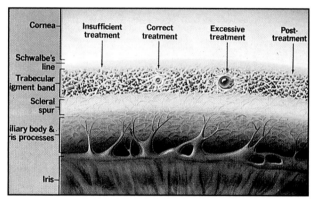

Figure 12-9. Correct level of energy delivered to the trabecular meshwork with argon laser generates a small steam bubble or blanching. The correct placement site is at the terminus of the arrow under the text "correct treatment." Adapted from Schwartz AL, Whitten ME, Bleiman B et al. Argon laser trabecular surgery in uncontrolled phakic open angle glaucoma. *Ophthalmology.* 1981;88:213.

coagulation of tissues is produced. Nevertheless, a cell with additional chromophore, such as melanin, will absorb an additional increment of laser energy thereby heating it to a temperature that denatures vital molecules and causes pigmented cell death. In addition to not creating thermal damage, IOP drops more rapidly when compared with traditional argon laser trabeculoplasty (Figure 12-10). The major problem with this procedure may be an economic one. Physicians may be unable to afford the financial penalty incurred to offer what may be an improved version of a technique that is effective and already widely available.

LASER SUTURE LYSIS

Laser suture lysis has had a profound effect on the performance and results of trabeculectomy. Sutures that are intended to be lysed postoperatively are placed during the trabeculectomy until a slow trickle of fluid is seen at the edges of the scleral flap. The surgeon should carefully note the location and the effect of the sutures placed at the time of surgery.

Patient Selection

Sutures are cut postoperatively according to the clinical course of the patient. Without antimetabolites, sutures may be cut within the first 2 weeks for maximum effect. When antimetabolites such as 5-fluorouricil or mitomycin-C are used, the period during which laser suture lysis can have an effect on filtering surgery is extended, and is longer for mitomycin-C than for 5-fluorouricil.

Preoperative Preparation

A patient undergoing laser suture lysis may have a drop of phenylephrine 2.5% placed on the eye to achieve vasoconstriction and to partially decongest the tissues. The laser procedure should be performed under topical anesthesia.

Contact Lenses

A variety of lenses are available for laser suture lysis. All lenses compress tissue and provide a viewing field. In a resident setting, the Mandelkorn laser suture lysis lens (Figure 12-11) offers the advantages of an increased viewing field and may be more durable than other available laser suture lysis lenses.

Surgical Technique

After the application of topical anesthesia, the patient is asked to look down. The laser should be preset to a 50-μm spot size and an exposure time of 0.1 seconds. The continuous wave power should start low, approximately 300 mW and be increased as needed. If an argon dye laser is available, a wave length in the orange region (595 nm) minimizes interaction with free hemoglobin or red blood cells present in the subconjunctival space. Krypton or diode lasers also are good choices for suture lysis. If an argon laser is utilized, great care should be taken not to apply laser energy in areas that have collections of subconjunctival blood. Sutures closest to the limbus should be cut first (Figure 12-12). Apical sutures should be lysed only on an as needed basis. Premature lysis of an apical suture may produce profound hypotony.

Postoperative Care

Postoperatively, the conjunctiva should be inspected for any microperforations produced by the laser beam. If present, these may be treated by patching the eye. In general, only one suture per day should be cut. In an emergent situation with elevated pressure, however, additional sutures should be cut leaving an interval between each suture lysis to assess the effects of the lysis of each suture.

CYCLODESTRUCTIVE PROCEDURES

Cyclodestructive procedures are the last choice in surgical intervention in the glaucoma patient. They create pain, inflammation, and visual loss. The ease of application of these procedures should not, in any way, increase the enthusiasm with which they are utilized in the care of the end stage glaucoma patient.

Patient Selection

These procedures may be offered to patients in whom trabeculectomy and aqueous drainage devices are either not an option or have been tried and have failed.

Preoperative Preparation

Cyclodestructive procedures are done under retrobulbar anesthesia. Although laser-based cyclodestructive procedures produce less pain than cyclocryotherapy, a prescription for a moderate strength analgesic such as oxycodone or acetaminophen with codeine (30 mg) should be given to the patient to treat postoperative discomfort.

Contact Lenses

The Shields contact lenses is available for the performance of non-contact Nd:YAG laser cyclophotocoagulation (Figure 12-13). In the case of the diode laser

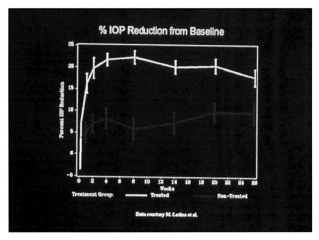

Figure 12-10. Trabeculoplasty with the Selectra laser results in IOP drops, which occur more rapidly when compared with traditional argon laser trabeculoplasty. Courtesy of Coherent Laser Corporation, Palo Alto, Calif.

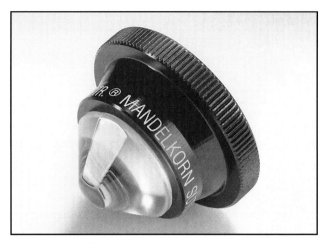

Figure 12-11. The Mandelkorn laser suture lysis lens has a wide viewing area which compresses tissue allowing better visualization of sutures. The optics of the lens reduce a 50-µm laser spot to 38 µm and increase irradiance by 1.7X at the focal point. Courtesy of Ocular Instruments, Bellevue, Wash.

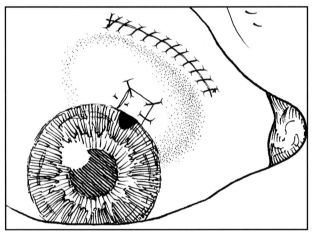

Figure 12-12. Laser suture lysis; the sutures closest to the limbus should be cut first. The surgeon should record the effects of placement of each suture at surgery. Sutures are generally melted in the order indicated. Lysis of the more posterior sutures may cause profound hypotony which may be exacerbated by the use of mitomicin-C.

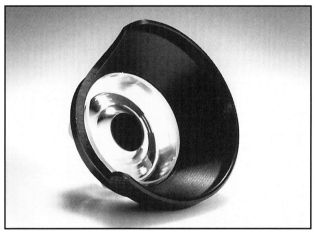

Figure 12-13. The Shields Lens for cyclophotocoagulation. This lens acts as a lid speculum and corneal light shield. It also compresses tissues to minimize conjunctival burns, and facilitates energy transfer to the ciliary body. A millimeter scale assists in accurate placement of laser spots. Courtesy of Ocular Instruments, Bellevue, Wash.

used for cyclophotocoagulation, the contact probe functions as the contact lens. It facilitates correct placement of the laser spot and compresses tissues, which increases optical transmission (Figure 12-14).

Surgical Technique: Non-Contact Nd:YAG Therapy

Lasers employed for this purpose are primarily the Microrupter series Nd:YAG lasers. They are utilized in the free-running mode, which can deliver

multiple Joule 20-ms pulses. The focus offset button is set at nine to allow the Nd:YAG beam to focus at a tissue level below the surface and disrupt the ciliary processes (Figure 12-15). A Shields contact lens may facilitate the procedure by compressing tissues and decreasing conjunctival burns. In addition, convenient marks are placed on this lens so that the laser energy may be placed 1 to 1.5 mm posterior to the limbus. Preoperatively, the operator may wish to localize the ciliary body by transillumination. Eight to 10 spots should be placed per quadrant, sparing the 3 and 9

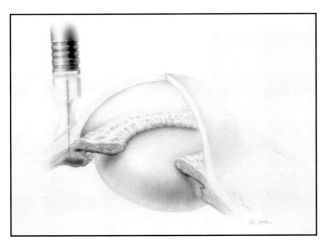

Figure 12-14. The G-probe for use with the Oculight SLX diode photocoagulator. The contact probe functions as the contact lens. It allows correct placement of the laser spot and compresses tissues which increases optical transmission. Photograph courtesy of Iris Medical, Mountain View, Calif.

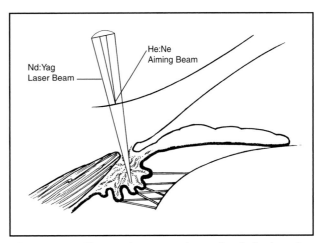

Figure 12-15. To treat tissue at a deeper level, the focusing offset is set to 9 on the Microrupter series lasers. This allows the He:Ne aiming laser to focus on the ocular surface and the Nd:YAG laser to converge at the level of the ciliary body.

o'clock positions to avoid injury to the long posterior ciliary arteries. Pulses in the 4 to 6 Joule range are usually suggested at the present time.

Surgical Technique:
Contact Laser Cyclophotocoagulation

Contact diode or Nd:YAG laser techniques maybe utilized with equal efficacy and morbidity. Currently, the most widely utilized lasers for cyclophotocoagulation are diode lasers. A representative example of this is the Oculight SLX (Iris Medical, Mountain View, Calif). These lasers use a contact probe delivery system. By compressing sclera, a localized dessication is created which increases optical transmission. These lasers use a much longer burn at a much lower power compared with non-contact techniques. The G-probe, which is available on the Iris unit (see Figure 12-14), has a convenient marking to allow delivery to the appropriate position posterior to the limbus. Although, initially 2 seconds at 1750 mW was suggested, recent studies have shown that a longer duration (4 seconds) at lower power (1250 mW) may result in fewer retreatments without any statistical significance in treatment outcomes. A number of treatment strategies are available, one of which treats 270 degrees sparing 90 degrees around the 3 or 9 o'clock position, or treating 360 degrees with 8 to 10 spots per quadrant, sparing the 3 and 9 o'clock positions.

Postoperative Care

Postoperatively, these patients are placed on a potent topical corticosteroid frequently (every 2 hours). In addition, atropine 1% is offered to these patients to treat ciliary spasm. A prescription for a moderate strength analgesic such as oxycodone or acetaminophen with 30 mg of codeine should also be provided. In treating patients with aqueous drainage devices, if a non-valved device or a device that has a very large drainage field is present, it is recommended that conservative treatment initially be employed to minimize the chances of hypotony after cyclodestructive therapy.

BIBLIOGRAPHY

Arden GB, et al. A survey of color discrimination in German ophthalmologists. Changes associated with the use of lasers and operating microscopes. *Ophthalmology.* 1991;98:567.

Berringer TA, et al. Using argon laser blue light reduces ophthalmologists' color contrast sensitivity. Argon blue and surgeons' vision. *Arch Ophthalmol.* 1989;107:1453.

Blok MDW, et al. Scleral flap sutures and the development of shallow or flat anterior chamber after trabeculectomy. *Ophthalmic Surg.* 1993;24:309.

Brancato R, Carassa R, Trabucchi G. Diode laser compared with argon laser for trabeculoplasty. *Am J Ophthalmol.* 1991;112:50.

Brown RH, et al. ALO 2145 reduces the IOP elevation after anterior segment laser surgery. *Ophthalmology.* 1988;95:378.

Brown SVL, Higginbotham E, Tessler H. Sympathetic ophthalmia following Nd: YAG cyclotherapy (letter). *Ophthalmic Surg.* 1996;21:736.

Campbell DG. Improvement of pigmentary glaucoma and healing of transillumination defects with miotic therapy. *Invest Ophthalmol Vis Sci.* 1983;23(suppl):173.

Campbell DG. Pigmentary dispersion and pigmentary glaucoma: a new theory. *Invest Ophthalmol Vis Sci.* 1979;20(suppl):25.

Chopra H, et al. Early postoperative titration of bleb function: argon laser lysis and removable sutures in trabeculectomy. *J Glaucoma.* 1992;1:54.

Cyrlin, et al. *Invest Ophthalmol Vis Sci.* 1998;32(suppl):2155.

Del Priore LV, Robin AL, Pollack IP. Neodymium:YAG and argon laser iridotomy. Long-term follow-up in a prospective, randomized clinical trial. *Ophthalmology.* 1988;95:1207.

Drake MV. Neodymium:YAG laser iridotomy. *Surv Ophthalmol.* 1987;32:171.

Edward DP, et al. Sympathetic ophthalmia following neodymium: YAG cyclotherapy. *Ophthalmic Surg.* 1989;20:544.

Gandolfi SA; Vecchi M. Effect of a Nd:YAG laser iridotomy on intraocular pressure in pigment dispersion syndrome. *Ophthalmology.* 1996;Oct:1693-1695.

The Glaucoma Laser Trial Research Group. The Glaucoma Laser Trial (GLT). 2. Results of argon laser trabeculoplasty versus topical medicines. *Ophthalmology.* 1990;97:1403.

Hampton C, et al. Evaluation of a protocol for transscleral neodymium: YAG cyclophotocoagulation in one hundred patients. *Ophthalmology.* 1990;97:910.

Hawkins TA, Stewart WC. One year results of semiconductor transscleral cyclophotocoagulation in glaucoma patients. *Arch Ophthalmol.* 1993;111:488.

Haynes WL, Alward WLM, Tello C, et al. Incomplete elimination of exercise induced pigment dispersion by laser iridotomy in pigment dispersion syndrome. *Ophthalmic Surg Lasers.* 1995;26:484-486.

Karickhoff JR. Pigmentary dispersion syndrome and pigmentary glaucoma: a new mechanism concept, a new treatment, and a new technique. *Ophthalmic Surg.* 1992;23:269-277.

L'Esperance Fa Jr. *Ophthalmic Lasers: Photocoagulation, Photoradiation, and Surgery.* 3rd ed. St Louis, Mo: CV Mosby; 1989.

Lieberman MF. Suture lysis by laser and goniolens. *Am J Ophthalmol.* 1983;95:257.

Melamed S, et al. Tight scleral flap trabeculectomy with postoperative laser suture lysis. *Am J Ophthalmol.* 1990;109:303.

Migliazzo CV, Shaffer RN, Nykin R, Magee S. Long-term analysis of pigmentary dispersion syndrome and pigmentary glaucoma. *Ophthalmology.* 1986;93:1528-1536.

Minckler DS. Does Nd: YAG cyclotherapy cause sympathetic ophthalmia? (editorial). *Ophthalmic Surg.* 1989;20:543.

Mittra RA, Allingham RR, Shields MB. Follow-up of argon laser trabeculoplasty: is a day-one postoperative IOP check necessary? *Ophthal Surg Lasers.* 1995;26:410-413.

Nelson JS, Berns MW. Basic laser physics and tissue interactions. Contemporay Dermatology. 1988;2:2.

Pavlin CJ, Ritch R, Foster FS. Ultrasound biomicroscopy in plateau iris syndrome. *Am J Ophthalmol.* 1992;113:390.

Potash SD et al. Ultrasound biomicroscopy in pigment dispersion syndrome. *Ophthalmology.* 1994;101:332.

Potash SD, Tello C, Liebmann J, Ritch R. Ultrasound biomicroscopy in pigment dispersion syndrome. *Ophthalmology.* 1994;Feb:332-339.

Ritch R. A new lens for argon laser trabeculoplasty. *Ophthalmic Surg.* 1985;16:331.

Ritch R. Argon laser peripheral iridoplasty: an overview. *J Glaucoma.* 1992;1:206.

Ritch R, Campbell DG, Camras C. Initial treatment of pigmentary glaucoma. *J Glaucoma.* 1993;2:44-49.

Ritch R, Potash SD, Liebmann JM. A new lens for argon laser suture lysis. *Ophthalmic Surg.* 1994;25:126.

Robin AL, et al. Effect of ALO 2145 on intraocular pressure following argon laser trabeculoplasty. *Arch Ophthalmol.* 1987;105:656.

Robin AL, Pollack IP, DeFaller JM. Effects of topical ALO 2145 (p-aminoclonidine hydrochloride) on IOP rise following argon laser iridotomy. *Arch Ophthalmol.* 1987;105:1208.

Savage JA, Simmons RJ. Staged glaucoma filtration surgery with planned early conversion from scleral flap to full-thickness operation using argon laser. *Ophthalmic Laser Ther.* 1986; 1:201.

Schuman JS ,et al. Contact transscleral Nd: YAG laser cyclophotocoagulation: midterm results. *Ophthalmology.* 1992;99: 1089.

Schwartz AL, Love DC, Schwartz MA. Long-term follow-up of argon laser trabeculoplasty for uncontrolled open angle glaucoma. *Arch Ophthalmol.* 1985;103:1482.

Shields MB, Wilkerson MH, Echelman DA. A comparison of two energy levels for noncontact transscleral neodymium-YAG cyclophotocoagulation. *Arch Ophthalmol.* 1993;111:484.

Shingleton BJ, et al . Long-term efficacy of argon laser trabeculoplasty, a ten-year follow-up study. *Ophthalmology.* 1993; 100:1324.

Simmons RB et al. Transscleral Nd: YAG laser cyclophotocoagulation with a contact lens. *Am J Ophthalmol.* 1991;112:671.

Spaeth GL, Baez K. Argon laser trabeculoplasty controls one third of cases of progressive, uncontrolled, open angle glaucoma for 5 years. *Arch Ophthalmol.* 1992;110:491.

Speakman JS. Pigmentary dispersion. *Br J Ophthalmol.* 1981;65:249-251.

Tomlinson CP, Brigham M, Belcher CD III. Suture manipulation with the argon laser. *Ophthalmic Laser Ther.* 1987;2:151.

Trope GE, Ma S. Mid-term effects of neodymium: YAG transscleral cyclocoagulation in glaucoma. *Ophthalmology.* 1990; 97:73.

Wise JB. Ten-year results of laser trabeculoplasty. *Eye.* 1987;1:45.

Chapter Thirteen

INCISIONAL SURGICAL TREATMENT OF GLAUCOMA

Robert F. Rothman, MD
Jeffrey M. Liebmann, MD
Robert Ritch, MD

INTRODUCTION

It has long been known that elevated intraocular pressure (IOP) is a significant risk factor for the development of glaucomatous optic neuropathy and visual field loss,[1-5] and that reducing the IOP in patients at risk can preserve visual function.[6-10] Although ophthalmologists have known about this association between elevated IOP and glaucoma since the early 1600s, surgical attempts at lowering the pressure did not originate until the 1800s when MacKenzie performed both a sclerotomy and paracentesis, which transiently lowered the IOP.[11-14]

The goal of filtering surgery for glaucoma is the creation and maintenance of a patent fistula from the anterior chamber to the subconjunctival space. The indications for performing glaucoma surgery are complex and varied. Although different procedures and techniques will be discussed in this chapter, the unifying goal of all procedures is to lower IOP to preserve visual function.

In general, incisional glaucoma surgery is performed on patients for whom medical or laser therapy has failed to control IOP. Factors that influence the choice of surgical technique include disease severity, the desired pressure reduction, and the patient's quality of life.[15-17] The long-term application of topical antiglaucoma medications has been reported to reduce the success of filtration surgery.[18-21] Therefore, earlier surgery may be indicated in certain patients.[22-25] The Collaborative Initial Glaucoma Treatment Study, a nationwide, prospective, randomized clinical trial sponsored by the National Eye Institute comparing the outcomes of newly diagnosed open-angle glaucoma patients treated initially with either medication or surgery, will help determine the relative risks of early surgery. The purpose of this chapter is to provide clinicians with an overview of incisional glaucoma surgery from the preoperative evaluation to the management of postoperative complications.

SURGICAL DECISION MAKING

As with any surgery, the preoperative evaluation of the glaucoma patient is a multi-faceted process,which may span many patient visits or may occur at a single examination. The patient's diagnosis (ie, type of glaucoma), previous surgical history, severity of disease, target IOP, and the status of the fellow eye are important factors in patient assessment. A thorough investigation should be made to determine the extent of glaucomatous optic neuropathy and visual field loss, loss of functional ability, and the rate of disease progression.

Once the decision to perform surgery has been made, a careful history and examination need to be performed so that the appropriate procedure can be planned. Factors that have been reported to affect the outcome of glaucoma surgery include younger age, black race,[26-28] glaucoma diagnosis,[29-39] and previous surgical history.[40-43] For example, older patients have a higher success rate than younger ones[44-47] due to a less intense fibroproliferative reaction and healing response. African-Americans appear to respond less favorably to standard filtering surgery due to increased scarring of the conjunctiva and Tenon's capsule.[48-50] While the success rate of filtration surgery is high for patients with chronic, non-inflammatory open-angle or angle-closure glaucoma who have not undergone previous surgery, a history of prior incisional surgery, neovascular glaucoma, or inflammation decreases surgical success. Each of these factors must be considered when contemplating surgical intervention.

The preoperative surgical examination begins with a careful assessment of the conjunctiva and periocular tissues. Conjunctiva that is scarred from cicatricial disease or previous incisional surgery may be difficult to manipulate for creation of a filtration bleb or may suggest the use of a fornix-based rather than a limbus-based conjunctival flap. Severe conjunctival scarring may preclude successful filtering surgery. Eyes that have significant peripheral anterior synechias may require an anterior placement of the sclerostomy, or an alteration in the position of the surgical site to enhance success. The presence of active inflammation or neovascularization often leads to a decision to perform surgery that relies less on the presence of healthy conjunctiva (ie, tube-shunt implantation). Adjunctive antifibrosis may be applied both during and after trabeculectomy in high-risk patients, or when a low postoperative IOP is desired.

Other necessary information to be identified during the examination includes the presence of concomitant ocular disease. Conditions such as cataract often cause an alteration in the choice of procedure. Combined cataract and glaucoma surgery may eliminate the need for multiple trips to the operating room while maximizing visual rehabilitation. Patients who require concomitant vitrectomy may undergo implantation of an aqueous tube-shunt into the vitreous cavity rather than the anterior chamber.

Once the history and examination have been completed, an assessment must be made as to the overall prognosis of the eye. Eyes with severely elevated pressure and poor visual potential should be managed with less invasive procedures, if possible. These eyes often respond to single or multiple attempts at ciliary body ablation with cyclocryotherapy or cyclophotocoagulation.

PREOPERATIVE PREPARATION

Informed consent must be obtained prior to surgical intervention and should include a discussion of the risks, benefits, and alternatives of the planned procedure. The discussion should be in language understandable to the patient, and all questions regarding the preoperative, operative, and postoperative routine should be answered. This includes both minor and major risks of the surgical procedure, postoperative restrictions, and anticipated medical regimen. This discussion should not be rushed and should be carried out by the person who will be performing the surgery.

It is often necessary for patients to discontinue certain medications prior to performing glaucoma surgery. Oral anticoagulants such as warfarin, persantine, and aspirin should be discontinued if possible. Effective anticoagulation can lead to hyphema from iris manipulation or even suprachoroidal hemorrhage from a precipitous drop in IOP. These medicines should not be discontinued if their discontinuation poses significant risk to the general health of the patient.

For patients who can tolerate a short period of IOP elevation, it is often advantageous to discontinue certain topical antiglaucoma medications as well. Long-acting miotics such as echothiophate iodide and demecarium bromide should be discontinued a minimum of 2 to 4 weeks prior to surgery with planned general anesthesia because of the potential systemic interaction between these medications and medications used during general anesthesia.[51] These topical agents have been shown to deplete plasma pseudocholinesterase, which also is responsible for the degradation of succinylcholine, a medication commonly used to induce paralysis prior to intubation during general anesthesia administration. Therefore, patients may experience prolonged muscle relaxation, respiratory depression, and apnea if succinylcholine is used in the presence of these agents.[52]

Aqueous suppressants should be continued until the day of surgery. This is especially true for patients with advanced glaucomatous optic neuropathy who are at risk for losing fixation due to an IOP rise. Miotics cause a breakdown in the blood-aqueous barrier and promote inflammation.[53-55] Discontinuing their use prior to intraocular surgery might decrease the amount of postoperative inflammation. If concomitant cataract or other intraocular surgery that requires an adequate view of the posterior segment is planned at the time of glaucoma surgery, discontinuation of miotics also may facilitate pupillary dilation. In addition, the prolonged stimulation of the ciliary body and pupillary sphincter induced by miotics can be counterproductive when attempting to manage a shallow anterior chamber or malignant glaucoma. Epinephrine agents should be discontinued because of their effects on conjunctival vasculature.

In general, patients who are to undergo intraocular surgery should have a preoperative general medical history and physical examination.[56-58] Even with the advent and implementation of topical anesthesia, intravenous sedation usually is administered regardless of the procedure. The presence of concomitant medical problems such as hypertension, diabetes, cardiac disease, and pulmonary disease are significant both in terms of anesthetic and sedative risk, and surgical positioning and tolerance. It is imperative that the ophthalmologist be aware of the medical status of his or her patient. Other medical problems that require the use of systemic medications for control also are important. Patients who regularly use anti-coagulants or steroids often have adjustments made to their medical regimen prior to surgery in an attempt to correct for possible missed doses and to overcome the stress that surgery places on the body.

Many surgeons prescribe broad spectrum topical antibiotics for several days prior to intraocular sur-

gery. Others use several drops 1 or 2 hours prior to the procedure. Nevertheless, several studies have shown that the only medication that causes a statistically significant reduction in the incidence of early postoperative endophthalmitis is topical 5% povidone-iodine used as a preoperative wash.[59,60]

Anesthesia

General anesthesia for glaucoma surgery is used primarily for infants and children. It also is appropriate, however, for those adult patients who are unable to remain in a comfortable, lying position due to musculoskeletal or respiratory difficulties, are extremely nervous, confused, or cannot cooperate under local anesthesia.[61-64] Other advantages of general anesthesia include elimination of the risk of orbital or ocular complications from the local anesthetic, and creation of better operating conditions for the surgeon. Ocular effects of inhalation anesthesia include a significant rise in IOP during endotracheal intubation[65,66] and a possible role in the formation of delayed suprachoroidal hemorrhage due to increased episcleral venous pressure, which occurs during extubation or secondary to postoperative nausea and emesis.[67]

Retrobulbar, peribulbar, subconjunctival, or topical anesthesia may be considered for glaucoma surgery.[68,69] Some individuals believe that retrobulbar anesthesia should be avoided, if possible, because of its many associated complications. It has been shown that the potential exists for a sudden, often extreme, elevation of IOP that can occur with retrobulbar injection.[70,71] The fluid bolus may also cause direct compression of the optic nerve, or its blood supply. Finally, the risk of retrobulbar hemorrhage, which also can compromise the optic nerve, and the risk of ocular perforation are removed.[69,72-75] Dilute concentrations of epinephrine used in an attempt to enhance the efficacy of local anesthesia should not be included, and may be harmful to patients with advanced glaucoma. The vasoconstriction caused by epinephrine not only counteracts the vasodilatory effect of local anesthetics, but theoretically, may compromise optic nerve blood flow.

Although peribulbar anesthesia is generally considered to be safer than retrobulbar anesthesia, the increased volume of fluid administered in the peribulbar space may be associated with slightly higher postinjection IOPs.[76] Sub-Tenon's anesthesia has very lit-

tle associated risk and has been shown to be efficacious in patients undergoing trabeculectomy.[72] In
addition, by injecting anesthesia into the sub-Tenon's
space superiorly, the associated fluid dissection can
facilitate the creation of limbus-based conjunctival
flaps. Finally, topical anesthesia can be used in those
patients who are able to cooperate during the planned
procedure or who are at increased risk from the
administration of other types of anesthesia. It also
should be mentioned that regardless of the type of
ocular anesthesia used, we routinely perform a lid
block in nearly every case to avoid blepharospasm
during the procedure.

SURGICAL TECHNIQUE

Trabeculectomy

Most patients with glaucoma who require a lowering of their IOP not attainable with the use of medication or laser therapy require trabeculectomy.

Surgical Exposure

Adequate exposure is critical for glaucoma surgery, particularly if a limbus-based conjunctival flap is
planned. Achieving such exposure involves properly
placing a sterile eye drape to remove the lashes from
the surgical field, and the use of an appropriately sized
lid speculum that exerts minimal pressure on the
globe. In an effort to have more control over the eye
during surgery, we routinely place a corneal traction
suture instead of a superior rectus bridle suture. This
technique involves placing an 8-0 Vicryl suture on a
cutting needle to the depth of the mid-corneal stroma
for approximately 3 mm at the limbus directly anteri-
or to the proposed scleral flap (Figure 13-1a and b).
The suture is then placed on gentle traction inferiorly.
This suture allows for excellent control of eye movement during surgery and avoids rectus muscle hemorrhage, most cases of postoperative ptosis,[77,78] and the
diplopia[79] that can occur with bridle sutures.

Conjunctival Flap

Creation of a conjunctival flap is critically important during glaucoma filtering surgery. Either a fornix-
or limbus-based approach can be used because both
have been shown to produce similar results in eyes not
receiving adjunctive antifibrosis therapy.[80-84] If a lim-

bus-based flap is to be used, the entry should be 8 to
10 mm posterior to the limbus to avoid placing the
conjunctival incision over the scleral flap (Figure 13-
2, a-c). The conjunctiva should be grasped with
anatomic or non-toothed forceps approximately 12
mm posterior to the limbus and elevated off of the eye.
The assistant should grasp the tissue approximately 1
to 2 mm anterior to the surgeon to create a tent in the
conjunctiva. Blunt Westcott scissors are then used to
incise the conjunctiva parallel to the limbus for
approximately 10 to 15 mm. The same procedure is
repeated for the incision of the Tenon's capsule. The
incision through Tenon's capsule and down to episclera should be at a point anterior to the conjunctival
incision. Blunt dissection should be used to reach the
conjunctival insertion at the limbus. Tenon's capsule
may be relaxed with circumferential incisions to permit adequate exposure. These relaxing incisions make
exposure of the surgical limbus much easier but care
must be taken to avoid accidental incision of the conjunctiva. When performing these dissections, both the
surgeon and the assistant should try to grasp only
Tenon's capsule when possible for traction. The conjunctiva should not be handled, if possible. Once the
dissection has reached the limbus, episcleral tissue
should be gently removed by scraping the sclera with
a surgical blade. Hemostasis should be obtained prior
to the scleral incision with cautery utilizing a fine tip
(0.25 mm) to minimize tissue contraction and shrink-
age.

The procedure for creation of a fornix-based conjunctival flap is technically easier than creation of a
limbus-based flap (Figure 13-3, a-d). A peritomy
encompassing approximately 2 clock hours is made at
the limbus with sharp scissors while grasping the tissue with anatomic or non-toothed forceps. The sub-
Tenon's space is then entered with blunt dissection.
Again, care must be taken to avoid tearing or macer-
ating the free conjunctival end so that a watertight closure can be performed. The technique for cautery and
exposure of the scleral bed are identical to that for the
limbus-based flap. The decision to perform either a
limbus- or fornix-based flap is one of surgical exposure, anatomy, and surgeon's preference.

Scleral Flap

After the scleral bed has been prepared, the globe
should be stabilized with a toothed forceps and the

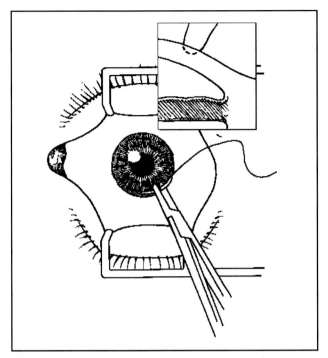

Figure13-1a. The needle is passed mid-stroma for approximately 3 mm.

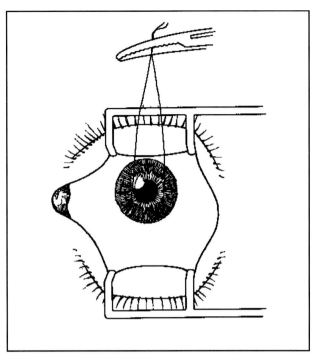

Figure13-1b. The needle is removed and the suture is placed on gentle inferior traction.

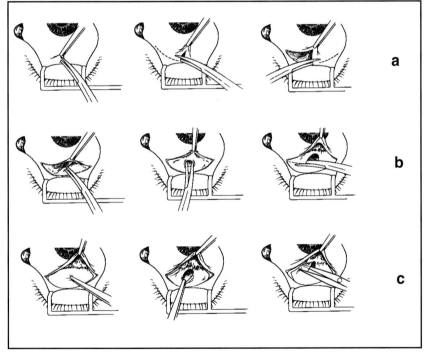

Figure13-2. (a) Conjunctival incision for limbus-based flap is begun 8 to 10 mm posterior to limbus and extended for several millimeters nasally and temporally. (b) Tenon's capsule is then entered more anteriorly and the opening is enlarged. (c) Blunt and careful sharp dissection are used as necessary to expose the surgical limbus.

outline of the scleral flap should be created (Figure 13-4). A one half thickness scleral flap then should be dissected into clear cornea utilizing a lamellar technique. If an intraoperative sponge application of antifibrosis agent is to be used, at this time it can be placed on the eye between Tenon's capsule and the scleral flap, and allowed to remain for the pre-determined period of time. After the sponge has been removed and copious irrigation performed, the procedure can continue. Care must be taken not to shred the flap during manipulation.

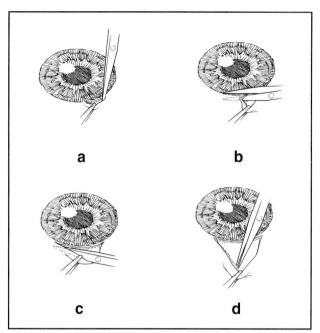

Figure13-3. (a) Conjunctival incision for a fornix-based flap is begun at the limbus with sharp scissors. (b and c) The incision is extended carefully for two clock hours. (d) Blunt and sharp dissection are used to expose the sub-Tenon's space.

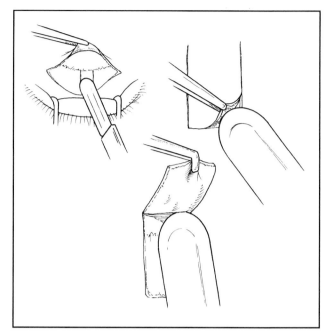

Figure13-4. A one-half thickness scleral flap is outlined with a surgical blade. Careful lamellar dissection is then used to elevate the flap.

Paracentesis

Following the scleral flap dissection, a paracentesis should be made in the temporal, peripheral cornea. This incision provides access to the anterior chamber for intra- and postoperative management of anterior chamber depth and IOP. Irrigation through the paracentesis aids in assessment of the outflow pathway. Conjunctival wound leaks and buttonholes also can be detected. If possible, the paracentesis should be placed so that the internal entry is over the iris and the wound angled toward the 6 o'clock position so that instrumentation placed into the eye will not cross over the pupil and lens.

Sclerostomy

For creation of the internal ostium (Figure 13-5a and b), the globe is grasped with toothed forceps adjacent to the scleral flap while the assistant gently lifts the flap out of the way. The anterior chamber should be entered at the base of the scleral flap and an internal section of clear cornea with or without trabecular meshwork should be excised with a knife or punch. The scleral flap should be able to fully cover the entire internal ostium.

Iridectomy

An iridectomy is performed in nearly all trabeculectomies. The purpose of iridectomy is to prevent iris from incarcerating into the internal ostium. The iris tissue is grasped with small-toothed forceps through the sclerostomy while the assistant gently lifts the scleral flap (Figure 13-6a and b). The role of the assistant is critical at this time because adequate exposure must be obtained while utilizing care not to distort the wound, which might result in excessive aqueous outflow and anterior chamber shallowing. The size of the iridectomy should be larger than the sclerostomy at its basal aspect and should not extend centrally. The iris tissue then is reposited into the eye with irrigation. The excised iris specimen should be examined to ascertain that a full-thickness piece of iris was removed. Gently rubbing the specimen against the surgical drape produces a dark streak of pigment if full-thickness iris tissue is present. If there is a small amount of bleeding from the iris root, it usually stops spontaneously within a few moments. Prolonged bleeding may require instillation of viscoelastic into the anterior chamber for tamponade. Cauterization rarely is necessary, and should only be done in extreme cases of prolonged bleeding not responsive to

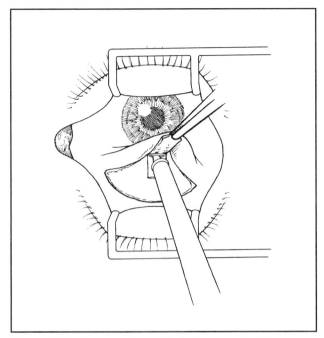

Figure13-5a. A super-sharp blade is passed into the anterior chamber at the base of the scleral flap.

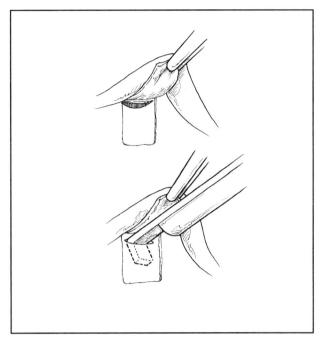

Figure13-5b. Once the ostium is created, a punch is placed behind the corneo-scleral tissue.

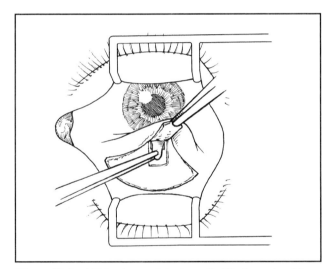

Figure13-6a. While the assistant gently lifts the scleral flap, the posterior iris is grasped with a small-toothed forceps.

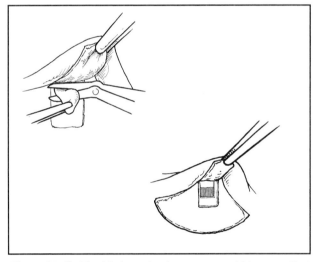

Figure13-6b. The iris is excised to create an iridectomy that is at least as large as the ostium.

conservative measures. The anterior chamber should be reformed with balanced salt solution as necessary.

Scleral Flap Closure

Closure of the scleral flap should be performed promptly and with little distortion of the globe. Excessive flow through the ostium can result in significant anterior chamber shallowing. Two or three nylon sutures usually suffice to re-approximate the

scleral flap to the scleral bed (Figure 13-7). The eye should be inflated with balanced salt solution to an appropriate IOP prior to securing the knots. Once the first suture is placed, the remaining sutures should be placed with similar tension. A notation should be made as to which is the tightest suture for subsequent laser suture lysis. Flow should be assessed again and the sutures adjusted, removed, and replaced as necessary to be certain that the flow rate is adequate.

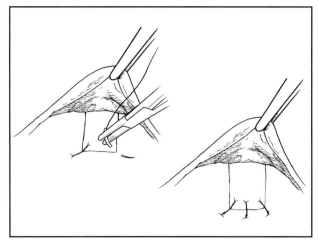

Figure13-7. Closure of the scleral flap with multiple monofilament sutures. The knots should be buried to avoid erosion of the suture ends through the bleb wall.

Conjunctival Closure

Once the scleral flap is secure and the anterior chamber is of appropriate depth, conjunctival closure can take place. Careful creation of a watertight seal helps prevent postoperative hypotony. Leakage at the wound edge predisposes to hypotony and its associated complications, delayed wound closure, and formation of localized blebs with poor pressure control. Many sutures and techniques for conjunctival closure have been described. When closing a limbus-based flap, we use either 9-0 polyglactin in a running and locked fashion or 10-0 nylon with a running, mattress technique (Figure 13-8). Non-toothed forceps are used to approximate the wound edges and relax any tension that may have developed from tissue retraction. The suture is then placed through both sides of the wound at one end and tied with a surgeon's knot (3:1:1). When using polyglactin, the suture is placed from the anterior to posterior wound edges and reverse locked to secure the tension. Each throw should be placed approximately 0.5 mm apart for the entire length of the wound. The suture is then tied at the distal end and cut long enough so as not to cause lid irritation. In an attempt to create a more watertight closure, Tenon's capsule should be incorporated into the closure on the posterior aspect of the wound. This also helps to prevent anterior migration of the wound. A non-locking mattress suture technique should be used with non-absorbable sutures because it is extremely tedious to remove a locked suture.

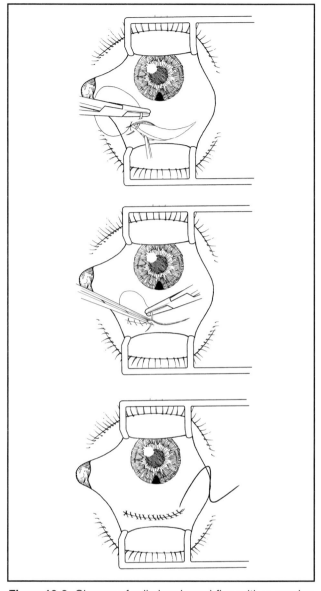

Figure13-8. Closure of a limbus-based flap with a running and locked polyglactin suture.

Closure of a fornix-based flap involves reattaching the conjunctiva to its limbal insertion. This is accomplished by placing a 10-0 nylon on a vascular needle through the conjunctiva and Tenon's fascia on its posterior surface and then distally through the cornea, back toward the scleral flap, and out the corneal tissue (Figure 13-9). The needle should be placed mid-stroma through the cornea and the bite should be at the peripheral limbus and approximately 2 mm long. By passing the suture in this manner, the knot can be moved to a location beneath the conjunctiva, reducing subsequent corneal irritation. Some sur-

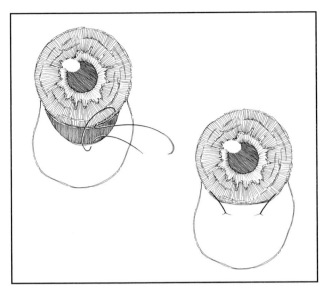

Figure 13-9. Closure of the fornix-based flap. The suture should be anchored into corneal tissue.

geons debride the corneal epithelium to enhance adherence of the conjunctiva or place an additional nylon suture in a mattress fashion centrally.

Once watertight closure has been achieved, the anterior chamber should be reformed with balanced salt solution to an appropriate IOP and the degree of flow through the sclerostomy assessed. The bleb should be checked with a fluorescein strip to detect for the presence of leaks, which should be closed before leaving the operating room. A subconjunctival injection of antibiotic and steroid usually is given in a location opposite the filtering site and additional combination antibiotic/steroid ointment is placed on the eye. A gentle patch is placed on the eye, which is taped shut and covered with a protective (eg, Fox) shield.

Full Thickness Procedures

Prior to the advent of trabeculectomy, full thickness procedures were routinely performed in the surgical management of glaucoma. The creation of a direct channel from the anterior chamber to the subconjunctival space was extremely effective at lowering IOP, but was associated with significant complications including hypotony, flat anterior chambers, ciliochoroidal detachments, endophthalmitis, and cataract formation.[47,85,86]

All full-thickness surgeries share the similar feature of the creation of a direct channel for free-flow of

fluid from the anterior chamber to the subconjunctival space. The procedure for posterior lip sclerectomy[87,88] involves creating a circumlinear incision of approximately 3 mm in length with a sharp knife immediately posterior to the conjunctival insertion. A punch is then used to take several pieces of full-thickness sclera from the posterior lip of the wound so that the approximate size of the sclerotomy is 1.5 to 2 mm long by 1 mm wide. A peripheral iridectomy then is performed followed by conjunctival closure.

Thermal sclerostomy[89-93] is a variation of posterior lip sclerectomy in which cautery is used to outline the linear incision in the sclera, which overlies the anterior chamber. Alternating cautery and sharp incisions are used to penetrate the eye wall. The heat of the cautery causes tissue contracture and mild gaping of the wound which allows for free flow of fluid from the eye.

Iridectomy for Angle Closure

The primary indication for performing iridectomy is to relieve angle-closure glaucoma due to pupillary block. Since the advent of both argon and Nd:YAG lasers, surgical iridectomy has become supplanted by these newer, non-invasive, and lower cost techniques.[94-96] In rare cases, however, where an inadequate view of the anterior segment and iris (eg, corneal edema) precludes successful laser treatment, surgical iridectomy may be indicated. In addition, one might perform an iridectomy as a primary procedure to remove a possible malignant iris lesion or to perform a biopsy.[97] With the exception of these two indications, iridectomy almost always is performed as part of another intraocular procedure.

Peripheral iridectomy involves the removal of a small piece of iris tissue from an area outside of the visual axis and, preferably, beneath the eyelid. A sector iridectomy involves the removal of a pie-piece shaped segment of iris tissue, which includes the iris sphincter and pupillary margin. Sector iridectomies have been advocated for enlargement of a miotic or corectopic pupil that inhibits adequate light from falling on the retina, or for removal of iris lesions. Complications of sector iridectomy include photophobia, glare, and hyphema.

Although a limbal incision can be used, a clear corneal incision is preferable to preserve conjunctiva for future filtering surgery. In creating the limbal wound, a conjunctival peritomy is made superiorly followed by the creation of a 2 to 3 mm beveled incision at the surgical limbus (Figure 13-10). This is analogous to a miniature cataract wound. If a clear corneal wound is to be placed, the 3-mm incision should be made perpendicular to the corneal plane just anterior to the limbus and central to the limbal arcade. In both cases, the groove should be beveled. The wound should be placed to facilitate performing a basal iridectomy, which is less visually significant and less likely to be occluded by synechias from the iris to the lens.

After removal of a full-thickness iris specimen, the wound is then closed with a single or multiple 10-0 nylon sutures with rotation of the knot into the tissue to avoid irritation. The wound should be watertight. The conjunctiva can be closed separately with absorbable suture if a limbal wound was used. If the anterior chamber shallowed during the procedure, it is best to reform it prior to suture placement to avoid overly tight sutures. The procedure is completed with subconjunctival injections of steroid and antibiotic followed by placement of a cycloplegic agent to help prevent ciliary spasm, synechia formation, and malignant glaucoma. Patients then can be placed on a standard regimen of frequent topical steroids, antibiotics, and cycloplegics during the postoperative period.

Complications of surgical iridectomy include bleeding and hyphema, flat anterior chamber from wound leakage,[98,99] malignant glaucoma, and failure to perform a complete iridectomy with persistence of pupillary block. Late complications include photophobia, glare and diplopia from large iridectomies,[100] cataract formation,[101-103] and subconjunctival fistula formation. Finally, all of the associated risks of intraocular surgery including endophthalmitis, wound incarceration, and vitreous loss must be considered.

Cataract and Glaucoma

The first step in the management of coexistent cataract and glaucoma is to determine the choice of surgical procedure. In patients who have early optic neuropathy and good IOP control, cataract extraction alone might be appropriate with monitoring of the IOP postoperatively. In patients with moderate to severe glaucoma, who also have a visually significant cataract, a combined procedure (one-site or two-site) often is indicated.[104-109] Finally, for patients with uncontrolled IOP and advanced visual field loss, con-

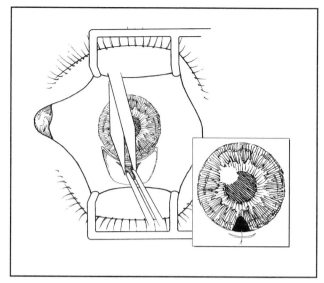

Figure13-10. Surgical iridectomy performed through a limbus incision. Conjunctival peritomy is made in an identical fashion as for trabeculectomy.

sideration can be given to a staged procedure (trabeculectomy first to allow for stabilization of the IOP followed by cataract extraction at a later date). The indications for performing cataract extraction are a topic beyond the scope of this chapter.

The preferred method of cataract extraction to be used in combination with trabeculectomy is phacoemulsification.[110-112] The smaller wound size promotes less inflammation and allows for greater success of the trabeculectomy. We usually employ a fornix-based conjunctival flap, although many surgeons use limbus-based flaps.[113,114] After creation of the conjunctival flap and preparation of the scleral surface, a linear incision is made in the sclera approximately 2 mm posterior to the limbus. The length of this incision should be long enough to accommodate both the phacoemulsification handpiece and the proposed intraocular lens. Dissection with a crescent blade then is carried into clear cornea just beyond the limbal arcade utilizing a lamellar technique. Particular attention should be directed to the thickness of the corneoscleral flap. If an antifibrotic agent is to be used, it is applied at this time. An effort should be made to avoid having the sponge contact the limbal conjunctiva as this may predispose to wound leakage. After the sponge is removed and thorough irrigation is performed, a paracentesis is made for placement of the second instrument used during phacoemulsifica-

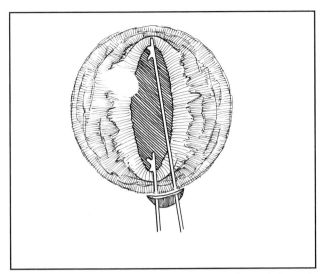

Figure13-11a. Vertical pupil stretching performed through cataract wound.

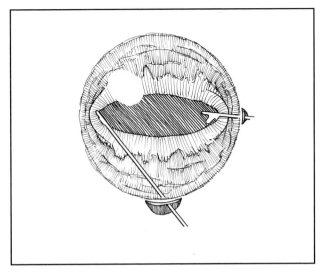

Figure13-11b. Horizontal pupil stretching with one instrument in cataract wound and one instrument through paracentesis.

tion. A keratome then is used to enter the anterior chamber through the corneoscleral wound.

Occasionally, patients who have been on miotics for an extended period of time or who have a history of inflammatory eye disease have an extremely miotic pupil that precludes adequate access to the lens. In these patients, freeing of the posterior synechiae with an iris sweep and placement of viscoelastic over the pupil may enlarge the opening enough for lens removal. If this is not sufficient, pupil stretching can be performed by placing two iris hooks through the wound and directing force both inferiorly and superiorly to physically open the pupil (Figure 13-11a and b). The same procedure is then performed nasally and temporally by placing one of the hooks through the paracentesis. When this procedure is not sufficient, we often employ iris retractors to artificially create a larger pupil.[115] Four, small retractors are placed through stab incisions at the 10, 2, 4, and 8 o'clock positions and effectively create a square pupil (Figure 13-12a and b). If iris retractors are not available to stretch the pupil, small sphincterotomies created with scissors often suffice.[116] Cataract extraction then is performed in the usual fashion.

Particular attention should be placed on thorough cortical clean-up and removal of all nuclear fragments because any residual lens material incites a significant inflammatory reaction, which may jeopardize the success of the filtration procedure. Lens insertion can be performed after the anterior chamber and capsular bag are inflated with viscoelastic. Once this procedure is

complete, a Kelly-Descemet punch is placed into the corneoscleral wound and a sclerostomy is performed with several bites to create a rounded opening. An iridectomy is then performed as usual, and the posterior aspect of the wound closed with 10-0 nylon sutures as necessary. If additional filtration is required, some surgeons create winged incisions at the lateral aspect of the scleral flap to create a more standard scleral flap, rather than a linear incision, and place their scleral flap sutures appropriately. If the method of cataract extraction needs to be converted to a standard extracapsular technique, this can easily be performed by extending the linear incision toward the limbus with a beveled blade and opening the tissue with corneoscleral scissors. The sclerostomy should be performed as usual at the conclusion of the case and meticulous suture technique must be employed to avoid leakage from the wound. This should be confirmed with irrigation through the paracentesis.

Glaucoma Implants

In cases where satisfactory filtration surgery may not be possible due to poor quality conjunctiva, glaucoma implants offer a viable option. These devices are designed to reduce IOP by shunting aqueous through a tube to an encapsulated area surrounding an explant located on the scleral surface approximately 10 mm posterior to the limbus. The long history of attempting to drain aqueous through a tube has led to the modern-day surgical device. Although there are many styles of

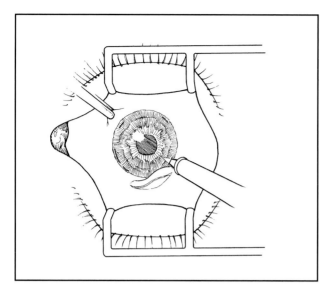

Figure13-12a. Placement of paracentesis for iris-hook insertion. The blade should be oriented vertically, being careful not to puncture the iris or lens capsule.

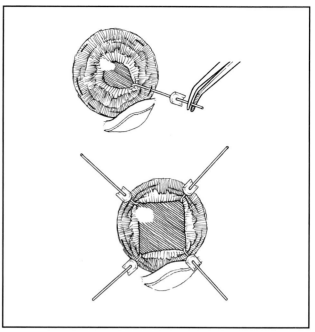

Figure13-12b. After four paracenteses are created, iris hooks are inserted beneath the iris and retracted to create a square pupil.

drainage implants,[117-122] modern devices all consist of a silastic tube attached to an external reservoir. Because the major determinant of IOP reduction with these devices is the resistance of the capsular wall to aqueous flow at the explant site,[123-125] surface area is of critical importance. Larger plates allow for a greater area of encapsulation and theoretically, lower IOP[118,126-128] although this relationship is not a direct one. The main difference between the currently available devices is the presence or absence of a valve designed to limit the flow of aqueous. The presence of a valve mechanism in the Krupin and Ahmed implants allows for restriction to flow particularly in the early postoperative period when this is most desirable. Non-valved implants require some form of ligature to control flow until encapsulation has occurred or staged implantation where the plate is placed on the sclera primarily and the tube is inserted into the anterior chamber approximately 6 weeks later during a second procedure.

The indications for performing implantation of an aqueous shunt are varied. Patients usually have elevated IOP despite maximal medical and laser therapy, and have either failed previous filtration surgery or have anatomic factors that limit the potential for successful filtration surgery. They have been used in all types of glaucoma, and have indications for primary insertion in patients with neovascular or other inflammatory glaucomas where the intense inflammatory nature of the disease most likely would cause irreparable scarring of a sclerostomy and scleral flap.[129-134]

Information about the design and flow characteristics of each implant is available elsewhere. Our preferred implant at this time is the Baerveldt 350 mm[2] implant. Many of the components of the surgical technique are identical between implants and vary only in the need to place some implants beneath rectus muscles, and methods of restricting flow through the tube in the early postoperative period.

The first part of the procedure is the creation of a fornix-based conjunctival flap (Figure 13-13). Limbus-based flaps should be avoided as they may lead to late dehiscence and erosion.[135] A relaxing incision at one side of the peritomy enhances surgical exposure. The conjunctiva is then undermined using blunt dissection, and a scleral pocket is created between the superior and lateral rectus muscles. A muscle hook then engages each muscle in succession to identify their insertions. The device is then placed on the surgical field and the tube is irrigated with balanced salt solution to ensure patency and to prime the valve on restrictive implants. In a non-restricted device, such as the Baerveldt, a 7-0 or 8-0 polyglactin ligature is placed around the tube near its base and tied tightly with needle holders. The tube should then

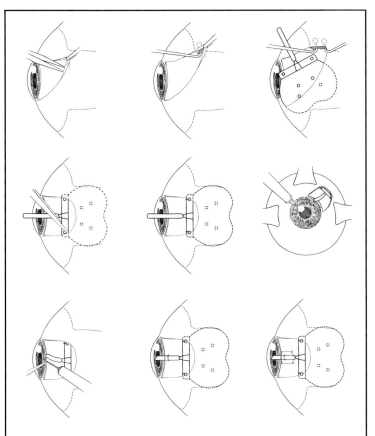

Figure13-13. After creation of a fornix-based flap, the implant tube is ligated to restrict fluid flow. The implant is then placed beneath the rectus muscles and secured to the sclera. The tube is then cut to an appropriate length, placed into the anterior chamber, and covered with a tissue graft.

be irrigated again to be certain that there is no flow through the tube. An absorbable suture should be used because this will dissolve in 4 to 6 weeks, after encapsulation has occurred. Alternatively, laser suture lysis or releasable suture techniques can be employed if earlier flow is required.[136-138] Once the flow has been completely restricted, the plate is positioned between the sclera and Tenon's capsule and between the two rectus muscles. This is accomplished by pushing the plate posteriorly until it lies behind the muscle insertions, about 10 mm from the limbus. This process is facilitated by using the muscle hook to first identify the superior rectus insertion, placing the plate behind it, and then identifying the lateral rectus insertion. The implant is then attached to the sclera with two nonabsorbable nylon sutures placed through anchoring eyelets on the device. The drainage tube should then be positioned over the limbus at the proposed site of entry into the anterior chamber. Scissors should be used to cut the tube to a length that will allow it to extend for 2 to 3 mm into the anterior chamber while not obscuring the visual axis. The tube should be cut with a bevel-up configuration that will limit the possi-

bility of tube blockage from iris tissue or vitreous. A paracentesis incision is then created temporally to allow for anterior chamber access. If vitreous is present, a thorough automated anterior vitrectomy should be performed through the paracentesis prior to placement of the tube.

A 23-gauge needle is then used to create the tube entry site. In pseudophakic or aphakic patients, the anterior chamber is entered approximately 0.5 to 0.75 mm posterior to the limbus with the incision made at an oblique angle, the needle being parallel to the iris plane. In phakic patients, the incision is made 0.5 mm posterior to the limbus with the needle angled a slightly flatter plane to avoid injury to the lens. The plane of the incision should be sufficient to keep the tube positioned close to the iris and away from the corneal endothelium. The tube is then placed through the entry track and into the anterior chamber. If it is too long, it can be removed, trimmed, and re-introduced. It is better to have a tube that is slightly long than one that is too short. Tube movement can be minimized by gently securing it to the eye wall with a nonabsorbable 10-0 nylon suture placed beneath the tube

4 or 5 mm from the limbus. The knot should be tied without creating tension on the tube and is then buried to avoid conjunctival erosion.

The tube should then be covered with a connective tissue graft[135,139,140] (processed pericardium, sclera, dura) that measures approximately 5 x 5 mm. This graft should cover the tube entry site and helps prevent erosion of the tube through the conjunctiva. The graft usually is secured to the sclera with 8-0 absorbable sutures. The conjunctiva then is closed with multiple absorbable sutures as necessary. The relaxing incision should be closed with a running, absorbable suture. Typical subconjunctival and topical medications are then applied.

Modifications of this procedure relate to methods of restricting flow through the tube[136,138,141-145] and to the position of tube insertion. The tube can be placed into the pars plana if a pars plana vitrectomy is planned or has been previously performed.[146-151] This position limits the potential risk to the cornea from tube migration or anterior entry. Furthermore, a two-stage implantation technique can be employed for nonrestrictive implants to avoid excessive flow and hypotony when immediate pressure reduction is not essential. In this situation, the plate is attached to the eye in the usual fashion but no ligature is placed around the tube. Instead, the tube is placed behind the muscle insertions and secured to the eye wall with nonabsorbable suture to prevent its anterior migration. Encapsulation is allowed to occur for 4 to 6 weeks and a second procedure is then performed, which locates the tube and places it within the anterior or posterior segment as previously discussed. Flow through the tube is established immediately, and because encapsulation already has occurred, there is little chance for hypotony. This technique is advantageous for patients who are predisposed to the development of choroidal hemorrhage or flat anterior chambers.

Aqueous shunt devices greatly expand the surgical options for the treatment of glaucoma. Modifications of this technology, hopefully, will lead to the development of a device with prolonged efficacy and low potential for hypotony.

ANTIFIBROSIS THERAPY

The major cause of glaucoma filtration surgery failure is external scarring of the conjunctival bleb.[152,153] The use of antifibrosis agents both during and after the operative procedure has greatly increased the success of this procedure.[154-175] These agents are applied with the intent of limiting fibroblast proliferation at the site of the surgical fistula in eyes that are presumed to be at a higher risk for failure. Risk factors for increased scarring include younger age, black race, previous incisional surgery, conjunctival scarring, active inflammation, eyes with neovascular or uveitic glaucoma, and eyes with a long history of chronic topical medication usage. The two agents commonly employed in current filtration surgery are 5-fluorouracil (5-FU) and mitomycin-C (MMC). The use of these medications has increased the success of filtration surgery, increased the level of IOP reduction, and decreased the need for additional postoperative pressure lowering therapy.

5-FU

5-FU works by selectively interfering with the synthesis phase (S phase) of the cell cycle. This agent is converted into a nucleotide analogue (5-fluoro-2-deoxyuridylate monophosphate), which competitively inhibits an enzyme involved in DNA synthesis. Abnormal protein products are produced within the cell, leading to death.[176,177] All actively dividing cells that come into contact with this agent are affected.

Numerous studies have shown a positive effect of 5-FU on success of filtration surgery. The initial method of application of this chemotherapy was to administer frequent subconjunctival injections in the immediate postoperative period consisting of 5 mg of 5-FU per injection for a cumulative dose of approximately 100 mg.[170-172] The occurrence of significant side effects including severe corneal epitheliopathy, however, led to many patients receiving a lower amount of medication. 5-FU can also be administered intraoperatively with a sponge application[161,178,179] and/or in the postoperative period. When administering 5-FU in the operating room, the technique involves preparation of the scleral bed and outlining of the scleral flap. A cellulose sponge is cut to create a rectangular piece of material approximately 3 x 2 mm. The sponge is placed in undiluted 5-FU (50 mg/mL) and then directly onto bare sclera. Tenon's capsule and conjunctiva should cover the sponge for 5 minutes. The sponge is then removed from the eye and discarded as chemotherapy by trained operating room staff. Copious irrigation of the sclera, conjunctiva, and cornea is performed and instruments are rinsed thoroughly. If the anterior chamber is inadvertently entered during creation of the scleral flap, antifibrotic agents should be administered with care as there is severe toxicity associated with intraocular administration of these agents.[180-183] In addition, if an unusually thin scleral flap is created, adjunctive antifibrosis may not be indicated because excessive leakage can occur. Once the surgery has been successfully completed, many surgeons administer additional injections of 5-FU subconjunctivally in the immediate postoperative period. The decision to administer these injections is based on the appearance of the bleb and the level of IOP reduction desired. The cumulative dose should be titrated to the level of corneal toxicity. Finally, there is no unified consensus as to the best location to give these subconjunctival injections. Many surgeons place them directly adjacent to the bleb in the hope of exerting a more local effect, while others believe that because the subconjunctival space is continuous, the injection can be given anywhere and still have an effect at the site of filtration. Those who give the injections inferiorly, away from the bleb, feel that there is less corneal toxicity from leakage and less chance of inadvertent injection into the bleb with subsequent intraocular spread. We routinely irrigate the eye with sterile eye wash after any injection to lessen the chance of topical toxicity. The procedure for injection is identical regardless of location and employs a 30-gauge needle on a tuberculin syringe placed at least 1 to 2 mm under the conjunctiva before injection to lessen the likelihood of leakage. Five mg can be administered per injection.

MMC

MMC is an antibiotic isolated from the bacteria *Streptomyces caespitosus*[176] and has been found to have antitumor activity. It is a cell cycle nonspecific alkylating agent, which interrupts DNA synthesis after short exposure to low concentrations of medication.[184-186] Many studies have shown a significant increase in the success rate of filtration surgery when intraoperative sponge application of MMC is used.[187-191] The efficacy of this medication appears to be greater than that of 5-FU[154,155] but there also is an increase in both the frequency and magnitude of complications. MMC is applied in the same manner as sponge 5-FU.

Various concentrations have been used, ranging from 0.2 to 0.5 mg/mL and have been applied from 30 seconds to 5 minutes.[189,191-202] We have had good results with 0.5 mg/mL applied for 3 minutes in most patients. These parameters, however, should be titrated based on the patient risk factors for surgical failure and on the status of the conjunctiva. No postoperative injections are required because a single topical application of MMC has been shown to have a continued anti-fibroblastic response.

Among the most common complications associated with the use of adjunctive antifibrosis are corneal toxicity from 5-FU,[170,172,203,204] and hypotony with both agents.[152,198,205-209] Both of these agents are designed to limit the fibroblastic response at the filtration site. Therefore, they also inhibit wound healing of the conjunctiva. Delayed wound closure can lead to prolonged hypotony and/or anterior chamber shallowing. In addition, hypotony maculopathy, defined as extremely low IOP, choroidal folds, decreased visual acuity, and disruption of the retinal pigment epithelium, can occur.[208,210-215] This condition also can occur without wound leakage when excessive filtration is present. Finally, there is an increase in the incidence of late bleb related infections when adjunctive 5-FU and MMC are used.[199,216-222] Such infections are believed to be related to the bleb characteristics which develop in these eyes.[193,223,224] The filtration blebs are usually thin, avascular, and cystic, and are prone to late leakage, which can predispose to infection.[47,218,225-227] The potential for early and late complications associated with the use of these medications should be weighed against the desired surgical outcome and the need for enhanced IOP reduction in certain patients.

COMPLICATIONS OF FILTERING SURGERY

Filtering surgery complications may occur during surgery or in the early or late postoperative period.

Intraoperative Complications

Both the local and systemic risks of anesthesia during glaucoma surgery have been discussed previously and will not be reiterated here.

Conjunctiva

The first tissue to be handled during glaucoma surgery is the conjunctiva. Careful handling of the conjunctiva is critical both for success of the procedure and for prevention of devastating complications. Conjunctival leakage in the early postoperative period may lead to hypotony, overfiltration, shallow anterior chamber, and failure to form a bleb. When the leak finally does seal, the conjunctiva may be scarred, with increased likelihood of filtration failure. For these reasons, intraoperative detection of conjunctival leakage is critical to maintaining bleb function and to enhancing bleb formation.

One of the easiest and often overlooked methods of eliminating conjunctival injury is to avoid the use of toothed forceps. During dissection, the conjunctiva should be manipulated with nontoothed forceps or surgical sponges to avoid accidental buttonhole injury. Scarred conjunctiva should be handled with particular care because adhesions may connect the conjunctiva to Tenon's capsule or episclera, increasing the possibility of inadvertent conjunctival perforation during blunt dissection. Lysis of adhesions should be done under direct observation of the external surface of the conjunctiva to avoid accidental incorporation of conjunctiva and subsequent buttonhole formation. At the conclusion of surgery, fluorescein dye should be applied to the conjunctival surface and the bleb expanded by anterior chamber irrigation to aid in the detection of previously unrecognized buttonhole defects or wound leaks.

A buttonhole detected intraoperatively should be closed in the operating room. The location of the conjunctival tear determines the method of repair. If a large buttonhole is noted during the early stages of a filtration operation, it is best to select a new surgical site. If it occurs at a later stage, tension at the wound edge must be relieved prior to closure to avoid excessive tension at the buttonhole. If the buttonhole is located in the center of the conjunctival flap or more posteriorly, a "purse string" ligature with 10-0 or 11-0 nylon can be attempted, either internally on the under surface of the conjunctiva or externally. A tapered atraumatic needle should be used to avoid creating a larger conjunctival defect, and Tenon's capsule should be incorporated into the repair if this tissue is present to provide added support. The most common location for a buttonhole is near the limbus, where it may either be oversewn with adjacent conjunctiva,

sutured directly to the cornea or sclera, closed as a "purse string," or sealed with the application of a tissue patch.[228] If the buttonhole is small at this location, creating a conjunctival peritomy and excising the buttonhole can repair it. The corneal epithelium in this area should be removed and the conjunctiva sutured to the cornea with mattress sutures to facilitate adhesion. We prefer 9-0 polyglactin or 10-0 monofilament nylon on a cardiovascular needle. Small buttonholes near the posterior edge of a limbus-based flap can also be removed in this manner as long as there is enough tissue to allow the wound to be closed without excessive tension. If a violation of the conjunctiva occurs prior to placement of adjunctive antifibrosis agents, consideration should be given to avoiding their use.

Scleral Flap

Most complications related to the scleral flap arise from inadequate thickness. Thin flaps may macerate, dehisce, or avulse during dissection, manipulation, or suture placement. If a hole is created in the scleral flap overlying the sclerostomy, excessive leakage can occur with resultant hypotony. Suturing with 10-0 nylon and attempting to incorporate a Tenon's plug if possible can repair this hole.[229] If necessary, a donor scleral or dura mater graft can be used to create a new scleral flap, which is sutured through the cornea to recreate a hinged flap. If a tear is created in the flap near its insertion, tight closure of the flap with nylon sutures prevents excessive flow. If the scleral flap is too thick, the anterior chamber can be entered prematurely at a posterior location. If this is the case, excessive outflow may occur due to an inability to adequately close the flap posteriorly. Injury to the ciliary body also can occur.

Anterior Chamber

Every attempt should be made to avoid excessive shallowing of the anterior chamber during surgery. Shallowing of the chamber can lead to endothelial damage from inadvertent lens-cornea touch. Preplaced scleral flap sutures may facilitate wound closure, and are particularly useful in aphakic, pseudophakic, vitrectomized, or highly myopic eyes. Some surgeons have advocated the use of intraoperative viscoelastic agents during routine filtering surgery. Potential advantages include maintenance of anterior chamber depth during surgery, tamponade of bleeding, and, in theory, decreased incidence of postoperative shallowing of the anterior chamber.[230-233] Several studies, however, have shown no benefit of these agents in maintaining anterior chamber depth and preventing hypotony in the early postoperative period.[234,235] In addition, they can cause significant elevation of IOP or can tamponade the surgical wound, thereby masking a previously undetected leak.[236]

Hyphema

Intraoperative anterior chamber hemorrhage most commonly occurs at the time of iridectomy from cut radial iris vessels or from a traumatized greater arterial circle within the ciliary body. Bleeding is best treated with observation, as most iris root/ciliary body bleeding spontaneously stops within minutes. The scleral flap should be held open while the pulsatile bleeding continues to allow the blood to exit the eye. This technique, and gentle irrigation, keeps the anterior chamber from filling with blood. It is important that the scleral flap not be sutured until all bleeding has stopped in order to prevent postoperative blockage of the internal ostium by the clotted blood. Persistent bleeding also may be treated with viscoelastic tamponade. Cautery is ill-advised, as it may lead to cataract formation in phakic patients, or vitreous loss from inadvertent involvement of the hyaloid face through the iridectomy. It is unnecessary to vigorously irrigate the anterior chamber to remove small amounts of blood as most hyphemas clear spontaneously without adverse sequelae.

Vitreous Loss

Vitreous loss is rare during glaucoma filtration surgery in phakic eyes but can complicate combined cataract extraction and trabeculectomy. In addition, vitreous may be present within the anterior chamber of aphakic and pseudophakic patients. Vitreous in the anterior chamber presents a problem because it can plug the sclerostomy and lead to surgical failure. Furthermore, vitreous can incarcerate within the scleral flap leading to delayed wound closure and, possibly, hypotony. A complete anterior vitrectomy should be performed in any eye where vitreous is present and threatens the success of filtration surgery.

Occasionally, viscoelastics also can be used intraoperatively to tamponade the movement of vitreous during the procedure, especially if the vitreous is present behind the iris plane. Viscoelastic can be used to move the vitreous posteriorly so that an iridectomy can be performed.

Choroidal Hemorrhage

Suprachoroidal hemorrhage can occur intraoperatively or postoperatively.[237-239] Patients often experience sudden, severe pain even with adequate local anesthesia at the time of surgery. During surgery, the anterior chamber shallows, the IOP rises and a dark posterior segment mass may become visible through the pupil. Intraoperative, expulsive choroidal hemorrhage is rare in phakic eyes undergoing trabeculectomy. Delayed choroidal hemorrhage occurs more commonly and is associated with postoperative hypotony.[240-243] Several risk factors have been associated with this condition and include advanced age, systemic vascular disease, aphakia, high myopia, previous vitrectomy, and elevated preoperative pressure.[241,244,245] The occasional bucking and straining associated with extubation after general anesthesia and postoperative coughing or vomiting also are risk factors.[246,247] Delayed choroidal hemorrhage often occurs in the situation of prolonged hypotony and choroidal effusion. Patients often describe a history of performing physical activities that are too strenuous for their recommended postoperative activity restrictions.

Choroidal hemorrhage usually occurs intraoperatively at a time of relative hypotony. When this condition is identified, the eye should be closed immediately.[248] The anterior chamber should be reformed with balanced salt solution, viscoelastic, or air. Often, posterior sclerotomies are performed to drain the choroidal hemorrhage when there is an inability to limit the spread of the bleeding within the posterior segment. Once the eye has been closed, intravenous acetazolamide and mannitol may be used to lower the IOP and stabilize the eye. The prognosis for recovery of vision remains fair as long as the eye can be closed without loss of uvea or retina. Later, drainage of the hemorrhage may be necessary. The most important factor related to a positive outcome is early recognition and immediate wound closure.

Delayed, postoperative choroidal hemorrhage is more common than intraoperative choroidal hemorrhage following glaucoma surgery. Acute onset of severe pain and decreased vision are the usual presenting symptoms. Patients should not be routinely placed on postoperative narcotics, because severe pain often means either a postoperative choroidal hemorrhage or markedly elevated IOP with corneal edema, both of which warrant immediate examination. Limited choroidal hemorrhages without retinal detachment or vitreous hemorrhage typically resolve, and are best treated with observation.[247,249] In cases where there is severe, intractable pain, retinal detachment, hypotony, or vitreous hemorrhage, surgical drainage often is performed.[250,251] Concurrent retinal therapy is performed at the same time, if necessary. It is helpful to delay the drainage for at least 7 to 14 days, if possible, because liquefaction of the clot during this period facilitates its removal.[239,252]

Avoiding prolonged hypotony is the best way to prevent this devastating complication both in the operating room and during the postoperative period.[241,243,247] We routinely prescribe stool softeners to all patients undergoing filtration surgery and educate patients regarding the avoidance of strenuous activities that involve bending or lifting.[243] Postoperative nausea and vomiting should be addressed.

Early Postoperative Complications

Early postoperative complications not already discussed are related specifically to the function of the trabeculectomy or operative technique. Many of these complications are related to pressure control within the eye and will be divided into those conditions associated with elevated IOP and those associated with decreased IOP.

Elevated IOP

Early, undetected rises in pressure after trabeculectomy occur with surprising frequency.[236] In susceptible eyes with advanced visual field loss, further visual field loss or loss of central fixation may occur, and could account for the so-called "snuff" phenomenon described following filtration surgery. There are many potential causes of elevated pressure. In the presence of a deep anterior chamber, the most common cause of elevated pressure is tight scleral flap sutures with inadequate filtration.[253] Also, blockage of the internal ostium by iris tissue, incompletely excised

Descemet's membrane, blood clot, fibrin, vitreous, lens capsule, or ciliary processes may also account for this situation. Retained viscoelastic material also can cause significant elevation of the IOP.

Management of elevated IOP depends on the specific etiology. Scleral flap suture release is possible with the aid of the argon laser or releasable suture techniques. The advantage of laser suture lysis is that the suture ends remain buried beneath the conjunctiva, whereas releasable sutures remain exteriorized and may protrude for an extended period of time if they do not need to be released. The disadvantage, however, is that extensive subconjunctival hemorrhage or thickened Tenon's capsule may prevent laser suture lysis in some eyes. Suture lysis should be completed within 7 to 10 days for trabeculectomy without anti-scarring medications, within 14 days for 5-FU trabeculectomy, and within 1 month for MMC trabeculectomy. We routinely make a postoperative notation as to flap suture tension and lyse the tightest suture first. In this manner, a desired reduction in IOP can be achieved while the remaining scleral flap sutures remain, providing support that decreases the likelihood of prolonged hypotony. If the IOP is elevated in the immediate postoperative period (ie, less than 5 days) we recommend conservative management with topical and systemic antiglaucoma medications, gentle bleb massage if appropriate, or paracentesis. Suture lysis should be avoided in the first 72 hours to reduce the risk of hypotony. In addition, only one suture should be cut at a time.

Laser suture lysis should be performed with as little conjunctival manipulation and laser energy as possible. Care must be taken to avoid a potential conjunctival burn or buttonhole injury. This may be accomplished by defocusing the beam posteriorly. In the presence of a subconjunctival hemorrhage, a diode or krypton laser should be used rather than the argon laser, because argon energy is absorbed by the blood and can result in a conjunctival burn or buttonhole. Settings of 0.05 seconds, 50 µm spot size, and 200 to 400 mW power usually are sufficient. Cautious digital massage or pressure to the edge of the scleral flap following suture lysis often helps to elevate the bleb if it does not do so spontaneously. If the bleb remains flat even with massage, it is a sign of impending bleb failure.

Gonioscopy is required to identify a blockage of the internal ostium and should be performed without injury to the conjunctiva. The etiology of the blockage dictates the course of therapy, which ranges from observation of retained viscoelastic to incisional surgery for removal of lens fragments. The Nd:YAG laser has been effective in cases in which surgery may have been indicated.[254-257]

The presence of a shallow anterior chamber associated with elevated IOP usually indicates the development of malignant glaucoma. The differential diagnosis includes pupillary block, choroidal hemorrhage, annular choroidal detachment with anterior rotation of the ciliary body causing angle closure, and malignant glaucoma. Posterior pooling of aqueous either within or behind the vitreous causes forward movement of the lens-iris or hyaloid-iris diaphragm, resulting in a flat anterior chamber with an elevated pressure. Medical treatment of aqueous misdirection is successful in about 50% of cases and consists of intense cycloplegia, aqueous suppression, and systemic administration of a hyperosmotic and a carbonic anhydrase inhibitor, if necessary.[258] Therapy also may include argon laser treatment of visible ciliary processes, and Nd:YAG anterior hyaloidectomy or posterior capsulotomy in aphakic and pseudophakic eyes.[259,260] Surgical therapy is necessary if these medical and laser techniques are ineffective, and usually consists of pars plana vitrectomy and lensectomy with rupture of the vitreous face in phakic eyes, and a limbal vitrectomy in aphakic eyes.[258,261-263]

Decreased IOP

Low IOP in the early postoperative period may be associated with a shallow anterior chamber. In this scenario, the etiology may be overfiltration, ciliochoroidal detachment with reduced aqueous production, a cyclodialysis cleft, or a wound leak.[35,264-267]

Overfiltration usually is caused by loose scleral flap sutures and is less common today with the trend towards tighter scleral flap sutures and early laser suture lysis. If an exuberant bleb has formed after guarded filtration surgery, the best management usually is external compression with a contact lens that compresses the bleb and/or scleral support from a Simmons shell or symblepharon ring. The utilization of these devices must be weighed against the potential for bleb failure. Consideration can be given to decreasing the level of postoperative anti-inflammatory medication in an attempt to promote wound healing, which may increase the resistance to flow, but this too has

potential for increasing the likelihood of long-term failure of the procedure. The use of external compression sutures also can be employed. This technique utilizes a nylon suture placed over a portion of the bleb in an attempt to cause localized scarring and an overall decrease in the effective size of the filtering bleb.

A wound leak is one of the most common causes of hypotony in the early postoperative period. Leakage may be from a conjunctival flap perforation not recognized at the time of surgery, an area of inadvertent, postcautery conjunctival necrosis, a wound dehiscence, or from a traumatized, thin filtration bleb.[268-270] Although the site of leakage often can be determined with a Seidel test,[271,272] gentle external pressure on the globe may be required to increase flow sufficiently to demonstrate a hole during times of decreased aqueous production. Early wound dehiscence when limbus-based conjunctival flaps are used, and retraction of the flap in fornix-based cases are the most serious wound-related complications, and generally require immediate surgical repair, particularly if the edge of the scleral flap becomes exposed. The administration of aqueous suppressants can enhance the closure of some leaks by decreasing flow across the leak.[273] Nevertheless, a further reduction in IOP can occur, which might cause an increased shallowing of the anterior chamber. Definitive therapy for all wound leaks is surgical closure. This procedure is often done in a minor surgical suite or even at the slit-lamp. A tapered, non-cutting cardiovascular needle should be used at all times, if possible, to avoid additional leakage at the suture tracks.[274] With thin, cystic blebs, a large diameter soft contact lens, symblepharon ring, or a Simmons shell often is successful in mechanically sealing the wound leak and reforming the anterior chamber.[275,276] Tissue adhesive also has been used. [277]

Choroidal effusions can occur in any situation in which there is decreased IOP.[278] This process further enhances hypotony by decreasing aqueous production due to abnormal positioning of the ciliary body. Hypotony leads to transudation of fluid into the potential space between the sclera and uveal tissues.[264,279] Development of an effusion in the absence of hypotony typically occurs in conjunction with inflammation because of protein accumulation in the ciliochoroidal space. When hypotony is present, it often is difficult to ascertain whether the hypotony caused the ciliochoroidal detachment, or vice versa. In cases in which choroidal effusions are isolated and not found in association with wound leaks or overfiltration, the detachment usually is transient and lasts for 10 to 14 days. In these cases, the only treatment required is frequent topical and possibly systemic steroid administration. Most cases of effusion resolve spontaneously and surgical drainage usually is indicated only for chronic effusions and for cases of prolonged "kissing choroidals" in which retinal apposition may lead to retinal tears upon separation. In the presence of flat anterior chamber with lens-cornea touch, reformation of the chamber with viscoelastic[280] or air often causes some resolution of the effusion.

Late Complications

Leaks

Although leaks that develop months to years after filtration surgery may be accompanied by an increased risk of endophthalmitis and hypotony maculopathy, they also may continue for prolonged periods without any adverse sequelae.[220,281,282] The decision to treat late leaks depends on the clinical situation. If there is compromise of the anterior chamber or complications of prolonged hypotony, then treatment should be initiated. Treatment options include patching, bandage contact lenses, focal cautery, laser photocoagulation, cryotherapy, tamponade shells, aqueous suppressants, tissue patches, cyanoacrylate, intrableb injection of autologous blood, and surgical revision.[283-294]

Hypotony

Chronic hypotony occurs more frequently when full-thickness procedures or trabeculectomy with 5-FU or MMC are used than in guarded procedures without antifibrosis agents. Although pressures of 4 to 10 mm Hg have not been shown to increase the incidence of visual compromise,[92] pressures of less than 4 mmHg more commonly have been associated with the development of vision threatening maculopathy.[212,295] The fundus changes associated with this condition include disc edema, choroidal and retinal folds, and retinal vascular engorgement. Often times, there is a failure to return to baseline visual acuity even with complete resolution of the maculopathy. Treatment for this condition revolves around treatment of the etiology of the hypotony.[296-298]

Cataract

Cataract progression has been reported after some filtration surgeries.[35,42,299-301] The incidence of progression has been reported to be from 2% to 53%. Such progression has been associated with multiple factors including increased postoperative steroid usage, hypotony, and flat anterior chamber.[32] There is no clear data linking the actual procedure itself to cataract progression, and there are a variety of associated factors that have not been thoroughly analyzed (ie, miotic usage and degree of pre-existing cataract).

Filtration Failure

Elevated IOP after filtration surgery with poor bleb function is the most common complication of filtering surgery. Risk factors associated with increased surgical failure include prolonged preoperative topical antiglaucoma medication usage,[18-21] neovascular glaucoma,[31,302] black race,[26,39,50,303] young age,[44,46,47] aphakia,[304-306] prior failed filtering surgery,[307,308] prior cataract surgery,[43] and uveitis.[29,30] The etiology of the failure may be due to multiple factors ranging from blockage of the internal or external ostium to bleb encapsulation. Early in the postoperative period, signs of potential problems preventing adequate filtration may develop. Early recognition of the signs, symptoms, and patterns of filtration failure allows for timely intervention to encourage filtration. Such recognition is particularly important during the first 2 weeks following surgery when the healing process is most active.

The appearance of the bleb is the most important factor in determining possible bleb failure.[309] Injection and vascularization of the bleb indicate the presence of inflammation, usually occur before an elevation of the IOP, and are poor prognostic signs.[310] In addition, decreased height of the bleb indicating poor flow and progressive loculation may indicate the development of bleb encapsulation. Although gonioscopy frequently can help to identify a blockage of the internal ostium, blockage of the external ostium often is a diagnosis of exclusion when no other signs of failure are present. If digital compression of the globe fails to elevate the bleb and the internal ostium is free of obstruction, the obstruction typically is at the level of the external ostium. Transient bleb formation, and a lowering of the IOP with compression suggest the presence of tight scleral flap sutures or loculation.[311]

Once the cause of the failure has been isolated, appropriate treatment may prolong the life of a failing filter. Because repeat filtration surgery often is unrewarding, it is best to maximize the effect of the initial surgery with all appropriate interventions.

Management of the failing filter requires therapy directed toward the level of blockage to aqueous flow and toward blocking the wound healing response to both the initial surgery and the planned intervention. For example, increased scarring of the bleb can be treated with intense anti-inflammatory medication and possibly with adjunctive 5-FU injections. Elevation of the conjunctiva with viscoelastic or balanced salt solution to reduce apposition of this tissue to the sclera also may decrease blockage at the level of the external ostium. Internal blockage of the ostium may be treated by laser revision or automated trephination, which effectively converts the procedure to a full-thickness trabeculectomy.[312,313] Bleb encapsulation, or Tenon's cyst formation, develops in approximately 10% to 28% of eyes undergoing trabeculectomy.[314-319] The encapsulation process consists of fibroblastic overgrowth that results in a tense, opalescent bleb with a thick wall in direct communication with the anterior chamber. There usually is loculation, thickening of the subconjunctival connective tissue, and elevated IOP. There is a spectrum of appearance ranging from incomplete loculation with mild hyperemia to complete encapsulation. The dome-like cyst is firm and often has mobile conjunctiva overlying it. The key to successful management is patience. In most cases, the pressure decreases within 2 to 4 months with the use of aqueous suppressants.[320] Extended use of aqueous suppressant following filtering surgery, however, may limit the extent of bleb formation by decreasing flow through the fistula. After resolution, the antiglaucoma therapy may be tapered.

Many encapsulated blebs, particularly those that are only partially loculated, may resolve spontaneously, or respond to intensive topical steroid therapy or digital compression. If resolution of the encapsulated bleb does not occur, and a cyst is present, the cyst can be punctured with a needle.[316,321-323] Bleb needling allows the surgeon to create an opening in the wall of an encapsulated bleb or to raise a flattened bleb at the slit-lamp via subconjunctival manipulation with a small gauge needle. The technique involves elevation of the conjunctiva off the surface of the globe with balanced salt solution or anesthetic utilizing a 30-gauge needle. The underlying episcleral/Tenon's capsule scarring then is incised with the needle. If this technique does not succeed in restoring filtration, the edge of the scleral flap may be elevated. Entry into the anterior chamber also can be performed in pseudophakic or aphakic patients but this action carries with it the increased risks of hyphema and infection. This procedure can be combined with a pre-needling injection of MMC or with a full post-needling course of 5-FU injections.[321,323-326] Many times, needle revision allows the patient to be spared another trip to the operating room.[309,327,328]

Bleb-Related Infection

Early postoperative endophthalmitis is caused by penetration of organisms at the time of surgery and is not related to the presence of a filtering bleb. Nevertheless, bleb related ocular infection can occur months to years after filtration surgery and has been reported to range between 0.2% and 9.6%.[216,220,282] The incidence of infection is greatest with full thickness procedures.[329] With the increased use of antifibrosis agents, producing blebs similar to those found after full-thickness procedures, however, the late bleb-related endophthalmitis rate once again is increasing. The route of infection is thought to involve migration of bacteria through the thin and cystic bleb walls of filters utilizing 5-FU and MMC. The potential for infection is greater in eyes with positive Seidel's test and in eyes that have had filtration surgery from below. Additional associations include diabetes mellitus, malnutrition, blepharitis, and a compromised immune system.

The clinical presentation of endophthalmitis usually is one of sudden onset of pain and redness, which often is localized to the filtration area, associated with photophobia and decreased visual acuity. Examination reveals bleb purulence and intraocular inflammation that may involve the posterior segment. When ocular involvement is limited to the anterior segment, treatment with topical, periocular, and systemic antibiotics is possible. If the vitreous is involved, more aggressive therapy is necessary and usually requires vitreous tap or pars plana vitrectomy with intravitreal antibiotics and steroids.

Surface cultures often do not yield the offending agent, and may yield results different from intraocular cultures.[226] Although a wide range of gram positive and gram negative organisms have been reported, staphylococcal and streptococcal species are the most common.

Patients should be instructed to report immediately any redness, pain, discharge, or decreased vision and should be treated intensively to avoid loss of vision, because good visual outcome depends upon early treatment. Although chronic antibiotic therapy has never been shown to effectively prevent the onset bleb-related endophthalmitis, consideration of such therapy in eyes at high risk for infection seems reasonable.[47] This includes eyes with thin, avascular, leaking blebs, or blebs located in the inferior quadrants.[216,226] Antibiotics should be alternated periodically to minimize the development of drug-resistant organisms.

Complications of Aqueous Shunts

Aqueous shunts are associated with the same operative and postoperative complications as trabeculectomy including hyphema, pupillary block, aqueous misdirection, choroidal hemorrhage, and infection.[330-337] Hypotony is usually related to leakage around the tube entry site or failure of a restrictive valve to regulate the IOP.[123,331,338] When leakage around the tube is present, it usually resolves spontaneously after 10 to 14 days. Choroidal hemorrhage occurs in up to 8% of eyes that receive glaucoma implants.[339,340]

Some complications, however, are unique to tube shunt implantation. Epithelial ingrowth can occur if the anterior chamber entry site is in the cornea rather than posteriorly.[341,342] This is an extremely difficult problem to battle, and should be avoided at all costs. In addition, improper tube placement can cause injury to the cornea, iris, and lens in phakic patients. Elevated IOP may occur from obstruction of the tube opening from blood, vitreous, fibrin, and even iris tissue. Various laser techniques have been employed to clear visible blockages[343-345] and flushing the tube with a cannula may be necessary when no obvious obstruction is visible.[346] Elevated IOP also can be related to encapsulation around the plate. The process is similar to that found with Tenon's cyst formation after trabeculectomy[347] and often responds to needling procedures.[348] Finally, migration of the tube against the cornea leading to corneal edema and bullous keratopathy from endothelial cell dysfunction can occur.

In rare cases, the tube can migrate completely out of the eye. Both of these situations require prompt repositioning of the tube, if possible, or removal of the implant.

The last unique complication of tube shunt implantation is transient or permanent diplopia.[349-357] Many patients have transient diplopia in the immediate postoperative period related to periocular edema and swelling. This is similar to the diplopia seen after scleral buckling. Permanent, restrictive diplopia is a much more significant problem and may occur from a large bleb causing compression against the orbital contents with decreased motility[353,358] or scarring between the plate and either the recti or oblique muscles. Strabismus appears to be more common with the Baerveldt implant[350] and is related to the placement of a large portion of the plate under a vertical and horizontal rectus muscle. If diplopia is intractable and not responsive to conservative therapy with prisms, the risks and benefits of removal of the device should be discussed with the patient.

POSTOPERATIVE MANAGEMENT OF FILTRATION SURGERY

Many of the postoperative recommendations and therapy strategies have already been discussed within this chapter. A few general principles, however, will be reviewed. First, it is important to remember that patients who undergo trabeculectomy require frequent follow-up visits during the early postoperative period. Patients should be informed of this prior to their surgery so that appropriate preparation can be made. If there are significant complications, daily visits may be required for some time. In addition patients should have severe restrictions placed upon their activity level. Valsalva maneuvers should be avoided. Anterior chamber shallowing also may occur with the presence of effusions in this circumstance. We routinely provide patients with stool softeners to be used during the early postoperative period as well.

All patients who undergo intraocular surgery are placed on a regimen of topical antibiotics and anti-inflammatory medication. The same holds true for filtration surgery. The regimen of postoperative anti-inflammatory medication usually is more vigorous than with other surgeries because an effort also is being made to prevent healing at the filtration site in addition to decreasing intraocular inflammation. Most patients require prednisolone acetate 1% every 1 to 2 hours while awake for the first 3 or 4 weeks.[359] This medication is tapered based on the patients' response and the use of additional therapy to control wound healing such as adjunctive antifibrosis injections. Antibiotics often are discontinued after the first 7 to 10 days unless there is a suspicion of any infectious process including active blepharitis. Cycloplegic agents usually are given to all phakic patients for control of pain and to lessen the likelihood and severity of any anterior chamber shallowing associated with hypotony, choroidal effusions, or aqueous misdirection. This medication also is tapered as the healing process continues.

Laser suture lysis, digital bleb compression, and needle revision all have been discussed previously as methods of lowering the IOP and preserving bleb function. The appropriate timing and sequence of these events is based on a thorough knowledge of filtration surgery, the patient's diagnosis, and extensive surgical experience.

The glaucoma surgery is only the beginning of the process. Intensive therapy and intervention are required to preserve bleb function, and it often takes many months before stabilization is achieved. The role of the glaucoma surgeon is to perform the appropriate surgery and to provide comprehensive postoperative care to ensure the success of that procedure. He or she must possess knowledge of advanced techniques, and must be able to identify and to treat all of the possible intra- and postoperative complications. It is this knowledge that provides patients with the best chance for preservation of their visual function.

Note: Supported by a grant from the New York Glaucoma Research Institute, New York, NY.

REFERENCES

1. David R, Livingston DG, Luntz MH. Ocular hypertension - a long-term follow-up of treated and untreated patients. *Br J Ophthalmol.* 1977;61:668.
2. Walker WM. Ocular hypertension: Follow-up of 109 cases from 1963 to 1974. *Trans Ophthalmol Soc UK.* 1974;94:525.
3. Gaasterland D, al e. Studies of aqueous humor dynamics in man. VI. Effect of age upon parameters of intraocular pressure in normal human eyes. *Exp Eye Res.* 1978;26:651.
4. Chauhan BC, Drance SM, Douglas GR, et al. Visual field damage in normal-tension and high-tension glaucoma. *Am J Ophthalmol.* 1989;108(6):636-42.
5. Kass MA, Hart WMJ, Gordon M, et al. Risk factors favoring the development of glaucomatous visual filed loss in ocular hypertension. *Surv Ophthalmol.* 1980;25:155-162.
6. Armaly MF. The visual field defect and ocular pressure level in open-angle glaucoma. *Invest Ophthalmol.* 1969;8:105.
7. Armaly MF. Ocular pressure and visual fields. A ten-year follow-up study. *Arch Ophthalmol.* 1969;81:25.
8. Mao LK, Stewart WC, Shields MB. Correlation between intraocular pressure control and progressive glaucomatous damage in primary open-angle glaucoma. *Am J Ophthalmol.* 1991;111:51-55.
9. Quigley HA, Maumenee AE. Long-term follow-up of treated open-angle glaucoma. *Am J Ophthalmol.* 1979;87:519.
10. Stewart WC, Chorak RP, Hunt HH, et al. Factors associated with visual loss in patients with advanced glaucomatous changes in the optic nerve head. *Am J Ophthalmol.* 1993;116:176.
11. MacKenzie W. *A Practical Treatise on Diseases of the Eye.* London, England: Longman, Rees, Orm, Brown & Green; 1830.
12. Kronfeld P. The rise of the filter operations. *Surv Ophthalmol.* 1972;17:168.
13. Spaeth GL. Guarded filtration procedure-not trabeculectomy. *Ophthalmic Surg.* 1992;23:583.
14. Sugar HS. Filtering operations: an historical review. *Glaucoma.* 1981;3:85.
15. Gutierrez P, Wilson MR, Johnson C, et al. Influence of glaucomatous visual field loss on health-related quality of life. *Arch Ophthalmol.* 1997;115(6):777-84.
16. Shin DH. Trabeculectomy. *Int Ophthalmol Clin.* 1981;21:47.
17. Smith RJ. Medical versus surgical therapy in glaucoma simplex. *Br J Ophthalmol.* 1972;56(3):277-83.
18. Broadway D, Grierson I, Hitchings R. Adverse effects of topical antiglaucomatous medications on the conjunctiva. *Br J Ophthalmol.* 1993;77:590-596.
19. Broadway DC, Grierson I, O'Brien C, et al. Adverse effects of topical antiglaucoma medication. II. The outcome of filtration surgery. *Arch Ophthalmol.* 1994;112:1446-1454.
20. Lavin MJ, Wormald RPL, Migdal CS, et al. The influence of prior therapy on the success of trabeculectomy. *Arch Ophthalmol.* 1990;108:1543-1548.
21. Sherwood MB, Grierson I, Millar L, et al. Long-term morphologic effects of antiglaucoma drugs on the conjunctiva and Tenon's capsule in glaucomatous patients. *Ophthalmology.* 1989;96:327-335.
22. Jay JL. Earlier trabeculectomy. *Trans Ophthalmol Soc UK.* 1983;103:35.
23. Migdal C, Hitchings R. The role of early surgery for open angle glaucoma. *Ophthalmol Clin N Amer.* 1991;4:853-861.
24. Sherwood MB, Migdal CS, Hitchings RA. Filtration surgery as the initial therapy for open-angle glaucoma. *J Glaucoma.* 1993;2:64-67.
25. Sherwood MB, Migdal CS, Hitchings RA, et al. Intial treatment of glaucoma: surgery or medications. *Surv Ophthalmol.* 1993;37:293-305.
26. Miller RD, Barber JC. Trabeculectomy in black patients. *Ophthalmic Surg.* 1981;12:46-50.

27. McMillan TA, et al. Histologic differences in the conjunctiva of black and white glaucoma patients. *Ophthalmic Surg.* 1992;23:762-765.

28. Freedman J, Shen E, Ahrens M. Trabeculectomy in a black American glaucoma population. *Br J Ophthalmol.* 1976;60: 573-574.

29. Hoskins HD, Jr. , Hetherington J, Jr. , Shaffer RN. Surgical management of the inflammatory glaucomas. *Perspect Ophthalmol.* 1977;1:173-181.

30. Jampel HD, Jabs DA, Quigley HA. Trabeculectomy with 5-fluorouracil for adult inflammatory glaucoma. *Am J Ophthalmol.* 1990;109:168-173.

31. Allen RC, Bellows AR, Hutchinson BT, et al. Filtration surgery in the treatment of neovascular glaucoma. *Ophthalmology.* 1982;89:1181-1187.

32. D'Ermo F, Bonomi L, Doro D. A critical analysis of the long-term results of trabeculectomy. *Am J Ophthalmol.* 1979;88: 829-835.

33. Eltz H, Gloor B. Trabeculectomy in cases of angle-closure glaucoma-successes and failures. *Klin Monatsbl Augenheilkd.* 1980;177:556.

34. Jerndal T, Kriisa V. Results of trabeculectomy for pseudoexfoliation glaucoma. *Br J Ophthalmol.* 1974;58:927.

35. Mills K. Trabeculectomy: a retrospective long-term follow-up of 444 cases. *Br J Ophthalmol.* 1981;65:790-5.

36. Tornqvist G, Drolsum LK. Trabeculectomies. A long-term study. *Acta Ophthalmol.* 1991;69(4):450-4.

37. Vesti E. Filtering blebs: follow up of trabeculectomy. *Ophthalmic Surg.* 1993;24:249-255.

38. Watson PG, Barnett F. Effectiveness of trabeculectomy in glaucoma. *Am J Ophthalmol.* 1975;79:831-845.

39. Watson P, Grierson I. The place of trabeculectomy in the treatment of glaucoma. *Ophthalmology.* 1981;88:175-96.

40. Gilvarry AM, et al. The management of post-keratoplasty glaucoma by trabeculectomy. *Eye.* 1983;3:713.

41. Shirato S, Kitazawa Y, Mishima S. A critical analysis of the trabeculectomy results by a prospective follow-up design. *Jpn J Ophthalmol.* 1981;26:468.

42. Jerndal T, Lundstrom M. 330 Trabeculectomies-a long time study (3-5 1/2 years). *Acta Ophthalmol.* 1980;58:947.

43. Gross RL, Feldman RM, Spaeth GL, et al. Surgical therapy of chronic glaucoma in aphakia and pseudophakia. *Ophthalmology.* 1988;95:1195-1201.

44. Gressel MG, Heuer DK, Parrish RK, II. Trabeculectomy in young patients. *Ophthalmology.* 1984;91:1242-1246.

45. Levene RZ. Glaucoma filtering surgery: factors that determine pressure control. *Trans Am Ophthalmol Soc.* 1984;82:282.

46. Cadera W, Pachtman MA, Cantor LB, et al. Filtering surgery in childhood glaucoma. *Ophthalmic Surg.* 1984;15:319-322.

47. Lamping KA, Bellows AR, Hutchinson BT, et al. Long-term evaluation of initial filtration surgery. *Ophthalmology.* 1986;93:91-101.

48. Ridgeway AEA. Trabeculectomy: A follow-up study. *Br J Ophthalmol.* 1974;58:680-6.

49. Ridgeway AEA, Rubinstein K, Smith VH. Trabeculectomy: a study of 86 cases. *Br J Ophthalmol.* 1972;56:511-516.

50. Schwartz PL, Ackerman J, Beards J, et al. Further experience with trabeculectomy. *Ann Ophthalmol.* 1976;8:207-17.

51. Ellis EP, Esterdahl M. Echothiophate iodide therapy in children: Effect upon blood cholinesterase levels. *Arch Ophthalmol.* 1967;77:598.

52. Barash PG, Cullen BF, Stoelting RK. *Handbook of Clinical Anesthesia.* Philadelphia, Pa: Lippincott; 1991.

53. Krohne SG. Effect of topically applied 2% pilocarpine and 0. 25% demecarium bromide on blood-aqueous barrier permeability in dogs. *Am J Vet Res.* 1994;55(12):1729-33.

54. Roberts CW. Intraocular miotics and postoperative inflammation. *J Cataract Refract Surg.* 1993;19:731-4.

55. Mori M, Araie M. Effect of apraclonidine on blood-aqueous barrier permeability to plasma protein in man. *Exp Eye Res.* 1992;54:555-560.

56. Bellan L. Preoperative testing for cataract surgery. *Can J Ophthalmol.* 1994;29(3):111-4.

57. Steinberg EP, Bass EB, Luthra R, et al. Variation in ophthalmic testing before cataract surgery. Results of a national survey of ophthalmologists [see comments]. *Arch Ophthalmol.* 1994;112(7):896-902.

58. Bruce AB, McGoldrick KE, Oppenheimer P. *Anesthesia for Ophthalmology.* Birmingham, Ala: Aesculapius; 1982.

59. Dereklis DL, Bufidis TA, Tsiakiri EP, et al. Preoperative ocular disinfection by the use of povidone-iodine 5%. *Acta Ophthalmol.* 1994;72(5):627-30.

60. Speaker MG, et al. Role of external bacterial flora in the pathogenesis of acute postoperative endophthalmitis. *Ophthalmology.* 1991;98:639.

61. Denha RF, Wraight WJ. Local or general anaesthesia for cataract surgery [letter; comment]. *Anaesthesia.* 1996; 51(12):1191-2.

62. Barker JP, Vafidis GC, Hall GM. Postoperative morbidity following cataract surgery. A comparison of local and general anaesthesia [see comments]. *Anaesthesia.* 1996;51(5):435-7.

63. Campbell DN, Lim M, Muir MK, et al. A prospective randomised study of local versus general anaesthesia for cataract surgery. *Anaesthesia.* 1993;48(5):422-8.

64. Vernon SA, Cheng H. Comparison between the complications of cataract surgery following local anaesthesia with short stay and general anaesthesia with a five- day hospitalisation. *Br J Ophthalmol.* 1985;69(5):360-3.

65. Magora F, Collins VJ. The influence of general anesthetic agents on intraocular pressure in man. *Arch Ophthalmol.* 1962;66:806.

66. Libonati MM, Complications of general anesthesia. In: Spaeth GL, Katz LJ, eds. *Current Therapy in Ophthalmic Surgery.* Philadelphia, Pa: BC Decker: 1989.

67. Cunningham AJ, Barry P. Intraocular pressure physiology and implications for anesthesia management. *Can Anaesth Soc J.* 1986;33:195.

68. Pinhas D, Liebmann J, Ritch R. Anesthesia for glaucoma surgery. In: Greenbaum S, ed. *Ocular Anesthesia.* Philadelphia, Pa: WB Saunders Co; 1997:109-124.

69. Ritch R, Liebmann JM. Sub-tenon's anesthesia for trabeculectomy. *Ophthalmic Surg.* 1992;23:502-504.

70. O'Donoghue E, Batterbury M, Lavy T. Effect on intraocular pressure of local anaesthesia in eyes undergoing intraocular surgery. *Br J Ophthalmol.* 1994;78(8):605-607.

71. Morgan CM, Schatz H, Vine AK, et al. Ocular complications associated with retrobulbar injections. *Ophthalmology.* 1988;95:660-665.

72. Buys YM, Trope GE. Prospective study of sub-tenon's versus retrobulbar anesthesia for inpatient and day-surgery trabeculectomy. *Ophthalmology.* 1993;100:1585.

73. Furuta M, Toriumi T, Kashiwagi K, et al. Limbal anesthesia for cataract surgery. *Ophthalmic Surg.* 1990;21:22-25.

74. Petersen WC, Yanoff M. Subconjunctival anesthesia: an alternative to retrobulbar and peribulbar techniques. *Ophthalmic Surg.* 1991;22:199-201.

75. Greenbaum S. Parabulbar anesthesia. *Am J Ophthalmol.* 1992;114(6):776.

76. Sanford DK, Minoso y de Cal OE, Belyea DA. Response of intraocular pressure to retrobulbar and peribulbar anesthesia. *Ophthalmic Surg Lasers.* 1998;29(10):815-817.

77. Singh SK, Sekhar GC, Gupta S. Etiology of ptosis after cataract surgery. *J Cataract Refract Surg.* 1997;23(9):1409-1413.

78. Loeffler M, Solomon LD, Renaud M. Postcataract extraction ptosis: effect of the bridle suture [see comments]. *J Cataract Refract Surg.* 1990;16(4):501-504.

79. Catalano RA, Nelson LB, Calhoun JH, et al. Persistent strabismus presenting after cataract surgery. *Ophthalmology.* 1987;94(5):491-594.

80. Brincker P, Kessing SV. Limbus-based versus fornix-based conjunctival flap in glaucoma filtering surgery. *Acta Ophthalmol.* 1992;70:641-644.

81. Luntz MH, Freedman J. The fornix-based conjunctival flap in glaucoma filtration surgery. *Ophthalmic Surg.* 1980;11: 516.

82. Reichert R, Stewart W, Shields MB. Limbus-based versus fornix-based conjunctival flaps in trabeculectomy. *Ophthalmic Surg.* 1987;18:672-676.

83. Shuster JN, Krupin T, Kolker AE, et al. Limbus v. fornix-based conjunctival flap in trabeculectomy. A long-term randomized study. *Arch Ophthalmol.* 1984;102:361-2.

84. Traverso CE, Tomey KF, Antonios S. Limbal- vs fornix-based conjunctival trabeculectomy flaps. *Am J Ophthalmol.* 1987;104:28.

85. Blondeau P, Phelps CD. Trabeculectomy vs thermosclerostomy. A randomized prospective clinical trial. *Arch Ophthalmol.* 1981;99:810-816.

86. Shields MB. Trabeculectomy vs. full-thickness filtering operation for control of glaucoma. *Ophthalmic Surg.* 1980;11:498-505.

87. Iliff CE, Haas JS. Posterior lip sclerectomy. *Am J Ophthalmol.* 1962;54:688.

88. Marion JR, Shields MB. Thermal sclerostomy and posterior lip sclerectomy: a comparative study. *Ophthalmic Surg.* 1978;9:67-75.

89. Scheie HG. Retraction of scleral wound edges: A fistulizing procedure for glaucoma. *Am J Ophthalmol.* 1958;45:220-229.

90. Bounds GW, Jr. , Minton LR. Peripheral iridectomy with scleral cautery. *Am J Ophthalmol.* 1964;58:84.

91. Drance SM, Vargas E. Trabeculectomy and thermosclerostomy: a comparison of two procedures. *Can J Ophthalmol.* 1973;8:413-415.

92. Hovanesian JAD, Higginbotham EJ, Lichter PR, et al. Long-term visual outcome of ocular hypotension after thermosclerostomy. *Am J Ophthalmol.* 1993;115:603-607.

93. Lewis RA, Phelps CD. Trabeculectomy vs thermosclerostomy-a five year follow-up. *Arch Ophthalmol.* 1984;102:533-536.

94. Abraham RK, Miller GL. Outpatient argon laser iridectomy for angle-closure glaucoma: a two-year study. *Trans Am Acad Ophthalmol Otol.* 1975;79:OP529.

95. Gieser D, Wilensky J. Laser iridectomy in the management of chronic angle-closure glaucoma. *Am J Ophthalmol.* 1984;98:446.

96. Ritch R, Podos SM. Argon laser treatment of angle-closure glaucoma. *Perspect Ophthalmol.* 1980;4:129.

97. Margo CE, Groden L. Balloon cell nevus of the iris. *Am J Ophthalmol.* 1986;102:282.

98. Douglas WHG, Strachan IM. Surgical safety of prophylactic peripheral iridectomy. *Br J Ophthalmol.* 1967;51:459.

99. Luke S-K. Complications of peripheral iridectomy. *Can J Ophthalmology.* 1969;4:346.

100. Allen JC. Incidence of photophobia in peripheral and sector iridectomy. *Am J Ophthalmol.* 1976;82:316.

101. Floman N, Berson D, Landau L. Peripheral iridectomy in closed angle glaucoma--late complications. *Br J Ophthalmol.* 1977;61:101.

102. Godel V, Regenbogen L. Cataractogenic factors in patients with primary angle-closure glaucoma after peripheral iridectomy. *Am J Ophthalmol.* 1977;83:180.

103. Krupin T, Mitchell KB, Johnson MF, et al. The long term effects of iridectomy for primary acute angle-closure glaucoma. *Am J Ophthalmol.* 1978;86:506.

104. Shingleton BJ, Jacobson LM, Kuperwaser MC. Comparison of combined cataract and glaucoma surgery using planned extracapsular and phacoemulsification techniques. *Ophthalmic Surg Lasers.* 1995;26(5):414-9.

105. Caprioli J, Park HJ, Weitzman M. Temporal corneal phacoemulsification combined with superior trabeculectomy: a controlled study. *Trans Am Ophthalmol Soc.* 1996;94:451-463.

106. Park HJ, Weitzman M, Caprioli J. Temporal corneal phacoemulsification combined with superior trabeculectomy. A retrospective case-control study. *Arch Ophthalmol.* 1997; 115(3):318-23.

107. Wyse T, Meyer M, Ruderman JM, et al. Combined trabeculectomy and phacoemulsification: a one-site vs a two-site approach. *Am J Ophthalmol.* 1998;125(3):334-9.

108. Zacharia PT, Schuman JS. Combined phacoemulsification and trabeculectomy with mitomycin-C. *Ophthalmic Surg Lasers.* 1997;28(9):739-44.

109. Weitzman M, Caprioli J. Temporal corneal phacoemulsification combined with separate-incision superior trabeculectomy. *Ophthalmic Surg.* 1995;26(3):271-3.

110. Wedrich A, Menapace R, Hirsch U, et al. Comparison of results and complications following combined ECCE- trabeculectomy versus small-incision-trabeculectomy and posterior chamber lens implantation. *Int Ophthalmol.* 1996;20(1-3):125-9.

111. Stewart WC, Crinkley CMC, Carlson AN. Results of trabeculectomy combined with phacoemulsification versus trabeculectomy combined with extracapsular cataract extraction in patients with advanced glaucoma. *Ophthalmic Surg.* 1994;25:621-627.

112. Wishart PK, Austin MW. Combined cataract extraction and trabeculectomy: Phacoemulsification compared with extracapsular technique. *Ophthalmic Surg.* 1993;24:814-821.

113. Tezel G, Kolker AE, Kass MA, et al. Comparative results of combined procedures for glaucoma and cataract: II. Limbus-based versus fornix-based conjunctival flaps. *Ophthalmic Surg Lasers.* 1997;28(7):551-7.

114. Berestka JS, Brown SVL. Limbus- versus fornix-based conjunctival flaps in combined phacoemulsification and mitomycin C trabeculectomy surgery. *Ophthalmology.* 1997;104:187-196.

115. Nichamin LD. Enlarging the pupil for cataract extraction using flexible nylon iris retractors. *J Cataract Refract Surg.* 1993;19(6):793-6.

116. Fine IH. Pupilloplasty for small pupil phacoemulsification. *J Cataract Refract Surg.* 1994;20(2):192-6.

117. Krupin Eye Valve Filtering Surgery Study Group T. Krupin eye valve with disk for filtration surgery. *Ophthalmology.* 1994;101:651-658.

118. Lloyd ME, et al. Intermediate-term results of a randomized clinical trial of the 350-mm2 vs. the 500-mm2 Baerveldt implant. *Ophthalmology.* 1994;101:1456.

119. Schocket SS, Lakhanpal V, Richards RD. Anterior chamber tube shunt to an encircling band in the treatment of neovascular glaucoma. *Ophthalmology.* 1982;89:1188-1194.

120. Tam MYM, et al. Preliminary results of glaucoma valve implant clinical trial. *Invest Ophthalmol Vis Sci.* 1994;35(Suppl):1914.

121. White TC. Clinical results of glaucoma surgery using the White glaucoma pump shunt. *Ann Ophthalmol.* 1992;24:365.

122. Joseph NH, Sherwood MB, Trantas G, et al. A one-piece drainage system for glaucoma surgery. *Trans Ophthalmol Soc UK.* 1986;105:657-664.

123. Minckler DS, al e. Experimental studies of aqueous filtration using the Molteno implant. *Trans Am Ophthalmol Soc.* 1987;85:368.

124. Wilcox MJ, Minckler DS, Ogden TE. Pathophysiology of artificial aqueous drainage in primate eyes with Molteno implants. *J Glaucoma.* 1994;3:140.

125. Francis BA, Cortes A, Chen J, et al. Characteristics of glaucoma drainage implants during dynamic and steady-state flow conditions. *Ophthalmology.* 1998;105(9):1708-14.

126. Molteno ACB. The optimal design of drainage implants for glaucoma. *Trans Ophthalmol Soc NZ.* 1981;33:39.

127. Wilson RP, et al. Aqueous shunts. Molteno vs Schocket. *Ophthalmology.* 1992;99:672.

128. Smith MF, Sherwood MB, McGorray SP. Comparison of the double-plate Molteno drainage implant with the Schocket procedure. *Arch Ophthalmol.* 1992;110:1246.

129. Hodkin MJ, Goldblatt WS, Burgoyne CF, et al. Early clinical experience with the Baerveldt implant in complicated glaucomas. *Am J Ophthalmol.* 1995;120(1):32-40.

130. Lloyd MAE, Baerveldt G, Heuer DK, et al. Initial clinical experience with the Baerveldt implant in complicated glaucomas. *Ophthalmology.* 1994;101:640-650.

131. Freedman J, Rubin B. Molteno implant as a treatment for refractory glaucoma in black patients. *Arch Ophthalmol.* 1991;109:1417-1420.

132. Cooper RL. Molteno implant surgery in refractory glaucoma [letter; comment]. *Surv Ophthalmol.* 1991;35(5):403.

133. Lieberman MF, Ewing RH. Drainage implant surgery for refractory glaucoma. *Int Ophthalmol Clin.* 1990;30(3):198-208.

134. Downes RK, et al. The Molteno implant in intractable glaucoma. *Eye.* 1988;2:250.

135. Lotufo DG. Postoperative complications and visual loss following Molteno implantation. *Ophthalmic Surg.* 1991; 22:650.

136. El-Sayad F, et al. The use of releasable sutures in Molteno glaucoma implant procedures to reduce postoperative hypotony. *Ophthalmic Surg.* 1991;22:82.

137. Egbert PR, Lieberman MF. Internal suture occlusion of the Molteno glaucoma implant for the prevention of postoperative hypotony. *Ophthalmic Surg.* 1989;20:53.

138. Kooner KS, Goode SM. Removable ligature during Molteno implant procedure [letter]. *Am J Ophthalmol.* 1992;114(1):102-103.

139. Raviv T, Greenfield DS, Liebmann JM, et al. Pericardial patch grafts in glaucoma implant surgery. *J Glaucoma.* 1998;7(1):27-32.

140. Brandt JD. Patch grafts of dehydrated cadaveric dura mater for tube-shunt glaucoma surgery. *Arch Ophthalmol.* 1993;111:1436.

141. Whitson WE, Price FW, Jr. Reducing hypotony after Molteno procedure [letter; comment]. *Ophthalmic Surg.* 1992;23(6):434.

142. Valimaki J, Tuulonen A, Airaksinen PJ. Outcome of Molteno implantation surgery in refractory glaucoma and the effect of total and partial tube ligation on the success rate. *Acta Ophthalmol.* 1998;76(2):213-9.

143. Stewart W, Feldman RM, Gross RL. Collagen plug occlusion of Molteno tube shunts. *Ophthalmic Surg.* 1993;24:47.

144. Sherwood MB, Smith MF. Prevention of early hypotony associated with Molteno implants by a new occcluding stent technique. *Ophthalmology.* 1993;100:85.

145. Henderson BC. Modification of slip-knot suture for Molteno shunt tube occlusion [letter]. *Ophthalmic Surg.* 1991;22(2):113.

146. Luttrull JK, Avery RL. Pars plana implant and vitrectomy for treatment of neovascular glaucoma. *Retina.* 1995;15(5):379-387.

147. Smiddy WE, Rubsamen PE, Grajewski A. Vitrectomy for pars plana placement of a glaucoma seton. *Ophthalmic Surg.* 1994;25(8):532-535.

148. Azuara-Blanco A, Katz LJ, Gandham SB, et al. Pars plana tube insertion of aqueous shunt with vitrectomy in malignant glaucoma [letter] [see comments]. *Arch Ophthalmol.* 1998;116(6):808-810.

149. Varma R, Heuer DK, Lundy DC, et al. Pars plana Baerveldt tube insertion with vitrectomy in glaucomas associated with pseudophakia and aphakia. *Am J Ophthalmol.* 1995;119:401-407.

150. Gandham SB, Costa VP, Katz LJ, et al. Aqueous tube-shunt implantation and pars plana vitrectomy in eyes with refractory glaucoma. *Am J Ophthalmol.* 1993;116(2):189-95.

151. Lloyd M, et al. Combined Molteno implantation and pars plana vitrectomy for neovascular glaucoma. *Ophthalmology.* 1991;98:1401.

152. Costa VP, Spaeth GL, Eiferman RA, et al. Wound healing modulation in glaucoma filtraion surgery. *Ophthalmic Surg.* 1993;24:152.

153. Skuta GL, Parrish RK, II. Wound healing in glaucoma filtering surgery. *Surv Ophthalmol.* 1987;32:149-170.

154. Smith MF, Doyle JW, Nguyen QH, et al. Results of intraoperative 5-fluorouracil or lower dose mitomycin-C administration on initial trabeculectomy surgery. *J Glaucoma.* 1997;6(2):104-110.

155. Singh K, Egbert PR, Byrd S, et al. Trabeculectomy with intraoperative 5-fluorouracil vs mitomycin C. *Am J Ophthalmol.* 1997;123(1):48-53.

156. Wilson RP, Steinmann WC. Use of trabeculectomy with postoperative 5-fluorouracil in patients requiring extremely low intraocular pressure levels to limit further progression. *Ophthalmology.* 1991;98:1047-52.

157. Whiteside-Michel J, Liebmann JM, Ritch R. Initial 5-fluorouracil trabeculectomy in young patients. *Ophthalmology.* 1992;99:7-13.

158. Weinreb RN. Adjusting the dose of 5-fluorouracil after filtration surgery to minimize side effects. *Ophthalmology.* 1987;94:564-570.

159. Watanabe J, al e. Trabeculectomy with 5-fluorouracil. *Acta Ophthalmol.* 1991;69:455.

160. Ticho U, Ophir A. Regulating the dose of 5-fluorouracil to prevent filtering bleb scarring. *Ann Ophthalmol.* 1991;23:225.

161. Smith MF, al e. Results of intraoperative 5-fluorouracil supplementation on trabeculectomy for open-angle glaucoma. *Am J Ophthalmol.* 1992;114:737.

162. Ruderman JM, Welch DB, Smith MF, et al. A randomized study of 5-fluorouracil and filtration surgery. *Am J Ophthalmol.* 1987;104:218-224.

163. Skuta GL, al e. Filtering surgery in owl monkeys treated with the antimetabolite 5-fluorouracil 5' monophosphate entrapped in multivesicular liposomes. *Am J Ophthalmol.* 1987;103:714.

164. Rockwood EJ, Parrish RKI, Heuer DK, et al. Glaucoma filtration surgery with 5-Fluorouracil. *Ophthalmology.* 1987; 94:1071-1078.

165. Rabowsky JH, Ruderman JM. Low-dose 5-fluorouracil and glaucoma filtration surgery. *Ophthalmic Surg.* 1989;20:347.

166. Patitsas CJ, al e. Glaucoma filtering surgery with postoperative 5-fluorouracil patients with intraocular inflammatory disease. *Ophthalmology.* 1992;99:594.

167. Ophir A, Ticho U. A randomized study of trabeculectomy and subconjunctival administration of fluorouracil in primary glaucomas. *Arch Ophthalmol.* 1992;110:1072-1075.

168. Krug JH, Melamed S. Adjunctive use of delayed and adjustable low-dose 5-fluorouracil in refractory glaucoma. *Am J Ophthalmol.* 1990;109:412-418.

169. Kitazawa Y, et al. 5-fluorouracil for trabeculectomy in glaucoma. *Graefes Arch Clin Exp Ophthalmol.* 1987;225:403.

170. Heuer DK, Parrish RK, II, Gressel MG, et al. 5-fluorouracil and glaucoma filtering surgery, II, A pilot study. *Ophthalmology.* 1984;91:384-394.

171. Heuer DK, Parrish RK, II, Gressel MG, et al. 5-fluorouracil and glaucoma filtering surgery. III. Intermediate follow-up of a pilot study. *Ophthalmology.* 1986;93:1537-1546.

172. Fluorouracil Filtering Surgery Study Group T. Fluorouracil filtering surgery study one year follow-up. *Am J Ophthalmol.* 1989;108:625-35.

173. Fluorouracil Filtering Surgery Study Group T. Three-year follow-up of the fluorouracil filtering surgery study. *Am J Ophthalmol.* 1993;115:82-92.

174. Fluorouracil filtering surgery study group T. Five-year follow-up of the fluorouracil filtering surgery study. *Am J Ophthalmol.* 1996;121:349-66.

175. Dietze PJ, Feldman RM, Gross RL. Intraoperative application of 5-fluorouracil during trabeculectomy. *Ophthalmic Surg.* 1992;23:662.

176. Falck FY, Skuta GL, Klein TB. Mitomycin versus 5-fluorouracil antimetabolite therapy for glaucoma filtration surgery. *Semin Ophthalmol.* 1992;7:97.

177. Tahery MM, Lee DA. Review: Pharmacologic control of wound healing in glaucoma filtration surgery. *J Ocular Pharmacol.* 1989;5:155.

178. Egbert PR, Williams AS, Singh K, et al. A prospective trial of intraoperative fluorouracil during trabeculectomy in a black population. *Am J Ophthalmol.* 1993;116:612-616.

179. Lanigan L, Stürmer J, Baez KA, et al. Single intraoperative applications of 5-fluorouracil during filtraion surgery: early results. *Br J Ophthalmol.* 1994;78:33-37.

180. Letchinger SL, Becker B, Wax MB. The effects of subconjunctival administration of mitomycin C on intraocular pressure in rabbits. *Invest Ophthalmol Vis Sci.* 1992;33 (Suppl):736.

181. Derick RJ, et al. Potential toxicity of mitomycin-C. *Arch Ophthalmol.* 1991;109:1635.

182. Peyman GA, Greenberg BS, Fishman GA. Evaluation of toxicity of intravitreal antineoplastic drugs. *Ophthalmic Surg.* 1984;15:411-413.

183. Gupta S, Basti S. Corneoscleral, ciliary body, and vitreoretinal toxicity after excessive instillation of Mitomycin-C. *Am J Ophthalmol.* 1992;114:503.

184. Khaw PT, et al. Prolonged localized tissue effects from 5 minute exposures to fluorouracil and mitomycin-C. *Arch Ophthalmol.* 1993;111:263.

185. Khaw PT, et al. The long-term effects of 5-fluorouracil and sodium butyrate on human Tenon's capsule fibroblasts. *Invest Ophthalmol Vis Sci.* 1992;33:2043.

186. Khaw PT, et al. 5-minute treatments with fluorouracil, floxuridine and mitomycin have long-term effects on human Tenon's capsule fibroblasts. *Arch Ophthalmol.* 1992;110:1150.

187. Scott IU, Greenfield DS, Schiffman J, et al. Outcomes of primary trabeculectomy with the use of adjunctive mitomycin. *Arch Ophthalmol.* 1998;116(3):286-291.

188. Chen CW. Enhanced intraocular pressure controlling effectiveness of trabeculectomy by local application of mitomycin-C. *Trans Asia-Pacific Acad Ophthalmol.* 1983;9:172.

189. Skuta GL, Beeson CC, Higginbotham EJ. Intraoperative mitomycin versus postoperative 5-fluorouracil in high-risk glaucoma filtering surgery. *Ophthalmology.* 1992;99:438-444.

190. Beeson C, et al. Randomized clinical trial of intraoperative subconjunctival mitomycin-c versus postoperative 5-fluorouracil. *Invest Ophthalmol Vis Sci.* 1991;32:1122.

191. Kitazawa Y, Kawase K, Matsushita H, et al. Trabeculectomy with mitomycin: a comparative study with fluorouracil. *Arch Ophthalmol.* 1991;109:1693-1698.

192. Robin AL, Ramakrishnan R, Krishnadas R, et al. A long-term dose-response study of mitomycin in glaucoma filtration surgery [see comments]. *Arch Ophthalmol.* 1997;115(8):969-974.

193. Bank A, Allingham RR. Application of mitomycin-C during filtering surgery. *Am J Ophthalmol.* 1993;116:377.

194. Costa VP, Moster MR, Wilson RP, et al. Effects of topical mitomycin C on primary trabeculectomies and combined procedures. *Br J Ophthalmol.* 1993;77:693-697.

195. Kitazawa Y, Suemori-Matsushita H, Yamamoto T, et al. Low-dose and high-dose mitomycin trabeculectomy as an initial surgery in primary open-angle glaucoma. *Ophthalmology.* 1993;100:1624-1628.

196. Mermoud A, et al. Trabeculectomy with mitomycin-C for refractory glaucoma in blacks. *Am J Ophthalmol.* 1993;116:72.

197. Neelakantan A, et al. Effect of the concentration and duration of application of mitomycin C in trabeculectomy. *Ophthalmic Surg.* 1994;25:612-615.

198. Palmer SS. Mitomycin as adjunct chemotherapy with trabeculectomy. *Ophthalmology.* 1991;98:317-321.

199. Mietz H, Krieglstein GK. Three-year follow-up of trabeculectomies performed with different concentrations of mitomycin-C. *Ophthalmic Surg Lasers.* 1998;29(8):628-34.

200. Lee JJ, Park KH, Youn DH. The effect of low-and high-dose adjunctive mitomycin C in trabeculectomy. *Korean J Ophthalmol.* 1996;10(1):42-7.

201. Megevand GS, Salmon JF, Scholtz RP, et al. The effect of reducing the exposure time of mitomycin C in glaucoma filtering surgery. *Ophthalmology.* 1995;102(1):84-90.

202. Singh J, O'Brien C, Chawla HB. Success rate and complications of intraoperative 0. 2 mg/ml mitomycin C in trabeculectomy surgery. *Eye.* 1995;9:460-466.

203. Lee DA, Hersh P, Kersten D, et al. Complications of subconjunctival 5-fluorouracil following glaucoma filtration surgery. *Ophthalmic Surg.* 1987;18:187-190.

204. Manche EE, Afshari MA, Singh K. Delayed corneal epitheliopathy after antimetabolite-augmented trabeculectomy. *J Glaucoma.* 1998;7(4):237-9.

205. Chen C, Huang H, Bair JS, et al. Trabeculectomy with simultaneous topical application of Mitomycin-C in refractory glaucoma. *J Ocular Pharmacol.* 1990;6:175-82.

206. Franks WA, Hitchings RA. Complications of 5-fluorouracil after trabeculectomy. *Eye.* 1991;5:385-389.

207. Jampel HD, Pasquale LR, DiBernardo C. Hypotony maculopathy following trabeculectomy with mitomycin C. *Arch Ophthalmol.* 1992;110:1049-1050.

208. Stamper RL, McMenemy MG, Lieberman MF. Hypotonous maculopathy after trabeculectomy with subconjunctival 5-fluorouracil. *Am J Ophthalmol.* 1992;114:544-553.

209. Zacharia PT, Deppermann SR, Schuman JS. Ocular hypotony after trabeculectomy with mitomycin C. *Am J Ophthalmol.* 1993;116:314-26.

210. Dellaporta A. Fundus changes in postoperative hypotony. *Am J Ophthalmol.* 1955;40:781-5.

211. Gass JDM, Hypotony maculopathy. In: Bellows JG, ed. *Contemporary Ophthalmology.* Baltimore, Md: Williams and Wilkins: 1972.

212. Suner IJ, Greenfield DS, Miller MP, et al. Hypotony maculopathy after filtering surgery with mitomycin C. Incidence and treatment [see comments]. *Ophthalmology.* 1997;104(2):207-214; discussion 214-215.

213. Altan T, Temel A, Bavbek T, et al. Hypotonic maculopathy after trabeculectomy with postoperative use of 5-fluorouracil. *Ophthalmologica.* 1994;208(6):318-320.

214. Shields MB, Scroggs MW, Sloop MW, et al. Clinical and histopathologic observations concerning hypotony after trabeculectomy with adjunctive mitomycin-C. *Am J Ophthalmol.* 1993;116:673-683.

215. Costa VP, Wilson RP, Moster MR, et al. Hypotony maculopathy following the use of topical mitomycin-C in glaucoma surgery. *Ophthalmic Surg.* 1993;24:389-94.

216. Wolner B, Liebmann JM, Sassani JW, et al. Late bleb-related endophthalmitis after trabeculectomy with adjunctive 5-fluorouracil. *Ophthalmology.* 1991;98:1053-1060.

217. Mochizuki M, Jikihara S, Ando Y, et al. Incidence of delayed onset infection after tbcy with adjunctive mitomycin C or 5-fluorouracil treatment. *Br J Ophthalmol.* 1997;81:877-883.

218. Greenfield DS. Bleb-related ocular infection. *J Glaucoma.* 1998;7(2):132-6.

219. Ayyala RS, Bellows AR, Thomas JV, et al. Bleb infections: clinically different courses of "blebitis" and endophthalmitis. *Ophthalmic Surg Lasers.* 1997;28(6):452-60.

220. Greenfield DS, Suner IJ, Miller MP, et al. Endophthalmitis after filtering surgery with mitomycin C. *Arch Ophthalmol.* 1996;114:943-949.

221. Higginbotham EJ, Stevens RK, Musch DC, et al. Bleb-related endophthalmitis after trabeculectomy with mitomcyin C. *Ophthalmology.* 1996;103:650-656.

222. Phillips WB, Wong TP, Berger RL, et al. Late-onset endophthalmitis associated with filtering blebs. *Ophthalmic Surg.* 1994;25:88-91.

223. Yaldo MK, Stamper RL. Long-term effects of mitomycin on filtering blebs. Lack of fibrovascular proliferative response following severe inflammation. *Arch Ophthalmol.* 1993; 111:824-826.

224. Belyea DA, Dan JA, Stamper RL, et al. Late onset of sequential multifocal bleb leaks after glaucoma filtration surgery with 5-fluorouracil and mitomycin C. *Am J Ophthalmol.* 1997;124:40-45.

225. Brown RH, et al. Treatment of bleb infection after glaucoma surgery. *Arch Ophthalmol.* 1994;112:57-61.

226. Mandelbaum S, Forster RK, Gelende H, et al. Late onset endophthalmitis associated with filtering blebs. *Ophthalmology.* 1985;92:964-972.

227. Susanna R, Jr. , Takahashi W, Nicolela M. Late bleb leakage after trabeculectomy with 5-fluorouracil or mitomycin C. *Can J Ophthalmol.* 1996;31:296-300.

228. Iliff CE. Flap perforation in glaucoma surgery sealed by a tissue patch. *Arch Ophthalmol.* 1964;71:215-8.

229. Brown SVL. Management of a partial-thickness scleral-flap buttonhole during trabeculectomy. *Ophthalmic Surg.* 1994;25:732-733.

230. Alpar JJ. Sodium hyaluronate (HealonR) in glaucoma filtering procedures. *Ophthalmic Surg.* 1986;17:724.

231. Barak A, Alhalel A, Kotas R, et al. The protective effect of early intraoperative injection of viscoelastic material in trabeculectomy. *Ophthalmic Surg.* 1992;23:206-209.

232. Raitta C, Lehto I, Puska P, et al. A randomized, prospective study on the use of sodium hyaluronate (Healon) in trabeculectomy [see comments]. *Ophthalmic Surg.* 1994;25(8):536-539.

233. Wand M. Viscoelastic agent and the prevention of post-filtration flat anterior chamber. *Ophthalmic Surg.* 1988;19:523-524.

234. Hung SO. Role of sodium hyaluronate (Healonid) in trianglular flap trabeculectomy. *Br J Ophthalmol.* 1985;69:46-50.

235. Teekhasaenee C, Ritch R. The use of PhEA 34c in trabeculectomy. *Ophthalmology.* 1986;93:487-491.

236. Liebmann JM, Ritch R, DiSclafani M, et al. Early intraocular pressure rise after trabeculectomy. *Arch Ophthalmol.* 1990;108:1549-1552.

237. Spaeth GL. Suprachoroidal hemorrhage: no longer a disaster. *Ophthalmic Surg.* 1987;18:329.

238. Taylor DM. Expulsive hemorrhage: some observations and comments. *Trans Am Ophthalmol Soc.* 1974;82:157.

239. Welch JC, Spaeth GL, Benson WE. Massive suprachoroidal hemorrhage: Follow-up and outcome of 30 cases. *Ophthalmology.* 1988;95:1202-1206.

240. Speaker MG, Guerriero PN, Met JA, et al. A case-control study of risk factors for intraoperative suprachoroidal expulsive hemorrhage. *Ophthalmology.* 1991;98:202-210.

241. Canning CR, Lavin M, McCartney ACE, et al. Delayed suprachoroidal haemorrhage after glaucoma operations. *Eye.* 1989;3:327-331.

242. Givens K, Shields MB. Suprachoroidal hemorrhage after glaucoma filtering surgery. *Am J Ophthalmol.* 1987;103:689-694.

243. Gressel MG, Parrish RK, II, Heuer DK. Delayed nonexpulsive suprachoroidal hemorrhage. *Arch Ophthalmol.* 1984;102:1757-1760.

244. Fluorouracil Filtering Surgery Study Group T. Risk factors for suprachoroidal hemorrhage after filtering surgery. *Am J Ophthalmol.* 1992;113:501-507.

245. Ruderman JM, Harbin TS, Jr. , Campbell DG. Postoperative suprachoroidal hemorrhage following filtration procedures. *Arch Ophthalmol.* 1986;104:201-205.

246. Ariano ML, Ball SF. Delayed nonexpulsive suprachoroidal hemorrhage after trabeculectomy. *Ophthalmic Surg.* 1987;18:661-666.

247. Frenkel REP, Shin DH. Prevention and management of delayed suprachorodial hemorrhage after filtration surgery. *Arch Ophthalmol.* 1986;104:1459-1463.

248. Brubaker RF. Intraocular surgery and choroidal hemorrhage. *Arch Ophthalmol.* 1984;102:1753-1754.

249. Lambrou FH, Jr. , Meredith TA, Kaplan HJ. Secondary surgical management of expulsive choroidal hemorrhage. *Arch Ophthalmol.* 1987;105:1195-1198.

250. Lakhanpal V, Schocket SS, Elman MJ, et al. A new modified vitreoretinal surgical approach in the management of massive suprachoroidal hemorrhage. *Ophthalmology.* 1989;96:793-800.

251. Reynolds MG, Haimovici R, Flynn HW, Jr. , et al. Suprachoroidal hemorrhage. Clinical features and results of secondary surgical management. *Ophthalmology.* 1993;100:460-465.

252. Chu TG, et al. Massive suprachoroidal hemorrhage with central retinal apposition. A clinical and echographic study. *Arch Ophthalmol.* 1991;109:1575-1581.

253. Portney GL. Trabeculectomy and postoperative ocular hypertension in secondary angle-closure glaucoma. *Am J Ophthalmol.* 1977;84:145.

254. Cohn JH, Aron-Rosa D. Reopening blocked trabeculectomy sites ith the YAG laser. *Am J Ophthalmol.* 1984;102:1024.

255. Dailey RA, Samples JR, Van Buskirk EM. Reopening filtration fisutlas with neodymium-YAG laser. *Am J Ophthalmol.* 1986;102:491.

256. Ofner S, Smith TJ. Neodymium:YAG laser for the treatment of encapuslated blebs after filtration surgery. *Am J Ophthalmol.* 1988;106:232-234.

257. Praeger DL. The reopening of closed filtering blebs using the neodymium:YAG laser. *Ophthalmology.* 1984;91:373.

258. Ruben S, Tsai J, Hitchings RA. Malignant glaucoma and its management. *Br J Ophthalmol.* 1997;81(2):163-7.

259. Little BC, Hitchings RA. Pseudophakic malignant glaucoma: Nd:YAG capsulotomy as a primary treatment. *Eye.* 1993; 7:102-104.

260. Melamed S, Ashkenazi I, Blumenthal M. Nd-YAG laser hyaloidotomy for malignant glaucoma following one-piece 7 mm intraocular lens implantation. *Br J Ophthalmol.* 1991;75:501.

261. Tsai JC, Barton KA, Miller MH, et al. Surgical results in malignant glaucoma refractory to medical or laser therapy. *Eye.* 1997;11(Pt 5):677-681.

262. Johnson DH. Options in the management of malignant glaucoma [editorial; comment]. *Arch Ophthalmol.* 1998;116 (6):799-800.

263. Cekic O, Batman C. Pars plana vitrectomy in the treatment of phakic and pseudophakic malignant glaucoma [letter; comment]. *Arch Ophthalmol.* 1998;116(1):118.

264. Bellows AR, Chylack JR, Hutchinson BT. Choroidal detachment: Clinical manifestation, therapy and mechanism of formation. *Ophthalmology.* 1981;88:1107-1115.

265. Berke SJ, Bellows AR, Shingleton BJ, et al. Chronic and recurrent choroidal detachment after glaucoma filtering surgery. *Ophthalmology.* 1987;94:154-162.

266. Burney EN, Quigley MA, Robin AL. Hypotony and choroidal detachment as late complications of trabeculectomy. *Am J Ophthalmol.* 1987;103:685.

267. Newhouse RP, Beyrer C. Hypotony as a late complication of trabeculectomy. *Ann Ophthalmol.* 1982;14:685.

268. Greenfield DS, Liebmann JM, Jee J, et al. Late-onset bleb leaks after glaucoma filtering surgery. *Arch Ophthalmol.* 1998;116:443-447.

269. Cohen JS, Shaffer RN, Hetherington J, Jr. , et al. Revision of filtration surgery. *Arch Ophthalmol.* 1977;95:1612-1615.

270. Galin MA, Hung PT. Surgical repair of leaking blebs. *Am J Ophthalmol.* 1977;83:328-333.

271. Romanchuk KG. Seidel's test using 10% fluorescein. *Can J Ophthalmol.* 1979;14:253.

272. Cain WJ, Sinskey RM. Detection of anterior chamber leakage with Seidel's test. *Arch Ophthalmol.* 1981;99:2013.

273. Tomlinson CP, Belcher CDI, P. D. S, et al. Management of leaking filtration blebs. *Ann Ophthalmol.* 1987;19:405-411.

274. Petursson GJ, Fraunfelder FT. Repair of an inadvertent buttonhole or leaking filtering bleb. *Arch Ophthalmol.* 1979;97:926-7.

275. Melamed S, Hersh P, Kersten D, et al. The use of glaucoma shell tamponade in leaking filtration blebs. *Ophthalmology.* 1986;93:839-842.

276. Hill RA, Aminlari A, Sassani JW, et al. Use of a symblepharon ring for treatment of over-filtration and leaking blebs after glaucoma filtration surgery. *Ophthalmic Surg.* 1990; 21:707-710.

277. O'Sullivan F, Dalton R, Rostron CK. Fibrin glue: an alternative method of wound closure in glaucoma surgery. *J Glaucoma.* 1996;5(6):367-70.

278. Katz LJ. Ciliochoroidal detachment. *Ophthalmic Surg.* 1987;18:1775.

279. Brubaker RF, Pederson JE. Ciliochoroidal detachment. *Surv Ophthalmol.* 1983;27:281.

280. Osher RH, Cionni RJ, Cohen JS. Re-forming the flat anterior chamber with Healon. *J Cataract Refract Surg.* 1996; 22(4):411-5.

281. Hattenhauer JM, Lipsich MP. Late endophthalmitis after filtering surgery. *Am J Ophthalmol.* 1971;72:1097-1101.

282. Katz LJ, Cantor LB, Spaeth GL. Complications of surgery in glaucoma: early and late bacterial endophthalmitis following glaucoma filtering surgery. *Ophthalmology.* 1985;92:959.

283. Ritch R, Schuman JS, Belcher CD, III. Management of the leaking filtration bleb. *J Glaucoma.* 1993;2:114-118.

284. Blok MDW, Kok JHC, van Mil C, et al. Use of the Megasoft bandage lens for treatment of complications after trabeculectomy. *Am J Ophthalmol.* 1990;110:264-268.

285. Kirk HQ. Cauterization of filtering blebs following cataract extraction. *Trans Am Acad Ophthalmol Otolaryngol.* 1973;77:573.

286. Baum M, Weiss HS. Argon laser closure of conjunctival bleb leak. *Arch Ophthalmol.* 1993;111:438.

287. Hennis HL, Stewart WC. Use of the argon laser to close filtering bleb leaks. *Graefes Arch Clin Exp Ophthalmol.* 1992; 230:537-541.

288. Oz MC, Johnson JP, Parangi S, et al. Tissue soldering by use of indocyanine green dye-enhanced fibrinogen with the near infrared diode laser. *J Vasc Surg.* 1990;11:718-725.

289. Yannuzzi LA, Theodore FH. Cryotherapy of post-cataract blebs. *Am J Ophthalmol.* 1973;76(2):217-222.

290. Wright MM, Brown EA, Maxwell K, et al. Laser-cured fibrinogen glue to repair bleb leaks in rabbits. *Arch Ophthalmol.* 1998;116(2):199-202.

291. Kosmin AS, Wishart PK. A full-thickness scleral graft for the surgical management of a late filtration bleb leak. *Ophthalmic Surg Lasers.* 1997;28(6):461-468.

292. Asrani SG, Wilensky JT. Management of bleb leaks after glaucoma filtering surgery. Use of autologous fibrin tissue glue as an alternative. *Ophthalmology.* 1996;103(2):294-8.

293. Smith MF, Magauran RG, III, Betchkal J, et al. Treatment of postfiltration bleb leaks with autologous blood. *Ophthalmology.* 1995;102:868-871.

294. Wilson MR, Kotas-Neumann R. Free conjunctival patch for repair of persistent late bleb leak. *Am J Ophthalmol.* 1994;117:569-574.

295. Pederson JE, Ocular hypotony. In: Ritch R, Shields MB, Krupin T, eds. *The Glaucomas.* St Louis, Mo: CV Mosby Co; 1989.

296. Cohen SM, Flynn HW, Jr. , Palmberg PF, et al. Treatment of hypotony maculopathy after trabeculectomy. *Ophthalmic Surg Lasers.* 1995;26(5):435-441.

297. Schwartz GF, Robin AL, Wilson RP, et al. Resuturing the scleral flap leads to resolution of hypotony maculopathy. *J Glaucoma.* 1996;5(4):246-251.

298. Duker JS, Schuman JS. Successful surgical treatment of hypotony maculopathy following trabeculectomy with topical mitomycin C. *Ophthalmic Surg.* 1994;25(7):463-465.

299. Keroub C, Hyams SW, Rath E. Study of cataract formation following trabeculectomy. *Glaucoma.* 1984;6:117.

300. Sugar HS. Cataract formation and refractive changes after surgery for angle-closure glaucoma. *Am J Ophthalmol.* 1970;69:747.

301. Chen TC, Wilensky JT, Viana MA. Long-term follow-up of initially successful trabeculectomy. *Ophthalmology.* 1997;104(7):1120-1125.

302. Parrish RK, II, Herschler J. Eyes with end-stage neovascular glaucoma; natural history following successful modified filtering operation. *Arch Ophthalmol.* 1983;101:745-746.

303. Merritt JC. Filtering procedures in American blacks. *Ophthalmic Surg.* 1980;11:91-94.

304. Bellows AR, Johnstone MA. Surgical management of chronic glaucoma in aphakia. *Ophthalmology.* 1983;90:807-813.

305. Herschler J. Medically uncontrolled glaucoma in the aphakic eye. *Ann Ophthalmol.* 1981;13:909.

306. Heuer DK, Gressel MG, Parrish RK, II, et al. Trabeculectomy in aphakic eyes. *Ophthalmology.* 1984; 91:1045-1051.

307. Schwartz AL, Anderson DR, Glaucoma surgery in aphakia. In: Emery JM, Paton D, eds. *Current Concepts in Cataract Surgery.* St Louis, Mo: CV Mosby Co; 1974.

308. Shirato S, Kitazawa Y, Mishima S. A critical analysis of the trabeculectomy results by a prospective follow-up design. *Jpn J Ophthalmol.* 1982;26:468-480.

309. Liebmann J, Ritch R. Management of the failing filtering bleb. *Semin Ophthalmol.* 1991;6:1-6.

310. Stewart WC, Shields MB, Miller KN, et al. Early postoperative prognostic indicators following trabeculectomy. *Ophthalmic Surg.* 1991;22:23-26.

311. Wieland M, Spaeth GL. Use of digital compression following glaucoma surgery. *Ophthalmic Surg.* 1988;19:350-352.

312. Brown RH, Lynch MG. Ab-Interno filtering surgery, internal sclerectomy with the trabecuphine. *Ophthalmol Clin N Am.* 1988;1:199.

313. Brown RM, et al. Internal sclerectomy for glaucoma filtering surgery with automated trephine. *Arch Ophthalmol.* 1987;105:133-6.

314. Feldman RM, et al. Risk factors for the development of Tenon's capsule cysts after trabeculectomy. *Ophthalmology.* 1989;96:336-341.

315. Ophir A. Encapsulated filtering bleb. A selective review-new deductions. *Eye.* 1992;6:348-352.

316. Pederson JE, Smith SG. Surgical management of encapsulated filtering blebs. *Ophthalmology.* 1985;92:955-958.

317. Richter CU, et al. The development of encapsulated filtering blebs. *Ophthalmology.* 1988;95:1163-1168.

318. Sherwood MB, et al. Cysts of Tenon's capsule following filtration surgery. Medical management. *Arch Ophthalmol.* 1987;105:1517-1521.

319. Campagna JA, Munden PM, Alward WL. Tenon's cyst formation after trabeculectomy with mitomycin C. *Ophthalmic Surg.* 1995;26(1):57-60.

320. Scott DR, Quigley HA. Medical management of a high bleb phase after trabeculectomies. *Ophthalmology.* 1988;95:1169.

321. Ewing RH, Stamper RL. Needle revision with and without 5-fluorouracil for the treatment of failed filtering blebs. *Am J Ophthalmol.* 1990;110:254-259.

322. Potash SD, Ritch R, Liebmann J. Ocular hypotony and choroidal effusion following bleb needling. *Ophthalmic Surg.* 1993;24:279.

323. Shin DH, Juzych MS, Khatana AK, et al. Needling revision of failed filtering blebs with adjunctive 5-fluorouracil. *Ophthalmic Surg.* 1993;24:242-248.

324. Mardelli PG, Lederer CM, Jr. , Murray PL, et al. Slit-lamp needle revision of failed filtering blebs using mitomycin C. *Ophthalmology.* 1996;103:1946-1955.

325. Greenfield DS, Miller MP, Suner IJ, et al. Needle elevation of the scleral flap for failing filtration blebs after trabeculectomy with mitomycin C. *Am J Ophthalmol.* 1996;122:195-204.

326. Apostolov VI, Siarov NP. Subconjunctival injection of low-dose Mitomycin-C for treatment of failing human trabeculectomies. *Int Ophthalmol.* 1996;20(1-3):101-5.

327. Gillies WE, Brooks AMV. Restoring the function of the failed bleb. *Aust NZ J Ophthalmol.* 1991;19:49-51.

328. Morales J, Ritch R. Treatment of failing filtering blebs. *Clin Decisions Ophthalmol.* 1987;11:4-11.

329. Tabbara KF. Late infections following filtering procedures. *Ann Ophthalmol.* 1976;8:1228-1231.

330. Nguyen QH, Budenz DL, Parrish RK, 2nd. Complications of Baerveldt glaucoma drainage implants. *Arch Ophthalmol.* 1998;116(5):571-5.

331. Melamed S, et al. Postoperative complications after Molteno implant surgery. *Am J Ophthalmol.* 1991;111:319.

332. Dugel PR, Heuer DK, Thach AB, et al. Annular peripheral choroidal detachment simulating aqueous misdirection after glaucoma surgery. *Ophthalmology.* 1997;104:439-444.

333. Paysse E, Lee PP, Lloyd MA, et al. Suprachoroidal hemorrhage after Molteno implantation. *J Glaucoma.* 1996;5(3):170-5.

334. Heher KL, et al. Late-onset sterile endophthalmitis after Molteno tube implantation. *Am J Ophthalmol.* 1992;114:771.

335. Lieberman MF. Late infectious endophthalmitis from exposed glaucoma setons [letter; comment]. *Arch Ophthalmol.* 1992;110(12):1685.

336. Fanous MM, Cohn RA. Propionibacterium endophthalmitis following Molteno tube repositioning. *J Glaucoma.* 1997; 6(4):201-2.

337. Krebs DB, Liebmann JM, Ritch R, et al. Late infectious endophthalmitis from exposed glaucoma setons. *Arch Ophthalmol.* 1992;110:174-175.

338. Brown RD, Cairns JE. Experience with the Molteno long tube implant. *Trans Ophthalmol Soc UK.* 1983;102:51.

339. Minckler DS, et al. Clinical experience with the single-plate Molteno implant in complicated glaucomas. *Ophthalmology.* 1988;95:1181.

340. Sherwood MB, Joseph NH, Hitchings RA. Surgery for refractory glaucoma: results and complications with a modified Schocket technique. *Arch Ophthalmol.* 1987;105:562.

341. Sidoti PA, et al. Epithelial ingrowth and glaucoma drainage implants. *Ophthalmology.* 1994;101:872.

342. Traverso CE, Tomey KF, Al-Kaff A. The long-tube single plate Molteno implant for the treatment of refractory glaucomas. *Int Ophthalmol.* 1989;13:159.

343. Fiore PM, Melamed S. Use of neodymium:YAG laser to open an occluded Molteno tube. *Ophthalmic Surg.* 1989;20:201.

344. Oram O, Gross RL, Severin TD, et al. Opening an occluded Molteno tube with the picosecond neyodymium-yttrium lithium fluoride laser. *Arch Ophthalmol.* 1994;112:1023.

345. Tessler Z, Jluchoded S, Rosenthal G. Nd: YAG laser for Ahmed tube shunt occlusion by the posterior capsule. *Ophthalmic Surg Lasers.* 1997;28(1):69-70.

346. Krawitz PL. Treatment of distal occlusion of Krupin eye valve with disk using cannular flush. *Ophthalmic Surg.* 1994;25:102.

347. Classen L, Kivela T, Tarkkanen A. Histopathologic and immunohistochemical analysis of the filtration bleb after unsuccessful glaucoma seton implantation. *Am J Ophthalmol.* 1996;122(2):205-12.

348. Chen PP, Palmberg PF. Needling revision of glaucoma drainage device filtering blebs [published erratum appears in *Ophthalmology.* 1997;104(10):1532] [see comments]. *Ophthalmology.* 1997;104(6):1004-10.

349. Frank JW, Perkins TW, Kushner BJ. Ocular motility defects in patients with the Krupin valve implant. *Ophthalmic Surg.* 1995;26(3):228-32.

350. Smith SL, et al. Early clinical experience with the Baerveldt 350-mm2 glaucoma implant and associated extraocular muscle imbalance. *Ophthalmology.* 1993;100:914.

351. Munoz M, Parrish RK, II. Strabismus following implantation of Baerveldt devices. *Arch Ophthalmol.* 1993;111:1096.

352. Kooner KS, Cavanagh HD, Zimmerman CF, et al. Eye movement restrictions after Molteno implant surgery [letter]. *Ophthalmic Surg.* 1993;24(7):498-499.

353. Ball SF, Herrington RG, Liang K. Brown's superior oblique tendon syndrome after Baerveldt glaucoma implant. *Arch Ophthalmol.* 1992;110:1368.

354. Christmann LM, Wilson ME. Motility disturbances after Molteno implants. *J Pediatr Ophthalmol Strabismus.* 1992;29:44.

355. Prata JA, Jr. , Minckler DS, Green RL. Pseudo-Brown's syndrome as a complication of glaucoma drainage implant surgery. *Ophthalmic Surg.* 1993;24:608.

356. Dobler AA, et al. Acquired Brown's syndrome after a double-plate Molteno implant. *Am J Ophthalmol.* 1993;116:641.

357. Cardakli UF, Perkins TW. Recalcitrant diplopia after implantation of a Krupin valve with disc. *Ophthalmic Surg.* 1994;25:256-258.

358. Wilson-Holt N, et al. Hypertropia following inferiorly sited double plated Molteno tubes. *Ophthalmology.* 1990; 109(Suppl):143.

359. Roth SM, Spaeth GL, Starita RJ, et al. The effects of postoperative corticosteroids on trabeculectomy and the clinical course of glaucoma: five-year follow-up study. *Ophthalmic Surg.* 1991;22:724-729.

Chapter Fourteen

Visual Rehabilitation and Low Vision Therapy for the Patient with Glaucomatous Vision Loss

John S. Ray, OD, MS

INTRODUCTION

The management of patients with advanced glaucoma is one of the most challenging tasks encountered by the low vision specialist. Success in such therapy is more limited than for other low vision problems, such as central vision loss from macular degeneration. The evaluation of such patients deserves the expertise of a seasoned professional. The devices available are either prisms or minifiers, which either enhance peripheral awareness or expand one's peripheral field. Their suitability, however, competes with the normal adaptation of organized scanning developed by patients over the long course of their visual field loss. Some prisms decrease acuity and image quality, and alter spatial orientation. Minifiers alter depth perception, size constancy, and visual acuity. Careful evaluation, thorough instruction, and good patient education allow those patients who can most benefit from therapy to make educated decisions about the appropriateness of these devices for their needs.

GLAUCOMATOUS FIELD LOSS

Generally speaking, the most frequently encountered disability as a result of glaucoma is visual field loss. It most typically is characterized by peripheral constriction, decreasing the dimensions in all directions. Asymmetry and peripheral islands of spared vision are not uncommon, and may impact on one's candidacy for certain devices. Although this is generally a gradual process taking years to develop, patient education for low vision services should begin early in the disease process. Patients with glaucoma generally experience the greatest difficulty with daily tasks when they reach legal blindness, which is defined as 20 degrees of total visual field in the horizontal meridian in the better eye. It is at that time that their motivation and likelihood of success in a vision rehabilitation program are at their greatest. When the visual field is reduced to this level, patients may report difficulty with ambulation. It is likely because of the decreased awareness in the periphery that they will bump into objects on either side. A small visual field also causes the patient to lose his or her place while reading, making reading text difficult and frustrating. It is at this time that a patient is most appropriately referred for vision rehabilitation services.

DEFINITION OF VISION REHABILITATION

Visual Rehabilitation is the specialty within vision care whose practitioners prescribe optical devices and non-optical strategies to maximize the patient's visual functioning. Its aim is not to restore vision that has been lost, but to maximize a patient's ability to perform desired activities. These activities may include walking, reading, and activities of daily living (ADLs). In this way, the patient's independence can be maximized, decreasing dependence upon others for assistance with these tasks. This process often can increase or preserve a patient's self esteem, confidence, and quality of life. It is important that the expectations regarding vision rehabilitation services are realistic on the part both of the patient and the referring doctor in order to facilitate and to augment the patient's total rehabilitation outcome.

VISION REHABILITATION FOR GLAUCOMA

Patients with glaucomatous field loss from glaucoma can generally receive assistance for ambulation and reading. For ambulation there are optical devices that minify to expand ones visual field, and devices incorporating prism to displace objects in the blind field into the sighted field in order to enhance the patient's awareness of the periphery. In addition, there are other services that teach safe ambulation and travel. These techniques can be used in lieu of, or in conjunction with optical devices. For reading, the use of minification is limited because it decreases acuity. Instead, the use of a closed circuit television system (Figure 14-1) or a non-optical strategy is prescribed. In any case, there are options available for patients with advanced glaucomatous disease for both distance and near activities. These aids can be incorporated into the spectrum of management services for these patients in a cooperative relationship between treating vision care professionals.

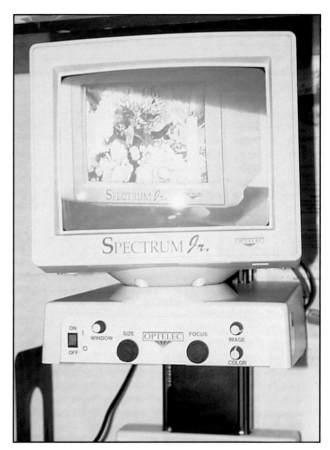

Figure 14-1. A closed circuit television. It greatly magnifies an object and the patient can vary his or her working distance from the apparatus.

REFERRING A PATIENT FOR LOW VISION THERAPY

When referring a patient for low vision or vision rehabilitation services, it is important that the referring doctor have identified the patient as having difficulties in functioning associated with the advanced disease. Documentation for such disabilities can be obtained at any visit, just by asking pointed questions of those patients with constricted fields to 20 degrees or less. The prognosis for the use of optical devices is also better when visual acuity is 20/100 or better, and the patient is well motivated. The referring clinician should develop a cooperative relationship with a low vision specialist. These doctors, most often are optometrists. They can be found in private practices, interdisciplinary clinics, academic institutions, or rehabilitation agencies. Local and state professional associations are excellent resources for locating these clinicians.

At the time of the referral, it is helpful to provide the low vision specialist with prior records, a summary report, and copies of the most recent visual field. In this way, the rehabilitation specialist is able to best assess the patient at the time of the appointment.

THE REHABILITATION SEQUENCE

The rehabilitation process often follows a sequence of events. It is common for the evaluation and treatment process to extend over several visits. Informing patients of this process at the onset of the evaluation is very important in order to provide them with a true picture of what will ensue during the course of rehabilitation. I often explain to my patients that one experiences loss of visual functioning over years, and that restoring that functioning is takes some time. In fact, the motivated patient must relearn to perform tasks that were once performed without difficulty.

Observation

Often, the first interaction of the patient with the low vision doctor is in the office at the time of the initial appointment. It is most helpful to meet the patient in the waiting room and to accompany him or her to the examination room. In this short distance, the doctor can observe the patient's skills in ambulation in an unfamiliar environment. One should note the degree of independence, mishaps on either side, head turns for compensation, speed of pace, and facility of walking. This brief period of observation can be valuable in assessing the patient's need for devices and services for ambulation. These observations are corroborated by more details when taking the patient history.

Patient History

The low vision history is broader in scope than a primary care history. It encompasses general information, health history, ocular history, educational level, living and social information, and functional information including the patient's problem areas and specific goals. All elements are key factors in assessing and treating the patient. The history is best performed by the doctor, patient and, if necessary, a corroborating source such as a friend or family member. If it seems that the patient is not the primary responder, it may be better to not include the corroborator.

General Information

This part of the history resembles any other history. Here patient demographics are confirmed. Contact information is important in case the doctor needs to contact the patient between visits. It assists the doctor in maintaining proper communication during the rehabilitation sequence.

Health History

This portion of the patient history includes the patient's health status in a "Review of Systems" format. This process may be facilitated by a pre-exam questionnaire completed by the patient possibly with the assistance of an accompanying individual. A checklist format is most helpful. This information provides the low vision doctor with information regarding mental state, energy level, cognitive status, medical alerts, and other information about the likelihood of the success of low vision rehabilitation.

Ocular History

Included in this section is information about the onset of the diagnosis of glaucoma. It also includes ocular medications, laser and incisional surgery, and information about coexisting ocular conditions. It is also important to ascertain the patient's understanding of glaucoma, its functional effects, and prognosis. The low vision doctor, at this time, may ask about the patient's understanding of why they presented for vision rehabilitation. Here one may ask about prior low vision evaluations.

Educational Information

The level of education is asked so that one knows the prior functioning status of the patient. It also provides the doctor with information on the patient's vocation and areas of interest.

Living and Social Information

The type of dwelling and the presence other individuals in the same household can impact rehabilitation. Knowing barriers in the dwelling (ie, stairs, elevators, and number of rooms) can guide the practitioner in identifying problems and in setting goals. Also, the presence of a supportive other may help motivate the patient and reinforce skills taught in rehabilitation.

Functional Information

This part of the history can inventory problems encountered in ADL caused by vision loss. Here a list of daily living skills is mentioned and problems are discussed. This part of the history identifies problems, sets and prioritizes goals, and develops realistic expectations for services.

THE LOW VISION EXAMINATION

The low vision examination evaluates several areas in order to improve the functioning of the glaucoma patient. Components of the examination are:
- Refraction
- Evaluation of magnification
- Evaluation of absorptive lenses
- Evaluation of field devices
- Evaluation of non-optical devices
- Networking with other professionals and services.

Refraction

Many patients with glaucoma have not been refracted to attain maximum visual acuity for a prolonged period of time (Figure 14-2). Particularly those with advanced field loss may have limited their ocular care to the management of the disease. Many patients feel that a change in glasses will not benefit them. Although it is true that a change in refraction will not impact the effect of peripheral field loss, increasing the corrected acuity to a maximum allows these patients to carry on desired tasks requiring detail discrimination. (ie, reading, watching television, and recognizing faces).

Using a low vision cardboard chart (Figures 14-3a and b) rather than a projector type better evaluates visual acuity. These charts are superior to a projector chart because they:
- Exhibit a wider range of optotype
- Provide higher contrast
- Allow more increments of acuity
- Can easily be moved for better viewing.

Because the patient with advanced glaucoma possesses a small conical shaped field, it is important not to present a character larger than the linear dimension

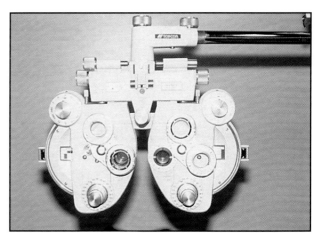

Figure 14-2. A phoropter. It is used to refract patients in many doctor's offices.

of their visual field dimensions. It is also important to adjust room illumination to patient preference in order to maximize the accuracy of the test.

Refracting the low vision patient is better performed using the trial frame (Figure 14-4) rather than a phoropter. The trial frame allows more light to enter the eye, is a more natural experience, and allows the doctor to observe the patient's eyes. In this way the practitioner is able to see eye movements and squinting. Halberg clips also are helpful in this regard. Retinoscopy is an excellent way to start the process of refractive error determination. The distance used can be closer than the conventional 20 to 26 inches used in primary care as long as the doctor notes the working distance and compensates for it. For example, if a reflex is attained at 20 cm, one would subtract 5D from his gross findings. This is called "radical retinoscopy." For patients with opaque media, a stenopaic slit can be used. Ophthalmometry can assist the clinician in determining the major meridians of the eye.

Determination of Binocularity

A discussion of refraction of patients with overall constricted fields is not complete without accounting for the patient's binocular status. This should be considered when the corrected visual acuity is within 2 lines of acuity between the eyes. For example if a patient's acuity is 20/30, 20/50 it is likely that the patient is using both eyes simultaneously. Conversely, the patient is not binocular if the acuities are 20/30, 20/400. If in doubt, one can used a red lens (Figure 14-5) or hand-held maddox rod over one eye while the

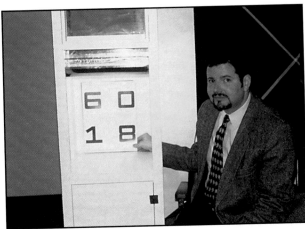

Figure 14-3a. A cardboard chart is used in low vision. Note the spacing of characters.

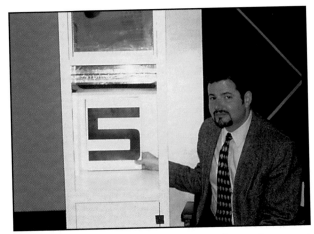

Figure 14-3b. Note the large optotype, larger than most conventional acuity charts.

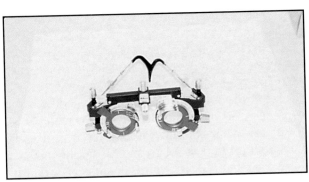

Figure 14-4. A trial frame with trial lenses used in the refraction of patients with low vision.

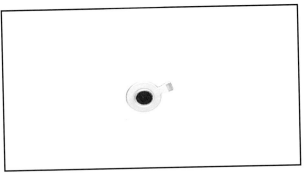

Figure 14-5. A Red Lens used to evaluate diplopia. This lens is inserted into a trial frame. (See Figure 14-4.)

patient views a penlight. If both the red image (a spot for the red lens and a red line for the maddox rod) and the white light are perceived simultaneously, then biocularity exists. Stereopsis might be absent, but the patient still uses both eyes simultaneously, thus biocularity is present. The implications for determining the presence of biocularity is to maximize the use of both eyes together by correcting visual acuity in both eyes, even though one may be less than the other.

Diplopia

Another reason for evaluating these patients for biocularity is that diplopia may result when only a small amount of central field remains in both eyes. This result is due to a misalignment or "drift " of the eyes from the object of regard. The explanation for this ocular drift might be the loss of peripheral fusion lock when there is profoundly constricted fields. The diplopia experienced by these patients is often tran-

sient and variable, inconsistent and difficult to reliably quantify. It also more commonly experienced at near while reading. I have observed similar diplopia in patients with retinitis pigmentosa (RP), which is not surprising because the field loss in patients with glaucoma is similar to that in patients with RP. Thus, diplopia is likely to be reported in both populations. Perception of double images from acquired misalignment of the eyes can only exist if the patient has biocularity.

Management of Diplopia

The management of diplopia is a formidable challenge. It is important that the doctor and patient understand the intractable nature of this kind of diplopia. It has been my experience that other entities causing diplopia may attain fusion with prismatic correction in over 50% of cases. Glaucomatous individuals, however, respond poorly to prism; encountering frustration while experiencing only glimpses of single vision with any magnitude of prism. For this reason, the preferred diplopia management is with occlusion. It is generally best to patch the non-dominant eye because it is less disruptive. This is the same principle utilized when prescribing monovision contact lenses where the near reading eye is the non-dominant eye.

When using occlusion, the most common patch is either one with an elastic headband ("pirate patch") or a clip-on patch (Figure 14-6). Another useful means of occlusion is the use of a small round piece of clear contact paper placed on a spectacle lens in front of the eye. A full-field patch is not necessary, and the contact paper should be only large enough to block the second perceived image. A piece the size of a quarter is often sufficient. If a more permanent patch is desired, the spectacle lens can be frosted. Clear nail polish applied to the spectacle lens and then stippled with a pointed object such as a pencil also is effective. Generally speaking, these patches are prescribed for prolonged near work.

Evaluation of Magnification

Because glaucoma can coexist with conditions that decrease visual acuity (ie, corneal degeneration, or cataracts), patients who have difficulty reading conventional print may need magnification. It is important that the minimum amount of magnification necessary to perform a task be used in individuals with extensive field loss. Otherwise, it is possible to overtake the dimensions of the patient's visual field, thus creating a more formidable obstacle than the patient's decreased acuity. Magnifying beyond the visual field would require a patient to scan each character in order for it to be recognized.

Besides limiting the amount of magnification, prescribed, it also is important to prescribe those magnifying devices that are used at more remote working distances. Microscopes (high powered, convex spectacle lenses) are not recommended because they often provide images larger than the patients field. The following devices are considered more appropriate. because the visual field is larger further from the patient:
- Hand-held magnifiers
- Stand magnifiers
- Closed circuit televisions.

Hand-held magnifiers come in a variety of powers (Figure 14-7). Their working distance can be varied to

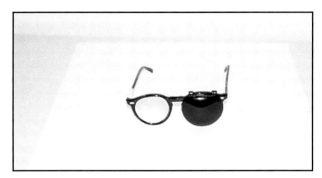

Figure 14-6. A clip-on style patch used for occlusion. It can easily be applied and removed. It is held in place by two overhanging clips which attach to the spectacle frame.

accommodate for a reduced field. Some models are illuminated. They are generally only appropriate for spot or short-term reading because holding them suspended in air can be fatiguing and tedious. They do have a fixed focal distance. Therefore, they are not recommended for patients with hand tremors, since the image quality is decreased by the tremor.

Stand magnifiers are a convex lens housed in a stand that rests on the reading material (Figure 14-8). They vary in power and working distance like the hand-held magnifiers. Many models are illuminated, decreasing the need for external lighting. Patients with hand tremors can use these because the base stabilizes the magnifier. They are difficult to maneuver around the binding of a book.

A closed circuit television (see Figure 14-1) is a device that electronically magnifies an object. It is composed of a camera and monitor. These devices deliver a wide range of magnification. The user can vary the working distance. There are also adjustments for color, reverse polarity (white text on a dark background), contrast, and a reading guide. These devices are among the most costly, but have been gaining popularity in low vision care.

Evaluation of Absorptive Lenses

Photophobia and light adaptation are particularly difficult for patients with decreased fields, particularly if media opacities coexist. Therefore, it is important to assess the patient's difficulty with illumination and to prescribe means to minimize resulting disability. Patients should be evaluated under conditions of both indoor and outdoor lighting because normal levels of illumination may be overwhelming to some patients.

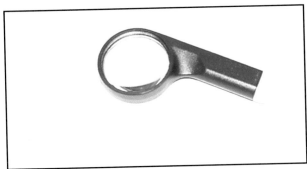

Figure 14-7. Two common hand-held magnifiers. They vary in size and magnification. The power dictates the focal distance.

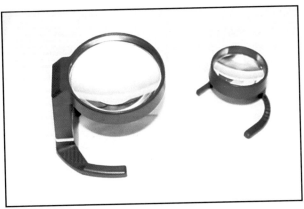

Figure 14-8. Two stand magnifiers. These rest on the reading material. The open base in these two examples allows them to be used for writing as well.

Sun lenses that shield from the top and sides like those manufactured by NOIR (South Lyon, Mich) (Figure 14-9) are very helpful because a great deal of extraneous light enters the eye from these locations. Conventional absorptive lenses do not provide this protection. These absorptive lenses can be worn over top of spectacles. Photochromatic lenses such as Corning Photochromatic Filters are particularly helpful for those patients who experience difficulty with light adaptation. The variability in absorption resulting from the degree of illumination makes these lenses most helpful for these patients. It has been my experience that some patients report increased contrast while wearing these lenses, which may incorporate the patient's refractive correction.

Evaluation of Field Devices

The evaluation of field devices involves assessing the patient's visual status and compensatory skills. The clinician should evaluate the patient's scanning and visual fields prior to the final evaluation and prescription of field devices.

Scanning

One of the most significant factors impacting upon the successful use of field devices is the patient's acquired compensation of scanning. Because the filed loss is a slow process in glaucoma compared to diseases such as stroke, the patient is able to develop an efficient means of scanning that may increase their functional field to several times the dimension of their static visual field. This result is attributed to efficient use of scanning. In fact, one study involving patients with retinitis pigmentosa showed that this process seemed to be performed with ease.[1] As noted previously, the similarity of fields between those with retinitis pigmentosa and those with glaucoma, make this noteworthy clinical information. The advantage here is that a patient who compensates without difficulty is still achieving increased functioning through his or her own rather than prescribed means.

Measuring Visual Fields

Prior to evaluating any patient for field devices is important to measure their full visual fields. Although visual fields that quantify the thresholds of the central 24-30 degrees are needed to properly medically manage of patients with glaucoma, the low vision practitioner also may need to perform other types of visual field testing. The two pieces of information needed by the low vision doctor for prescribing field devices are:

1. The absolute limits of the remaining central field in major meridians
2. The presence or absence of islands of vision in the periphery.

Knowing these data, the doctor can select those devices and powers that are most appropriate for a particular patient. Also, the presence of peripheral islands may decrease the likelihood of success with some devices, particularly those containing prism. These islands may cause increased confusion due to the displacement or relocation of images caused by the displacement from prism.

The most intriguing and challenging portion of the low vision management of patients with advanced glaucoma is the use of devices to enhance or expand the visual field. Generally speaking these devices are used for distance tasks such as ambulating and sighting objects. There are two major classifications of devices: field enhancers, which utilize prisms to relocate objects, and field expanders, which minimize to condense more environmental surroundings into the patients remaining field. Both types of devices have advantages, disadvantages and specific uses. It is important that the practitioner presents them to the patient, carefully explains their functions, and provides adequate instruction to maximize benefit and safety for the patient.

Prismatic Field Devices

Field enhancement devices recently have gained in popularity. In fact, there has been more development of these devices as indicated by the number of new products available. These devices contain prisms which shift an object's location from the non-sighted field into the sighted field. In this way, these devices increase the effective result of small amplitude saccades. Because patients with glaucoma experience a slow degradation of their visual field, they are afforded ample time to compensate with head and eye movements. The function of prismatic devices is to increase the amount of field viewed with the same or lower amplitude eye movements. In this way, the need for head movement or large amplitude saccades is greatly decreased. In fact, a patient achieves 1 degree of field awareness for every 2 prism diopters of prism. Thus, one may describe the effect as getting "more for less." Prisms increase awareness by projecting the image into visible field. They present the image in a location linearly displaced from its original location. These effects initially can cause confusion, and therefore, are not intended for crossing streets or for negotiating stairs. These devices generally are prescribed for ambulation because they are placed outside the patient's primary field of view and the patient only calls upon their use when performing a voluntary saccade. At all other times the patent looks through the carrier, which does not contain prism. The two types of visual field prismatic devices discussed in this chapter are Fresnel prisms and the Inwave Field Expanding Channel Lens.

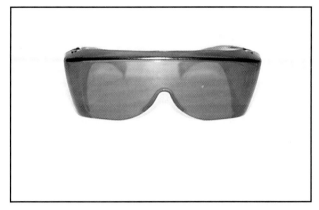

Figure 14-9. An example of a NOIR absorptive lens. These contain variable transmission and colors. They also have side shields and a top shields for additional protection.

Fresnel Prisms

Fresnel prisms (Figure 14-10) have been used in low vision for the remediation of visual field defects. They have been used for hemianopia, altitudinal defects, and constricted fields. They are composed of thin (1 mm) polyvinyl chloride material that is applied to the ocular surface of a spectacle lens using surface tension, water, or permanent clear adhesive. Their advantages are that they are lightweight, inexpensive, and come in a wide range of powers. The design of the prism incorporates small, serially placed prisms in one lens blank. Thus, a high powered prism in this format can be made lighter in weight and thinner than an equally powered ophthalmic prism. For constricted fields, the powers and corresponding enhancements most commonly used are 15 (7.5 degrees), 20 (10 degrees), and 30 (15 degrees) prism diopters. Their design, though, has several disadvantages, including acuity degradation, loss of contrast, and chromatic aberration. They can also easily fall off the spectacle lens, are difficult to clean, and become yellowed and brittle with age. For these reasons, they need to be replaced every several months.

Fitting

The prisms are prepared for mounting following a sequence of steps. The power used is dependent upon the degree of field loss, patient adaptation to the displacement effect, and tolerance of the aberration and distortion. I often use 15 prism diopters to start, and then increases power to a maximum level of accept-

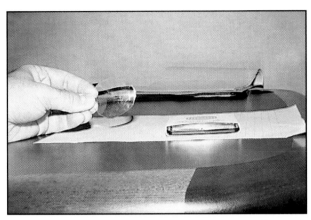

Figure 14-10. A Fresnel prism. They can be cut to fit a variety of spectacle lenses.

ance. Some patients, however, adapt quickly to the 30-prism diopter lens. As with any prism, the edge is placed just outside the patient's primary position of gaze. The prism base is placed towards the defect being treated. For example, with constricted fields, the greatest impediment to ambulation is the loss of the temporal fields. An initial placement would be base out placed in the temporal periphery of each lens. After, the patient has become accustomed to the effects of the Fresnel prism, more prism may be added to increase the awareness of the remaining fields. Because patients with advanced glaucoma generally have small, circular fields, each spectacle lens can be fitted with four prisms in a concentric design: base up, superiorly; base down, inferiorly; base in, nasally; and base out, temporally.[2] The prescribed sequence of fitting, once tentative power is determined, is as follows.

First, the doctor demonstrate the field loss to the patient. This can be done by showing them the printout of their visual field or through a functional field. The latter is preferred because it is more concrete and relates to visual functioning. It can be performed in a hallway. The patient faces an observer at least 10 feet straight ahead of them. Although the patient keeps his or her eyes stationary, the tester walks from behind the patient on either side. The patient then signals when the tester is first seen. The demonstration is repeated for the contralateral side. Eventually, the doctor demonstrates all the space that is not being viewed. The test can be varied using a dynamic functional field in which both the patient and tester are walking.

Second, one demonstrates the effect of the Fresnel prism on the visual field. A good screening method is to have the patient hold the prism in front of one eye, usually the eye with the smaller field. The patient observes the increased awareness by presenting the Fresnel in front of their eye, then removing it. In this way, they can compare the enhanced vs the unenhanced visual field and anticipate the potential benefit to be derived from the prism. It is also good at this time to educate the patient as to the effects of image displacement and acuity degradation.

Third, the edge placement of the prism is determined. One brings an opaque surface, such as paper, from the periphery towards the center of the eye. When the edge is first noted, the location is marked on the frame. This process is repeated several times and an average is determined. It is advisable to place the edge of the prism 1 to 2 mm peripheral to this location to insure that the prism is free of the patient's primary field of view. The prism then is cut and its edge placed at the appropriate location. The prism edge is cut in a straight line and the rest is cut to fit within the confines of the spectacle frame. To insure that it does not easily fall off the spectacle, the prism should not touch the frame. Rather, it should be one mm from it in all directions. If the patient later starts noticing the edge, an additional one mm is cut off and the prism is replaced.

Patient Instruction

Equally as important to the fitting of a Fresnel prism is the instructional sequence. The instruction increases the proper use, benefit, and safety to the patient. Here the patient needs to become familiar with the distortion, aberrations, scotoma at the edge of the prism, diplopia in certain directions of gaze, "jack in the box" effect, and image displacement caused by the prism. The four major steps for instruction are:
1. Stationary patient/stationary object
2. Stationary patient/moving object
3. Moving patient/stationary object
4. Moving patient/moving object.

Patients vary in their ability to acclimate to these effects. The instructional sequence may take up to several visits. Included in this instruction is teaching proper care for the prism such as removal, cleaning, and reapplication. At the completion of this instruction, the patient takes the prism home for a trial period. A follow-up visit occurs several weeks later to address problem areas and to determine the degree of success.

The Inwave Field Expanding Channel Lens

This particular device (Figure 14-11) is a spectacle lens that contains three prisms molded to a channel shaped carrier lens:

1. 12 prism diopters temporally
2. 12 prism diopters nasally
3. 8 prism diopters inferiorly.

As with Fresnel prisms, the patient perceives increased visual field awareness by performing a saccade in the desired direction. Using the clinical rule from above, this would enhance the visual field by 4 degrees vertically and 6 degrees horizontally. The lens is cosmetically pleasing, and the apex lines resemble executive bifocal or slab-off lines. It comes in a variety of refractive powers and also is available in a round 22 bifocal. It is recommended that it be incorporated in a frame no larger than a 54-eye size.

The manufacturer has a fitting set of trial lenses that can be purchased and used with a standard trial frame. The Channels available range from 6 to 14 mm. The patient's functioning visual field is to be centered within the channel in primary gaze. The trial lens is presented to the patient and the channel chosen is the minimum width that allows the patient not to experience diplopia in primary gaze. The inferior apex is generally at the same location as a bifocal.[3] The sequence for instructing the patient about the image displacement is similar to that for Fresnel prisms, except that the distortion, aberration, and acuity degradation are clinically unimportant.

Minimizing Field Devices

The second group of field devices are minifiers (Figure 14-12) that aim to condense information into the patient's field of view. As a result, these devices are composed either entirely or partially of concave lenses. They are intended for stationary observation rather than for ambulating. Examples of their uses include scanning a crowd in a room or looking for a particular person within a crowd of people. Their use is more transient than the prismatic systems. They are held by the patient and expand the breadth of their awareness as the patient pivots his or her head or body in the desired direction. These devices are incompatible with ocular scanning because they obstruct the view of the patient if the eyes are moved out of their alignment. Furthermore, the amplitude of scanning

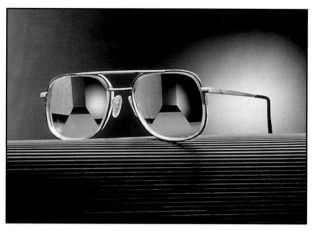

Figure 14-11. A finished Inwave Channel Lens used for constricted fields. Note the central channel surrounded by three prisms all combined into one spectacle lens.

often is greater than the width of the device. In addition, size constancy and depth perception is disrupted because objects appear further away than their actual location. In order to screen for those patients who may benefit from these devices, one can have the patient hold a concave trial lens (ie, –5.00 D) at arms length and view the expanded field through it. One also can use a low powered (2.5x or 2.8x) telescope (Figure 14-13) and view throughout its objective lens. If the response is positive in either of these situations, a minifying device should be investigated. The two minifying devices discussed here are the Ocutech Image Minifier and the Reverse Telescope. A third device, the New Horizon Lens, will be mentioned; however, as of the writing of this chapter it is no longer being manufactured.

The Ocutech Image Minifier

This is a single concave lens held at arm's length. This device, in conjunction with the patient's accommodative response, acts as a telescope in reverse. In order to increase its range, the patient and lens move as a combined unit much like turning a telescope. These devices minify in proportion to their power. For example, if a patient with 20/30 acuity holds a –10.00 D lens at 30 cm, the patient will need to accommodate 2.5 D. Therefore, the minification is 2.5/10x or 0.25x. The resulting acuity be 20/120. The power prescribed is the maximum power tolerated by the patient in terms of increased field and acuity degradation. The device can be mounted permanently mounted on a

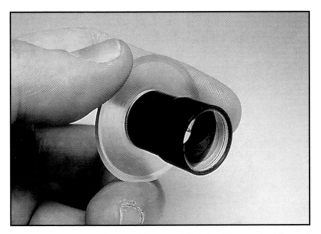

Figure 14-12. An Ocutech Image Minifier (Ocutech, Chapel Hill, NC) housed in a trial ring. This can be placed in a trial frame for patient evaluation.

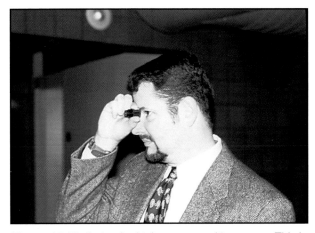

Figure 14-13. A standard telescope used in reverse. This is a useful screening method to investigate a patient's response to an actual reverse telescope.

spectacle lens or worn around the neck, suspended by a chain.[4] When using the later design, the device is used by picking it up when it is wanted for field expansion. It is concealed or worn around the patient's neck all other times.

The Reverse Telescope

As the name of this implies, it is a telescope constructed in reverse. In fact it can be either a Keplerian or Galilean design. The telescope is either hand-held or mounted into a spectacle frame. It is placed in the upper portion of the carrier lens (bioptic design) or in the center (full diameter design). With the bioptic design, the patient only spots through it when tilting the chin downward and moving the eyes upward needs it. At all other times, the patient looks through the carrier lens. Designs for Vision (Ronkonkoma, NY) is the manufacturer of these devices.

In response to the decreased acuity resulting from the use of minifiers, the late Dr. William Feinbloom invented the Amorphic or New Horizon lens. It consisted of a cylindrical concave lens system (axis 90), which only minified in the horizontal meridian. In this way the vertical dimension was unaffected, thus maintaining visual acuity. Objects appeared taller and thinner than their actual dimensions. The manufacturer has discontinued this device.

Evaluation of Non-optical Devices

There is a large number of non-optical devices available in catalogs such as those from The Lighthouse (New York, NY). In that catalog are lighting fixtures devices for ADLs and many others. Below is a list of common non-optical devices used for patients with low vision.

Typoscopes and Other Reading Guides

A typoscope is a reading guide (Figure 14-14). It consists of a plastic template about the size of an index card with a slot cut out of it. The patient positions the typoscope with the desired line of text in the slot. The patient then moves the typoscope to the end of the line, reads over the line just read backwards, then drops down to the next. The typoscope helps one keep his or her place while reading from left to right and assists in helping the patient negotiate the next line of text. Often, patients with decreased left field lose their place while using a diagonal saccade from the end of one line to the beginning of another. In some patients, the typoscope reduces glare from a white printed page as well as increases the contrast of the text on the page.

In addition, through the use of a typoscope, better accuracy and efficiency while reading may be accomplished by using a finger to move from word to word. The use of a rulers to underline lines of text also helps

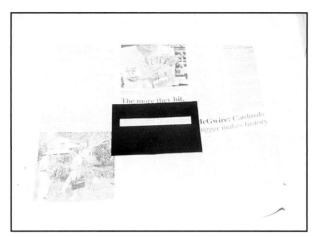

Figure 14-14. A typoscope selectively isolates portions of text while reading.

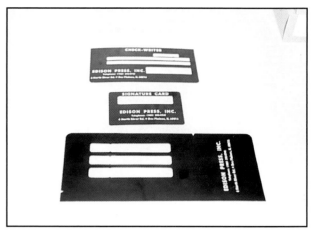

Figure 14-15a. There are also check writing guides (top), signature guides (center), and envelope writing guides (bottom).

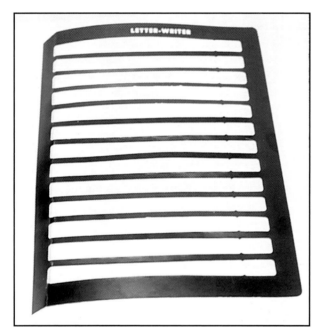

Figure 14-15b. A writing guide to enable a person to write in straight lines on a page.

one keep his or her place while reading. Using bold or bright borders at the right and left margins of printed material, or using one's arms as anchors on either side of a page, also may be helpful. Repositioning the printed page by centering in front of the favored eye, may place it better within the preferred field of view. This technique is particularly helpful with asymmetric visual file loss. Rotating text 45 to 90 degrees also may be beneficial, particularly for those patients having a horizontal field less than that of its oblique or vertical dimensions. In this way, matching the text orientation to the largest meridian of visual field attains the maximum field of view.

Writing Guides

These are plastic templates like the typoscope and are fashioned for specific uses (Figures 14-15a and 14-15b). There are guides designed for writing checks, signing one's name, addressing envelopes, and writing lines of text as in a letter. Bold line and raised line paper assist in writing letters. A bold line, felt tipped pen is also a writing guide because its ink is easier to see than that of a ballpoint pen.

Illumination

Proper task lighting is important to any activity. Gooseneck lamps (Figure 14-16) are recommended for reading because they provide intense direct lighting with little glare. Table lamps and ceiling fixtures only deliver a fraction of the illumination provided by a gooseneck even when they have a high wattage bulb. The inverse square law explains this phenomenon. Illumination decreases inversely by a square of the distance from the light source. For example, if a table lamp and gooseneck both have a bulb with the same wattage, and if the patient is twice as far from the table lamp as from the gooseneck, the light provided by the table lamp is one-fourth of that provided by the gooseneck.

There are also illumination sources that are bright and divergent for mobility at night. An example is the

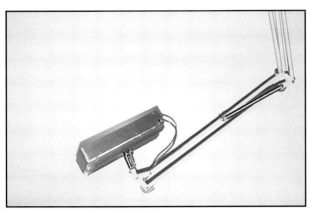

Figure 14-16. A gooseneck style lamp for task lighting. The adjustable arm allows for maximal illumination without excessive glare to suit an individual's lighting needs.

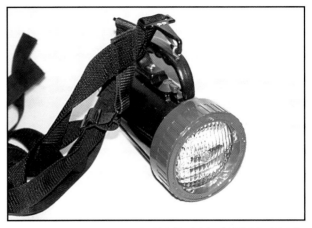

Figure 14-17. A Wide-Angle Mobility Light (WAML) which is used for night travel.

Wide-Angle Mobility Light (WAML) (Figure 14-17). This device allows patients to experience better vision at night. A mobility therapist is an appropriate professional to determine the patients who wish to gain independence while ambulating at night and who would most benefit from this device.

Networking with Other Professionals

This chapter has focused on the role of the low vision optometrist in rehabilitating patients with vision loss from glaucoma. Another important facet to the rehabilitation process is the proper referral to other professionals that can provide additional or supplemental services. These individuals can be found in public or private settings. Below is a description of some of the most common resources that may fill the needs of patients living with glaucomatous vision loss.

State Agencies

Each state has a vocational rehabilitation agency. Sometimes it is separate from that for blindness and vision impairment. In other states, it is housed within one agency serving persons with all types of physical challenges. These agencies are funded using public monies. They provide vocational counseling and restoration services for individuals seeking gainful employment and independent living. Within these agencies are service providers that can be networked for patients needing direct service.

Orientation and Mobility Therapy (O&M)

Orientation is knowing one's location within space. Mobility is traveling about through space. Specialists in these areas people who are blind or visually impaired to ascertain their location while traveling, and help them safely travel to a desired destination. The specialty of O&M developed out of the need to rehabilitate blinded World War II veterans. O&M therapists teach their clients to use optical devices prescribed by their doctor (field expanders and enhancers), canes, guide dogs, and mobility devices (Figure 14-18). Being able to travel increases an individual's independence. Refraining from travel due to a vision problem and fear of harm decreases one's quality of life. It is the philosophy of some low vision doctors that all persons with restricted fields be referred to an O&M therapist even if they don't admit to having problems with travel.[5] It is only after they discover what these individuals provide that patients realize the problems they have in these areas.

Rehabilitation Teaching

The rehabilitation teacher instructs the client in the use of Braille, which is an alternative means of communication and reading for people finding conventional print too difficult. Such reading difficulties occur when field loss is severe or when a person becomes blind from glaucoma. Rehabilitation teachers provide assistance with organizational skills for the home, such as arranging the kitchen and bathroom for ease of use. Other ADL areas in which the may be helpful include grooming, cooking, household cleaning, and shopping.

Counseling and Advocacy

Vision loss is associated with other concomitant challenges in other areas including job, independence, driving, self-esteem, and interpersonal relationships. Depression often occurs in response to such losses and challenges, and needs appropriate medical and psychotherapeutic services from individuals such as psychiatrists, psychologists, and psychotherapists. Most importantly suicidal ideation needs to be monitored by a trained professional. Any mention of taking one's life in any setting should be taken seriously and the patient needs an immediate psychiatric referral. Therefore, all doctors should have developed a referral relationship with a qualified mental health professional.

Adaptive Technology

Adaptive technology has grown in popularity with the widespread availability of computers. A qualified specialist can evaluate a patient with vision loss and recommend systems that magnify, use auditory output, or tactile output. In this way, these patients can learn alternative means for information processing. These services can be delivered by a state agency or contracted to an outside vendor.

CONCLUSION

The rehabilitation evaluation for a patient with glaucoma generally occurs in the presence of advanced visual field loss. The process attempts to identify problem areas, and to prescribes optical devices and strategies to achieve the patient's goals. Networking for other services also is a vital part of a patient's rehabilitation.

The slow process of vision loss in glaucoma allows the patient to develop compensatory strategies, making the rehabilitation process a challenging one for the low vision practitioner. The clinician providing medical treatment for a patient with glaucoma also should consider the functional losses encountered by their patients. By undergoing screening for these problems, the patient can receive low vision services

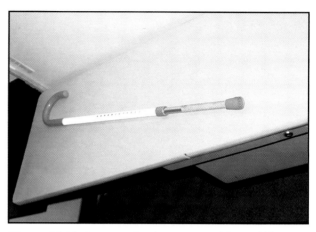

Figure 14-18. An example of a cane used for mobility.

when they are appropriate and potentially increase his or her independence and quality of life.

REFERENCES

1. Weiss NJ. The low vision management of retinitis pigmentosa. *J Am Optom Assoc.* 1991;62:42.
2. Weiss NJ, Brown WL. Uses of prism in low vision. In: Cotter SA, London RL, eds. *Clinical Uses of Prism—A Spectrum of Applications.* St Louis, Mo: Mosby; 1995.
3. *The InWave Fitting Guide.* Janesville, Wis: InWave Optics, Inc.
4. *The Ocutech Guide for the Ocutech Image Minifier.* Chapel Hill, NC: Ocutech, Inc.
5. Cohen J, Waiss B. Visual field remediation. In: Cole RG, Rosenthal BP, eds. *Remediation and Management of Low Vision.* St Louis, Mo: Mosby; 1996.

INDEX